Human Genetics: From Molecules to Medicine

Christian Patrick Schaaf, MD, PhD
Assistant Professor
Baylor College of Medicine, Houston, TX, USA
The Jan and Dan Duncan Neurological Research Institute, Houston, TX, USA

Johannes Zschocke, Dr.med.habil., PhD
Professor and Chair of Human Genetics
Medical University Innsbruck
Innsbruck, Austria

Lorraine Potocki, MD
Professor
Department of Molecular and Human Genetics
Baylor College of Medicine
Houston, TX

. Wolters Kluwer | Lippincott Williams & Wilkins
Health
Philadelphia · Baltimore · New York · London
Buenos Aires · Hong Kong · Sydney · Tokyo

Acquisitions Editor: Susan Rhyner
Product Manager: Jennifer Verbiar
Development Editor: Jennifer Maybin
Translators: Anna Taylor and Renate Winkler
Marketing Manager: Joy Fisher-Williams
Design Coordinator: Holly McLaughlin
Compositor: Aptara, Inc.

First Edition

351 West Camden Street   Two Commerce Square
Baltimore, MD 21201   2001 Market Street
                             Philadelphia, PA 19103

Printed in China

9 8 7 6

Library of Congress Cataloging-in-Publication Data

Schaaf, Christian Patrick.
   Human genetics : from molecules to medicine / Christian Patrick
Schaaf, Johannes Zschocke, Lorraine Potocki.
      p. ; cm.
   Includes bibliographical references and index.
   ISBN 978-1-60831-671-7 (alk. paper)
   1. Human genetics.   2. Medical genetics.   I. Zschocke, Johannes.
II. Potocki, Lorraine.   III. Title.
   [DNLM: 1. Genetic Phenomena.   2. Genetic Diseases, Inborn.
3. Genetics, Medical—methods.   QU 500]
   QH431.S3148 2011
   599.93'5—dc23
                                          2011018905

DISCLAIMER

Care has been taken to confirm the accuracy of the information present and to describe generally accepted practices. However, the authors, editors, and publisher are not responsible for errors or omissions or for any consequences from application of the information in this book and make no warranty, expressed or implied, with respect to the currency, completeness, or accuracy of the contents of the publication. Application of this information in a particular situation remains the professional responsibility of the practitioner; the clinical treatments described and recommended may not be considered absolute and universal recommendations.

The authors, editors, and publisher have exerted every effort to ensure that drug selection and dosage set forth in this text are in accordance with the current recommendations and practice at the time of publication. However, in view of ongoing research, changes in government regulations, and the constant flow of information relating to drug therapy and drug reactions, the reader is urged to check the package insert for each drug for any change in indications and dosage and for added warnings and precautions. This is particularly important when the recommended agent is a new or infrequently employed drug.

Some drugs and medical devices presented in this publication have Food and Drug Administration (FDA) clearance for limited use in restricted research settings. It is the responsibility of the health care provider to ascertain the FDA status of each drug or device planned for use in their clinical practice.

To purchase additional copies of this book, call our customer service department at (800) 638-3030 or fax orders to (301) 223-2320. International customers should call (301) 223-2300.

Visit Lippincott Williams & Wilkins on the Internet: http://www.lww.com. Lippincott Williams & Wilkins customer service representatives are available from 8:30 am to 6:00 pm, EST.

To our patients - past, present and future - who
continue to be the inspiration and motivation
for everything that we do.

Foreword

Human genetics by virtue of its inherent focus on how and why human beings differ from each other should have formed a central core of medical education. But for all too long, those who toiled on its behalf worked with one hand behind their backs. The key tool of most animal or plant geneticists, the making of genetic crosses between parents of well-defined phenotypes, was unavailable to reveal human genotypes. Human geneticists can only observe as opposed to arrange genetic crosses. When a disease-causing trait passes regularly from one generation to the next, the causative gene is likely a dominant allele, whereas a trait that preferentially appears after mating of closely related individuals is likely a recessive allele needing to be in two copies for its phenotype to be expressed.

Happily, the arrival of the powerful new recombinant DNA gene cloning techniques of the early 1980s soon led to the isolation and sequencing of several of the best-known human disease genes, including those responsible for cystic fibrosis, Duchenne muscular dystrophy, and Huntington disease. Each of their respective gene isolations, however, required almost heroic efforts, and human genetics could only move into high gear when completion of the Human Genome Project in 2003 revealed the DNA sequences of all 24 human chromosomes. By now the genes behind some 2500 different human medical disorders have been defined at the molecular level.

Relatively inexpensive "gene chips" bearing representative DNA sequences of known Mendelian diseases are just this year beginning to move into the public arena. For less than $500, an individual can be tested to see if he or she is the carrier of any of some 100 of the most common recessive human disease genes. Soon, it will be possible to provide early preparation, education, and options for the parents of children who fear that their offspring may be affected by the often challenging draws of the genetic dice.

Human genetics will move even faster following the introduction of personal genomes into medical practice. When my personal genome was sequenced just 4 years ago, $1 million was expended. Within the next 5 years, however, the cost of sequencing single personal genomes will be lowered to no more than $1,000. Soon the main obstacle for human geneticists will be how to handle the inherent great complexity of individual genomes. My genome still remains largely to be understood. Hundreds of thousands, if not millions, of human personal genomes may have to be examined before we have a good handle on what the 3×10^9 base pairs (bits) of information in our individual genomes portend about our futures. There will also be the nontrivial task of introducing this knowledge into medical practice. The better the medical profession itself understands medical genetics, the more useful will be the advice passed on to patients.

In Germany, *Basiswissen Humangenetik* has already well served students through its clear presentations of the molecular and cellular underpinnings of gene-based medical conditions. In its newly expanded English translation, *Human Genetics: From Molecules to Medicine*, Drs. Schaaf, Zschocke, and Potocki have produced a text that should greatly benefit a broad audience ranging from pure scientists to medical practitioners.

The best days of molecular medicine are yet to arrive. May this volume speed up their appearance!

James D. Watson, Ph.D.

Preface

Welcome to the exciting world of human genetics! Over the past several decades there have been tremendous discoveries in medical genetics and molecular biology, which have fundamentally changed our medical practice. Disease classifications are continually being revised according to new genetic data, treatment is individually tailored to molecular information, and genetic counseling helps patients to deal with health challenges. It is not an exaggeration to say that every practicing physician—irrespective of his or her specialty—will need a strong foundation in the science that is at the heart of molecular medicine. *Human Genetics: From Molecules to Medicine* is an ideal text for anyone studying medicine in the 21st century as it contains the essential facts as well as clinical scenarios that illustrate the application of molecular biology to the diagnosis and treatment of human disease.

The book has developed from *Basiswissen Humangenetik*, one of the most popular human genetics textbooks in Germany. It has been praised for the way it distills complex concepts, and students appreciate its brevity and applicability in the clinical setting. In addition to these features, *Human Genetics* also addresses many of the social and personal aspects of individuals who are diagnosed with inherited disorders, as we include many photographs and narrative accounts that demonstrate individuals *living* with these conditions. Rick Guidotti's exceptional photographs from the Positive Exposure initiative enhance the text while portraying the beauty of the diversity inherent in our human race.

All of the authors are practicing physicians. We designed *Human Genetics* to be as clinically useful as possible while providing the student with the necessary foundation in the most important genetic principles. Parts I and II of the book contain all that a physician really needs to know about molecular and clinical genetics, while Parts III and IV focus on the presentation and management of individuals with genetic disorders, using a systematic approach. Part V provides valuable insight into the lives of those living with genetic disorders.

We extend our appreciation and thanks to our patients and their families who have provided photographs for this edition and who have shared their stories. Heartfelt gratitude goes to our own families, who continue to patiently support us as we put forward our efforts related to this publication.

Christian P. Schaaf, MD, PhD
Johannes Zschocke, MD, PhD
Lorraine Potocki, MD

Acknowledgments

We gratefully acknowledge the assistance of several people who helped to make this volume possible: Martina Siedler, Rose-Marie Doyon, and Kathrin Nühse from Springer, and Susan Rhyner, Jenn Verbiar, Kelley Squazzo, and Jennifer Maybin from Wolters Kluwer.

We thank the following individuals who have provided photographs and images to this book: Gholamali Tariverdian, Theda Vogitländer, Bart Janssen, Hans-Dieter Hager, and Anna Jauch (all from the Institute of Human Genetics, University of Heidelberg, Germany); Georg F. Hoffmann, Andreas Kulozik, and Marcus Mall (all from the Department of Pediatrics, University of Heidelberg, Germany); Jens-Peter Schenk (Pediatric Radiology, University of Heidelberg, Germany); Martina Kadmon (Department of Surgery, University of Heidelberg, Germany); Matthias Kloor (Department of Pathology, University of Heidelberg, Germany); Volker Voigtländer (Klinikum Ludwigshafen, Germany); Raoul Hennekam (Institute of Child Health, London, UK); Richard A. Lewis (Department of Human and Molecular Genetics and Department of Ophthalmology, Baylor College of Medicine, Houston, TX, USA); Hansjakob Müller (Department of Biomedicine, University of Basel, Switzerland); and Rick Guidotti (Positive Exposure, New York, NY, USA).

About the Cover Art and Photography

The cover photo and many images in this text were generously contributed by award-winning fashion photographer Rick Guidotti of **POSITIVE EXPOSURE**.

Founded in 1997, **Positive Exposure** is a highly innovative visual arts organization that seeks to significantly impact the fields of genetics, mental health, and human rights by promoting positive images, self-esteem, and self-advocacy for people living with genetic difference.

Many individuals, families, and organizations have voiced the need to help physicians, and particularly medical students and trainees, learn how to best meet the concerns of people whose lives have been touched by genetic disorders. Each individual living with a genetic difference desires to be viewed *first and foremost as a human being* with his/her own special needs, rather than as a specific diagnosis or disease entity. Unfortunately, some clinical images illustrating genetic difference are experienced as dehumanizing or dispiriting for patients living with those conditions.

This text seeks to change that experience by including photographs donated from **Positive Exposure's** *Spirit of Difference* image data bank. We believe these photos serve as valuable clinical references for physicians and health care workers, yet still support and promote human dignity for our patients—particularly children—living with genetic conditions.

The authors and Publisher wish to thank **Positive Exposure** for their contributions to this text, as well as for their many photographic and interview workshops conducted in collaboration with people living with genetic conditions. We encourage those interested in the mission of **Positive Exposure** to explore their website at www.positiveexposure.org.

Contents

III   Clinical Genetics

IV   Approaches to Clinical Problems

V   Living with Genetic Disorders: Patient Reports

1 Introduction

LEARNING OBJECTIVES

1 Compare the prevalence of different types of genetic disorders in different age groups.

2 Discuss the clinical relevance of constitutional, somatic, and germline mutations for the affected individual

1.1 Genetics: A Key Discipline of Modern Medicine

In some way, each person is like all others
In some way like a few
In some way unique, like no other.
(Origin unknown)

All humans are equal, and yet so diverse. We share the same genetic information, with the exception of minute differences, yet we differ in our appearance, character, behavior, and health status. Our knowledge about the genetic bases of health status has rapidly changed over the last few years. The completion of the **Human Genome Project** provided us with a map of the 3 billion base pairs encoding the blueprint of human life. It is now possible to sequence the entire genome of an individual in a single day! However, while the DNA code of a single human may appear simple, the interpretation of this code for the purpose of understanding the intricacies of health and disease has proven to be tremendously complex. Advancements in molecular biology have determined that factors beyond the genetic code itself—for example, epigenetic regulation and noncoding RNAs—are integral to these processes. These discoveries, and the ever-expanding availability of clinical assays for genetic traits, have led to the emergence of the relatively new field of "**molecular medicine**" in which physicians and health care providers apply genetic information to maintain health, rapidly diagnose illness, and solve the problems associated with human disease.

All physicians in this age of molecular medicine must be well versed in the core principles of **human genetics**, which is the science of the mechanisms and principles through which genetic information determines health and disease. Searching for genetic changes and gene variants within a population, questioning the link between genotype and phenotype, probing the meaning of gene–gene and gene–environment interactions, investigating the role of somatic mutations in the formation of tumors, exploring the possibilities for prenatal diagnostics, and surveying the gene therapy for directed treatment strategies and preventative medicine are relevant for all fields of medicine. Human genetics serves as an important bridge between basic biology, on one hand, and practical clinical medicine, on the other. It is a "meta-discipline" that permeates all medical specialties. It helps with the diagnosis of a genetic predisposition to the development of a particular illness as well as the interdisciplinary care of affected individuals. It also serves to meet special needs for communicating information about the cause of an illness and its significance in the context of genetic counseling.

The 50 years that span the timeline of early genetic medicine, from the discovery of the DNA double helix by Watson and Crick (in 1953) to the publication of the sequence of 99.99% of the human genome (in 2003), can be thought of as the "pregenomic" period in medical history. As we approach the second decade of the "postgenomic" era, we have a greater appreciation of the complexities regulating the genomic sequence and the importance of understanding these complexities to promote health and cure disease.

1.2   Frequency of Genetic Diseases

Genetic diseases occur with varying frequency in all stages of life. It is estimated that, before a pregnancy, up to 50% of all **conceptions** are lost due to a numeric chromosomal disorder. Of all recognized **pregnancies**, one-sixth end in a miscarriage, mostly in the first trimester, and 50% to 60% of these are also attributable to a chromosomal aberration.

Genetic diseases contribute significantly to **childhood** mortality and morbidity rates. While in developing countries 95% of all pediatric hospital admissions are attributable to nongenetic causes (mostly infections), up to 25% of the hospitalized children in developed countries have a genetic disease. At least 50% of all learning disabilities (18 out of 1,000 school-age children) are attributable to genetic factors.

During **adulthood** cardiovascular diseases and cancer are the most frequent causes of death. Cancer can be considered a genetic disease that is caused by the accumulation of somatic mutations in conjunction with only tentatively known, nonspecific, hereditary genetic variants. In the development of cardiovascular diseases, the interaction of nongenetic and genetic factors plays a central role.

Chromosomal Disorders

Chromosome disorders occur in 0.5% of all newborns. As mentioned previously, this figure is merely "the tip of the iceberg" with regard to all conceptions. Every 10th sperm and every 4th egg cell have an abnormal set of chromosomes. The frequency of individual chromosome disorders varies considerably at different stages of embryonic development. Among aborted fetuses, trisomy 16 represents the most frequent autosomal trisomy; frequently there is a triploidy. Only three autosomal trisomies are viable: 13, 18, and 21. Autosomal monosomies are not viable, whereas monosomy X is viable (it leads to Turner syndrome). Monosomy X is estimated to occur in 1% of all conceptions, yet only 1 in 50 of these children is born alive.

Submicroscopic Chromosomal Anomalies

Many genetic syndromes are caused by losses and gains of chromosomal material below the detection level of light microscopy and involve several or many genes. The recent development of DNA arrays for the genome-wide analysis of copy number variations (CNVs) has led to the discovery of both many more pathogenic variants as well as frequent copy number polymorphisms of uncertain clinical relevance. Bridging the gap between single genes and whole chromosomes, and between polymorphisms and disease-causing mutations, will help bring to light the full impact of CNVs on health and disease.

Single Gene Defects

The data in ▫ Table 1.1 refer to the frequency at which these genetic defects become clinically significant. Numerous mutations remain clinically silent throughout an entire life span; however, they may be **risk factors** for diseases and thus play important roles in the development of multifactorial diseases. For example, it has been shown that 1% of the population carries a mutated allele in the gene coding for the von Willebrand Factor, but in most individuals this causes little or no symptoms. Some genetic variants can be advantageous for the carrier in certain situations; they are part of the normal genetic variability.

The frequency of monogenic diseases varies significantly between different geographic regions. Basically, all diseases occur in all populations, yet no disease has the same frequency in all populations. Furthermore, in different populations the same genetic disorder is usually caused by different mutations. The underlying mechanisms for these phenomena, such as new mutation, founder mutation, selection, or genetic drift, are covered in detail in Section 14.3.

☐ **Table 1.1.** Frequency of Genetic Diseases

Type of Disorder	Detection before Age 25	Detection after Age 25	Total Frequency
Chromosome disorders[a]	2:1,000	2:1,000	4:1,000
Single-gene defects[b]	3.5:1,000	16.5:1,000	20:1,000
Multifactorial disorders (with a genetic component)	46:1,000	600:1,000[c]	646:1,000
Somatic mutations	—	240:1,000	240:1,000[d]

[a]Without balanced translocations.
[b]Without the carriers of premutations.
[c]This is an estimate of the total prevalence.
[d]This number is based on the assumption that all types of cancer are caused by an accumulation of somatic mutations. Single-gene inherited disposition for cancer is included under the category of "single-gene defects."
(From Rimoin et al. 2007.)

Multifactorial Disorders

The vast majority of medical conditions is influenced by genetic factors. Examples of typical multifactorial diseases, where genetic and nongenetic factors work together to varying degrees, are arterial hypertension, rheumatoid arthritis, and dementia. Multifactorial diseases therefore represent the largest group of genetic disorders (during childhood as well as in adulthood).

Somatic Mutations

The genetic makeup of a cell potentially changes with each cell division. Mutations that occur in the germ line (i.e., the path from the zygote to the germ cell of the next generation [in human females not more than 30 mitoses]) are transmitted as new mutations to the offspring and, as the case may be, become visible. Many more mutations arise in somatic cells and contribute to illness. The best examples of these mutations are neoplastic diseases that typically occur only when several independent somatic mutations work together in one single cell (Section 7.1). Somatic mutations, by definition, are not demonstrable in the entire organism but only in individual tissues (e.g., in a tumor). Somatic mutations play an important role in aging processes and probably in autoimmune diseases.

Somatic mutation: A mutation that has arisen after conception in somatic cells. It may contribute to illness but is not inherited from the parents and is not passed on to children.

Germline mutation: A mutation that has arisen after conception in the germ line. It is not inherited from the parents and does not usually contribute to illness, but may be passed on to children (see also: germline mosaicism).

Constitutional mutation: A mutation that is inherited from the parents, is present in all cells of the body, and may be passed on to children.

The Biological Basis of Human Genetics

2 Molecular Basis of Human Genetics

LEARNING OBJECTIVES

1 Describe the structural and functional differences between DNA and RNA.

2 Outline the main functional elements of a gene and discuss the difficulties of an exact definition of a gene.

3 Describe the major steps of transcription and translation.

4 Describe the three main elements of pre-mRNA modification and their functional importance.

5 Give at least five different types of noncoding RNA and their functional roles.

6 Define chromatin and describe the differences between euchromatin and heterochromatin.

7 Describe the mechanism of X-inactivation and give three different examples that illustrate why understanding this mechanism is important for understanding genetic disorders.

What distinguishes the human from other mammalian species? It is not the nucleotides within our DNA sequence, the packaging of DNA into chromosomes, the mechanism of DNA replication, or the translation of genetic information into protein. These components of heredity are similar in all species, from human beings to chimpanzees, to axolotls to Mongolian gerbils. For decades it was thought that human complexity was attributable to a greater number of genes—once estimated at 100,000 to 150,000. The Human Genome Project, however, taught us differently: humans have 20,000 to 22,000 protein-coding genes and in this way do not differ from other higher forms of life. It is not the number of genes that makes human beings different but rather their intelligent interaction, or the regulation of their expression. The recent discovery of more than 8,000 noncoding RNA genes and the manifold functions of noncoding RNA made us realize that the complexity of these mechanisms had been largely underestimated.

2.1 DNA

Deoxyribonucleic acid (DNA) is the genetic code of humans. It is a strandlike macromolecule of numerous **nucleotides (nt)**, each composed of a base, a sugar, and a phosphate group. The sugar and phosphate groups give the macromolecule its structure, whereas the bases are the actual carriers of genetic information, the letters of the genetic text.

The sugar moiety of the nucleotide in the DNA is deoxyribose. The prefix "deoxy-" indicates that this sugar has one fewer oxygen atom than ribose, from which it originates. Ribose constitutes the sugar moiety of the nucleotide of RNA (ribonucleic acid).

The nitrogen-containing bases of DNA are derivatives of purines or pyrimidines. Purine bases in DNA are **adenine (A)** and **guanine (G)**; pyrimidine bases are **thymine (T)** and **cytosine (C)**. RNA also consists of adenine, guanine, and cytosine. In place of thymine, the pyrimidine base is **uracil (U)** (◻ Fig. 2.1).

DNA is a double strand of two **complementary** nucleotide chains. The sequence of the nucleotide bases of the one strand (in the 5′ to 3′ direction) complements the sequence of nucleotide bases on the other strand (in the 3′ to 5′ direction). The two nucleotide chains run **antiparallel**. They are coiled around a common axis, connected with one another by hydrogen bonds between the bases A and T (two hydrogen bonds) and between the bases G and C (three hydrogen bonds) and in this way form a **double helix**. A-T and G-C are called **complementary base pairs**. The ratio of A to T and of G to C is 1:1. From the proportion of a single nucleotide base it is therefore possible to determine the contribution of all other bases (◻ Fig. 2.2).

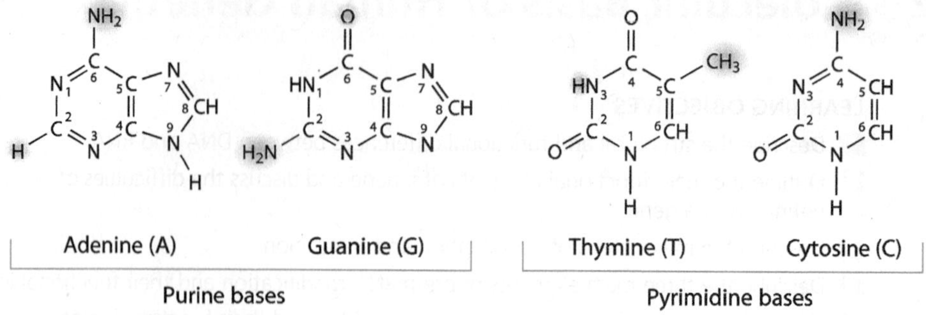

| Adenine (A) | Guanine (G) | Thymine (T) | Cytosine (C) |

| Purine bases | Pyrimidine bases |

Figure 2.1. Nucleotide Bases.

Example: With humans, the contribution of the nucleotide adenine is 29%. Thymine has the same share (i.e., 29%). Since $(A + T) + (G + C) = 1$, $(G + C) = 100\% - (29\% + 29\%) = 42\%$. G and C each contribute 21% of the nucleotide bases of human DNA.

The purine and pyrimidine bases face the inside of the double helix, whereas the sugar and phosphate moieties are on the outside. Because the spatial relationship of the opposing bases is fixed, the two chains of the double helix are exactly complementary. The diameter of the helix is 2 nm. Neighboring bases along the axis of the helix are 0.34 nm apart. A twist of the DNA double helix corresponds to 10 consecutive base pairs (i.e., 3.4 nm). Because the sugar and phosphate groups are placed on the outside, the double helix is not symmetrical. There are two forms: a right-turning form (B-form) and a left-turning form (Z-form). The DNA of the cell's nucleus is mainly of the (more stable) right-turning B-form (□ Fig. 2.3).

The length of DNA is measured by the number of base pairs (bp) or nucleotides (nt). Larger segments are measured in kilo bases (kb = 1,000 bp) or mega bases (Mb = 1 million bp). For obvious reasons, the length of (single-stranded) RNA is always given in nucleotides (nt).

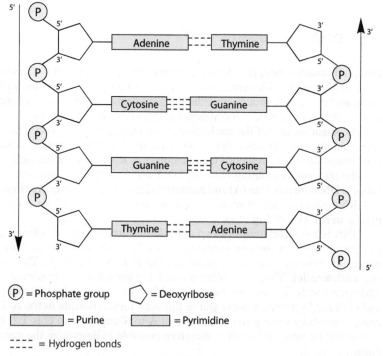

(P) = Phosphate group   ⬠ = Deoxyribose

▭ = Purine   ▭ = Pyrimidine

- - - - = Hydrogen bonds

Figure 2.2. Complementary Structure of the Double-Stranded DNA. (From Barsh et al., 2002.)

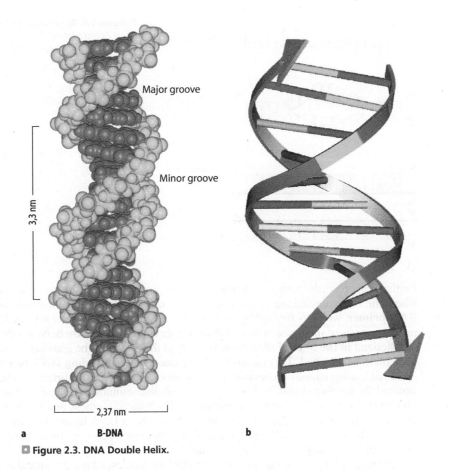

Major groove

Minor groove

3,3 nm

2,37 nm

a   **B-DNA**   b

□ **Figure 2.3. DNA Double Helix.**

Replication of DNA

In 1953 **James Watson** and **Francis Crick** recognized the three-dimensional structure of DNA from which they could deduce the mechanism of its replication that allows the reliable transmission of genetic information from one generation to the next.

During each cell division, replication provides for the creation of two identical copies of the cell's DNA molecules. It starts in parallel at more than 10,000 origins, which are recognized by specific replication initiation proteins; these origins separate the so-called replication units or replicons of the DNA. Replication proceeds with the aid of a multi-enzyme complex containing helicases, topoisomerases, various DNA polymerases, and other proteins. In this way, a single strand of DNA is prepared over a length of approximately 2,000 bp as a template for a new, complementary chain and in effect a new copy of the double helix.

Helicases: Enzymes that start replication by unwinding the DNA bidirectionally, leading to the separation of the hydrogen bonds and, in effect, the two chains. This results in the creation of two so-called replication forks.

Topoisomerases: Enzymes that prevent a supercoiling of the DNA helix during unwinding and separation because they are capable of cutting individual strands, permitting them to unwind.

Ligases: Enzymes that splice cut DNA pieces (e.g., during replication).

Polymerases: Enzymes that synthesize DNA or RNA strands.

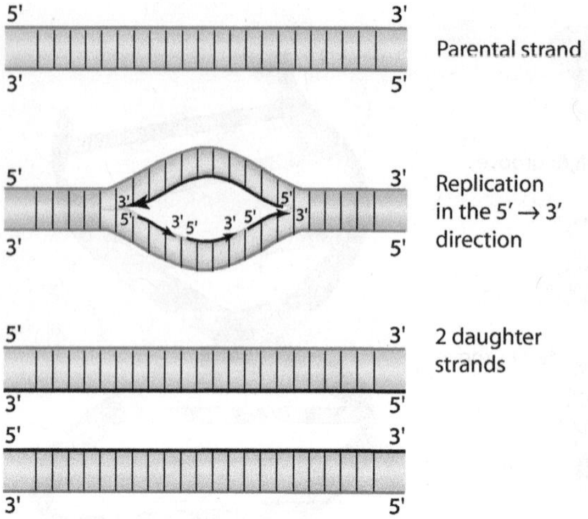

Figure 2.4. Replication of DNA. The so-called "parent strands" are shown in red, while black indicates the newly synthesized strands.

Replication proceeds from the starting point in both directions of the replicons, up to the point where the two approaching replication bubbles meet. It begins with a small complementary **RNA primer**, which is formed by **polymerase α** and later cut out and replaced by DNA. The main synthesis of the nucleotide strand occurs through **polymerase δ**. New DNA can only be **synthesized in the 5′ to 3′ direction**, for only at the 3′ end of the growing chain can the next nucleotide be attached. This means that only one of the unwinding DNA parent strands (the so-called leading strand) allows continuous synthesis in the 5′ to 3′ direction. The other strand, denoted the lagging strand, is 5′ to 3′ replicated discontinuously (quasi-backwards) in small 200-bp fragments called **Okazaki fragments**. Each such fragment needs a new RNA primer, and after replication, adjacent fragments are linked by a **DNA ligase**. During replication the *proofreading function* of DNA polymerase identifies errors, cuts out faulty bases, and replaces them with the correct bases (◻ Figs. 2.4 and 2.5).

The result of replication is two daughter DNA molecules, whose one strand is newly synthesized, while the other strand derives from the parent DNA. This **semiconservative** replication, aided by sophisticated repair mechanisms, enables the genome to copy itself with remarkable precision through millions of cell divisions over a lifetime.

2.2   Genes

The term gene as a name for a hereditary factor was first coined in 1909 by Wilhelm Johannsen. It derived from the Greek terms **genos** ("clan") and **genesis** ("origin"). Since then the definition has undergone several evolutions, many of which had to be modified or were dropped as new research became available. An example would be the "one gene one protein" hypothesis still familiar to students today but only partially applicable as it does not explain the occurrence of splice site variants, nor the diversity of RNA. The more we have learned about the structure and function of the human genome, the more cautious we have become in our definition of the term *gene*. For practical purposes, we can define a gene as a **functional unit** in the genome that contains the genetic information for one or more gene products; however, we should realize that this definition may be modified in the future. A typical protein-coding gene has three components: the coding sequence, regulatory sequences, and seemingly useless (some of them probably regulatory) sequences. Within the genomic DNA, a gene is defined by the direction of transcription in the **5′ to 3′ direction** and may be located on either strand of a chromosome. Different genes are not necessarily physically separated: some genes are located within other genes or contain regulatory sequences in genes far away; sometimes the complementary strands at a single locus contain two different genes.

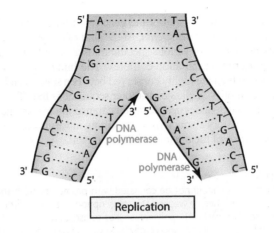

Replication

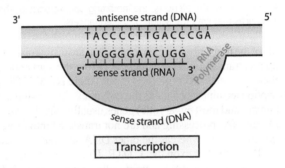

Transcription

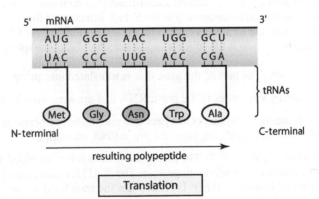

Translation

⬙ Figure 2.5. Flow of Genetic Information. Replication provides for the formation of identical DNA molecules within a cell. The concept of "transcription" refers to the transcription of DNA into a complementary RNA molecule. Subsequently, the language of the nucleic acids is translated into the language of a polypeptide sequence. (From Barsh et al., 2002.)

Gene: A functional unit in the genome that contains the genetic information for one or more gene products.

Pseudogenes: DNA sequences that have all the characteristics of a potential encoding transcription unit but which encode for no functional product.

The DNA strand, which (except for Ts and Us) corresponds to the RNA sequence, is called the *sense strand*; its complement (which serves as a template for RNA biosynthesis) is the *antisense strand*. The DNA before the 5′ start of the gene (the transcribed region) lies *upstream*, while the DNA beyond the 3′ end lies *downstream*. At the start of the gene lies the **promoter region,** which serves as a docking station for various specific transcription factors and an RNA polymerase that represents the transcription initiation complex. The human genome contains different kinds of promoters, many of which are highly conserved between species and contain various specific short (4 to 8 nt) sequence motifs. A classic promoter sequence is the "TATA box" (TATAAA or its variants). It is situated 25 nucleotides upstream of the transcription start site. Different types of promoters produce different regulatory characteristics, resulting in varying patterns of expression for the genes they direct in the course of the organism's development.

■■■ Enhancers Silencers, Insulators

Regulatory elements that should not be confused with promoters are **enhancers** or **silencers**. They are DNA segments that strengthen or weaken the transcription of a gene through a direct interaction with the transcription initiation complex (RNA polymerase II or transcription factors). While the promoters are always located 5′ upstream of the gene, enhancers may be at varying distances away from the gene whose transcription they regulate. Some of the enhancers are situated within the intron of a gene whose expression they regulate. The same is true for the silencers, the inhibiting counterparts of the enhancers. In addition, there are **insulator** sequences that limit the action of the enhancers.

Various segments of the transcribed sequence of a gene are distinguished according to their fate during RNA processing and translation. The sequences before the start codon and after the stop codon of the gene are called untranslated regions (UTRs); there is a 5′ UTR and a 3′ UTR. The sequence at which transcription terminates contains the polyadenylation signal AAUAAA (see Section 2.4). Transcripts of human (and most eukaryotic) genes usually contain segments that are removed during messenger RNA (mRNA) processing and are not translated into protein. These seemingly useless sequences are called introns, whereas the other DNA segments are called exons. The first exon(s) contain the 5′ UTR and the last exon the 3′ UTR. Human exons are usually short, with an average length of about 150 nt, whereas introns are usually longer than 10,000 nt (10 kb) long. Individual exons often correspond to structural and/or functional domains of the resulting protein. Exons and introns are numbered consecutively in the 5′ to 3′ direction of the transcript; exon 1 is followed by intron 1. Introns almost always begin with the nucleotides GT (or GU in RNA) and end with AG. The 5′ start of an exon is the splice acceptor site; the 5′ end, the splice donor site (◻ Fig. 2.6).

Coding region: The part of the gene that is translated into protein.

Exons: Coding sequences in the pre-mRNA that are separated by noncoding introns.

Introns: Noncoding sequences in a gene that are positioned between coding sequences (exons) and are removed by splicing from the pre-mRNA transcript.

Untranslated region (UTR): The part of the gene that is transcribed and included in the mature mRNA but is not translated into protein. The 5′ UTR denotes the translated sequences prior to the start codon, while the 3′ UTR denotes the translated sequences after the stop codon.

While still in the nucleus, introns are removed from the pre-mRNA by **RNA splicing**. Thus, introns do not contribute to the polypeptide product of a gene; however, they can have regulatory effects as noncoding RNAs (ncRNAs). The extent of this function (i.e., the full relevance of introns in the regulation of gene expression) remains to be clarified.

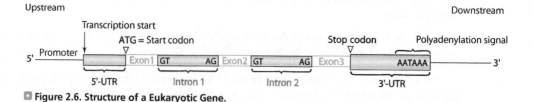

◻ **Figure 2.6. Structure of a Eukaryotic Gene.**

> **Important**
>
> **IN**trons remain **IN** the cell's nucleus. **EX**ons leave the nucleus of the cell and are **EX**pressed.

■■■ Pseudogenes

Pseudogenes are DNA sequences that have all the characteristics of a potential encoding transcription unit (promoter, encoding region, splice acceptor points, etc.) but do not encode for a **functional product**. Many pseudogenes were derived through **gene duplication** and subsequent mutation. A well-known example is a pseudogene that belongs to the family of α globins ("$\Psi\zeta$"). It has all the characteristics of a functional globin gene, yet one single-point mutation in the coding region prevents its expression as a complete globin. Sometimes a duplicated gene contains a residual function and may partly compensate for the deficiency of the "real" gene; examples are *SMN1* and *SMN2* in spinal muscular atrophy (Chapter 31.1.3).

Pseudogenes can also be created through **reverse transcription and subsequent integration**. In case the mRNA of a real gene accidentally gets transcribed by the enzyme reverse transcriptase into a complementary DNA (cDNA), it can be incorporated into the genomic DNA. In such cases the genomic DNA includes a gene without introns and with a poly A tail ("processed pseudogene").

2.3 Repetitive Sequences

In an attempt to explain structure and function of the human genome as well as various chromosomal or molecular aberrations, one might use the metaphor of 46 books (chromosomes) that contain many individual instruction manuals (genes). Unlike real books, however, the genome contains a lot of repetitive elements on all levels, from small sequences to large chunks of the chromosomes, with remarkable variation between individuals. Repetitive elements in the telomeres (Section 2.7) and **centromeres** (explained further in the next section) have important effects on chromosome function, but other elements are remnants of our evolutionary history or may simply be the result of replication errors. Variability of many repetitive elements has no functional impact, but some may contribute to differences among individuals or may be the cause for specific diseases (Chapter 3). There is a difference between **tandem repeats**, in which a number of identical elements are found in a row, and **interspersed repeats** that are linked to mobile genetic elements scattered throughout the genome.

Array-based genome quantification methods led to the identification of many chromosomal regions that occur in variable copy numbers in the general population. These **copy number variants** (CNVs) may range in size from 1 kb to more than 1 Mb and may represent both functional (disease-causing) mutations as well as genomic polymorphisms of uncertain relevance. These include **low copy repeats** (LCRs), duplicated or multiplicated chromosomal regions that facilitate the generation of chromosomal rearrangements through nonhomologous pairing and recombination during meiosis. The common microdeletion syndromes and some monogenic deletions or duplications are triggered by the presence of LCRs in the form of intrachromosomal segmental duplications often in the same chromosomal band.

Repetitive Elements in the Human Genome

Tandem repeats: The presence of a number of identical elements in a row.
- Short tandem repeats (STRs): Tandem repeats with a unit size of 2 to 6 nt.
- Minisatellites (variable number tandem repeats, or VNTRs): Tandem repeats with a unit size of 10 to 60 nt.
- Satellite DNA: Repetitive units of 60 to 200 nt that constitute important chromosomal structures, such as the centromeres.

Interspersed repeats: Identical elements linked to mobile genetic elements that are scattered throughout the genome.
- Retrotransposons: DNA sequence elements multiplied through reverse transcription of mRNA into cDNA.

— DNA-transposons: Mobile DNA fragments with a length of approximately 1.2 to 3 kb that encode for a transposase, which cuts out a transposon and inserts it elsewhere.

Multiple copies of chromosomal regions:

— Copy number variants (CNVs): Chromosomal regions with a size ranging from 1 kb to many Mb that occur in variable copy number in the general population.

— Low copy repeats (LCRs): Duplicated or multiplicated chromosomal regions of 1 to 400 kb; they facilitate the generation of chromosomal rearrangements through nonhomologous pairing and recombination during meiosis.

Satellite DNA

The term satellite DNA is not linked to the "satellites" of acrocentric chromosomes but is used for a relatively large proportion of the genome that consists mostly of repetitive sequences. The name derives from the behavior of these elements in density gradient electrophoresis where they form separate bands because of their particular nucleotide composition (a high percentage of adenine and thymine). Satellite DNA units have a size of 60 to 200 nt. The centromeres, for example, contain several 10,000 copies of 171-bp-long **α-satellite DNA**, which binds specific proteins that together with a large number of other proteins form the kinetochore. The kinetochore serves as the point of origin for the microtubules of the mitotic spindle.

The term *satellite* is also applied to two other types of repetitive sequences whose number is highly variable between individuals and mostly inherited. Minisatellites (variable number tandem repeats, or VNTRs) are repetitive sequences of 5 to 50 nucleotides. Repetitive sequences of 2 to 4 nucleotides are **microsatellites** (short tandem repeats, or *STRs*). Mini- and microsatellites usually have no functional significance. Since they are so variable and easily analyzable, they are used in numerous genetic analyses, ranging from genetic fingerprinting and paternity tests to linkage analyses within families. They play a special role in trinucleotide repeat disorders (Chapter 3.6).

Mobile Genetic Elements

The human genome contains large numbers of originally mobile DNA elements, so-called **transposons** or retrotransposons, also referred to as "jumping genes." These are DNA sequences that are able to leave a chromosome and to reenter the genome at nonhomologous points of the DNA. The mobile DNA fragments of the transposons have a length of approximately 1.2 to 3 kb and encode for a transposase that cuts out the transposon and inserts it elsewhere. In the case of retrotransposons the DNA sequence is multiplied through reverse transcription of mRNA into cDNA, which is then integrated into the genome at a different location; the necessary reverse transcriptase is typically encoded by the retrotransposon itself. More than 40% of the human genome is thought to be linked to mobile elements, although most such sequences have long lost the ability to jump.

■■■ Retrotransposons

We differentiate between *long terminal repeat* (LTR) retrotransposons of a length of approximately 5 to 10 kb whose central protein-encoding region is flanked *by long terminal repeats*, and non-LTR retrotransposons where this is not the case. The latter contains *long interspersed elements* (LINEs) of a length up to 7 kb, as well as *short interspersed elements* (SINEs) of up to 300 bp in length, including the so-called Alu sequences. The LINEs and SINEs make up approximately one-third of the total human genome.

Mobile genetic elements have a great influence on the structure of the genome. They probably also played an important role during evolution, and they can contribute in various ways to disease. Alu sequences, for example, can mediate an asymmetric recombination and thus cause genomic deletions and duplications; many frequent microdeletion syndromes are typically generated via this mechanism. The 1983 Nobel Prize for medicine was awarded to Barbara McKlintock for her work in identifying mobile elements.

2.4 From the Gene to mRNA

Most individual genes of the human genome are only expressed in certain tissues or only at certain times during prenatal and postnatal development. Our understanding of the delicate regulation of the expression of eukaryotic genes is still limited. Only a small portion of the human genome sequence (approximately 2%) encodes for proteins. The remaining ~98% was once presumed to be evolutionary "garbage"; however, this supposition, which is not based on scientific evidence, likely underestimates the value of the vast majority of the human DNA sequence. To determine the meaning of non-protein-encoding sequences is one of the major challenges of human genetics of the 21st century.

Regulation of Gene Expression

The expression of individual genes can be regulated on different levels, and many individual steps are necessary until the DNA sequence has turned into a functioning protein. These include unpacking of the chromatin at a certain gene locus, initiation of transcription through binding of transcription factors, and then the actual transcription, followed by the processing of the primary transcript, the transport of the modified transcript into the cytoplasm, the translation of the mature mRNA into a polypeptide, and finally degradation of the mRNA molecule. Each of these steps offers contact points for possible regulators. Above all, it is the **transcription** step itself that is intensively and differentially directed and regulated. Changes in chromatin structure and the binding of specific transcription factors are decisive for the timing and tissue specificity of genetic expression. Chromatin (Section 2.6) in transcriptionally active regions adopts an open conformation associated with extensive acetylation of histones. This allows easy access of transcription factors that can replace histones and nucleosomes for transcription. In contrast, methylation of cytosine in cytosine-guanosine (CpG) dinucleotides within the DNA sequence is associated with tight packing of nucleosomes and transcriptional inactivity. Many genes have clusters of CpG dinucleotides, particularly in their promoter regions, which allow effective silencing. DNA hypermethylation is mirrored by hypoacetylation on the histone level.

Most of the eukaryotic genes are only expressed after transcription factors have bound to the promoter region of the gene and have begun the formation of a large, multicomponent transcription initiation complex. Many transcription factors have structural elements for DNA binding, such as zinc finger, leucine zipper, or helix-loop-helix elements. Looping of the DNA permits the binding of the transcription initiation complex to promoters, enhancers, or other transcription signals that sometimes are several kilobases away from the start of the transcription.

> **Important**
>
> Genes whose gene product is essential for the metabolism of the cell and that are constantly expressed because they are needed in all cells and tissues are called *housekeeping genes*.

Transcription

Transcription: The process of transcribing the DNA into a complementary RNA molecule.

This first step in decoding genetic information takes place in the cell's nucleus. Transcription begins with the formation of the transcription initiation complex from transcription factors and RNA polymerase at the promoter region. Eukaryotes have three different RNA polymerases. The most important is RNA polymerase II, which transcribes protein-encoding mRNA; non-coding RNA as a rule is read by RNA polymerase I or III (⬛ Table 2.1).

Table 2.1. Eukaryotic RNA Polymerases

RNA Polymerase	Transcripts
RNA polymerase I	45S rRNA in the nucleolus, is then split into 18S, 5.8S, and 28S rRNA
RNA polymerase II	mRNA and others
RNA polymerase III	tRNA, 5S rRNA, and other noncoding RNA
rRNA, ribosomal RNA; mRNA, messenger RNA; tRNA, transfer RNA.	

■■■ Amantadine—Poison of RNA Polymerase II
Every year dozens of people die after eating *Amanita phalloides*, the green Death Cap fungus. It contains the poison α-amantadine that binds with strong affinity to RNA polymerase II and thus blocks RNA elongation and the formation of pre-mRNA in the cell. At high concentrations, amantadine also blocks RNA polymerase III.

RNA polymerase binds to the DNA double helix, unwinds it, and starts RNA synthesis (initiation). The template for this is the antisense strand since by definition the sequences of transcript and sense strand are identical. By traveling in the 3' to 5' direction along the antisense strand of the DNA, the RNA polymerase synthesizes RNA in the usual 5' to 3' direction (elongation). The transcribed DNA rewinds behind the RNA polymerase into the double helix.

During and after the transcription process, the emerging pre-mRNA (also called hnRNA or heterogeneous nuclear RNA) is further modified and processed into mature mRNA that is transported into the cytoplasm for translation. The three important steps of capping, splicing, and termination/polyadenylation are closely interconnected as part of the normal transcription process. Posttranscriptional modification of pre-mRNA is partly mediated by subunits of the RNA polymerase II but involves numerous other proteins, RNA molecules, and specific DNA sequences. Mutations affecting any of these processes may have a direct impact on post-transcriptional mechanisms such as mRNA release, export, abundance, and translation and thus may have medically relevant consequences. Monogenic disorders are frequently caused by mutations affecting correct splicing. For example, a common variant in the prothrombin gene that changes a CG sequence at the transcript cleavage site into a much more efficient CA sequence is an important risk factor for thrombosis (Chapter 21.7).

Capping and Polyadenylation

The first nucleotide of the RNA transcript is modified by binding 7-methylguanosine (m^{7}G, from GTP) in a special 5'-5' phosphodiester bond. This is called **capping** the RNA and protects the transcript from degradation through exonucleases, facilitates transport from the nucleus to the cytoplasm, and is required for the attachment to the ribosomes. Correct capping is also required for correct splicing and polyadenylation.

Termination of the RNA strand is mediated through specific sequences of the 3' UTR that are recognized by a large number of specific proteins. This termination is carried out through formation of an RNA loop, which is cut usually at a CA dinucleotide. There are two core elements of this process: the polyadenylation signal AAUAAA located 10 to 30 nt before the cleavage site, and a downstream sequence element up to 30 nt after the cleavage site. Once cleavage has occurred, about 200 adenylate (i.e., adenosine monophosphate, AMP) residues are sequentially added to form a poly(A) tail of the mature mRNA. This **polyadenylation** also increases the stability of the mature mRNA and protects it from intracytoplasmic exonucleases. It regulates the frequency with which an mRNA is read by being continually shortened during translation (a process called *deadenylation*) until the breakup of mRNA is initiated when the poly(A) tail has disappeared completely.

Capping: The attachment of 7-methylguanosine to the 5' start of mRNA.

Polyadenylation: The attachment of multiple adenylate residues to the 39 end of mRNA.

Splicing: Removal of noncoding introns positioned between coding exons in the pre-mRNA transcript.

Splicing

Splicing of RNA is a complicated process that is closely interconnected with the transcription process and is mediated through a large RNA protein complex, the so-called spliceosome. It consists of 5 different small RNA molecules (snRNAs) and more than 50 different proteins. Splicing takes place in three essential steps. First, the intron is cleaved at its 5′ end, that is, just after the preceding exon (**splice donor site**). Next, the G residue of the free 5′ end binds to an invariant adenine in the conserved **branch site** located 20 to 40 nt before the end of the intron, thereby forming the **lariat intermediate**. Finally, the intron is cleaved off at its 3′ end (**splice acceptor site**), and the two free ends of the neighboring exons are linked together. The free lariat is degraded or may fulfill other functions as noncoding RNA.

Several human genes permit so-called **alternative splicing** by supporting the use of different splice donor, splice acceptor, or branch sites. This means that exons of a single gene can be assembled differently and thus create different mRNAs that may encode for functionally different polypeptides. In this way alternative splicing greatly increases the repertoire of proteins in eukaryotes.

▪▪▪ mRNA Editing

Sometimes the information content of mRNA is further changed after transcription, a process called RNA editing. A well-known example is apolipoprotein B, which, as nonedited RNA, encodes for ApoB-100. Post-transcriptional deamination of a specific methylcytosine in the mRNA can change a C into a U and, consequently, a codon CAA (for glutamine) into UAA, a stop codon. This posttranscriptional change (catalyzed by the enzyme deaminase) leads to the replacement of the normal ApoB-100 with ApoB-48, a truncated version of the protein with a completely different function.

Nonsense-mediated decay: A quality-control mechanism that selectively degrades mRNAs that contain premature stop (nonsense) codons.

▪▪▪ Nonsense-mediated decay

Various "internal quality control" mechanisms have been identified that trigger early destruction of faulty mRNA in the cytosol. Most well known is the principle of nonsense-mediated decay (NMD), which is triggered by mutations that cause termination of translation before the last splice site in the mRNA has been reached. It is now understood that the splicing process in the nucleus leaves protein remnants at the mRNA, the so-called exon junction complex (EJC) 20 to 24 nt upstream of every exon junction, which is removed by the ribosome in the first round of translation. Failure to remove the EJC because of a premature stop codon (created by a nonsense mutation) at least 40 nt before the last exon—exon junction is detected by the cellular surveillance machinery and triggers immediate mRNA degradation. This phenomenon is also found with other types of mutations that cause premature termination of translation such as frameshift mutations or mutations that cause elongation of the 3′ UTR. NMD has an important cellular function since it increases the efficiency of translation and also protects from the accumulation of defective polypeptide fragments. Occasionally it can be disadvantageous in monogenic disorders—if, for example, a shortened protein would have residual function but is not produced because of mRNA degradation.

2.5 From mRNA to Protein

Genetic Code

After capping, polyadenylation, and splicing, the mature mRNA is translocated from the nucleus to the cytoplasm where its information is translated into a polypeptide sequence. The mediators between the mRNA sequence and the various amino acids are the **tRNAs** (transfer RNAs). Three nucleotide bases of the mRNA sequence (**codons**) bind to three nucleotide bases of the corresponding tRNAs (**anticodons**). Transfer RNAs are single-strand RNA chains of approximately 80 nucleotides, some of which are modified after transcription to contain unusual bases such as inosine, pseudouridine, or dihydrouridine. The human genome contains several hundred tRNA genes distributed over almost all human chromosomes, in addition to

22 tRNA genes in the mitochondrial genome. The individual strands of all known tRNAs form a clover leaf in which about one-half of the nucleotides are paired by way of hydrogen bonds. All tRNAs are L-shaped, with the anticodon at one end and the amino acid binding point at the other. Aminoacyl-tRNA-synthetases recognize the different tRNAs at the anticodons and at the acceptor arm. They catalyze the coupling of the amino acid to the appropriate tRNA.

The encryption of the amino acid sequence in the DNA sequence is called the **genetic code**. Each codon (of three bases) corresponds to one amino acid. In each codon there is a first, second, and third base, each defined as such. The genetic code additionally contains sequences for the beginning (start codon) and end (stop codon) of the translation. The genetic code is (virtually) **universal**; that is, the same codons are utilized by different organisms (from bacteria to Mongolian gerbils to humans). Exceptions are e.g. the human mitochondrial genome or the genome of the ciliates (paramecia).

Since three bases form a codon and four different bases (A, U, G, C) are present in mRNA, there are a total of $4^3 = 64$ possible combinations, resulting in 64 different codons (◻ Table 2.2). Sixty-one of these codons correspond to specific amino acids, and three codons (UAA, UAG, and UGA) are stop codons. Since there are a total of 20 amino acids and 61 codons, the

◻ **Table 2.2.** The Genetic Code

First Nucleotide	Second Nucleotide	Third Nucleotide	Codes for	Short Code
	A	A or G	Lysine	Lys, K
		U or C	Asparagine	Asn, N
	C	Any	Threonine	Thr, T
A	G	A or G	Arginine	Arg, R
		U or C	Serine	Ser, S
	U	U, C, or A	Isoleucine	Ile, I
		G	Methionine **(Start)**	Met, M
	A	A or G	Glutamine	Gln, Q
		U or C	Histidine	His, H
C	C	Any	Proline	Pro, P
	G	Any	Arginine	Arg, R
	U	Any	Leucine	Leu, L
	A	A or G	Glutamate	Glu, E
		U or C	Aspartate	Asp, D
G	C	Any	Alanine	Ala, A
	G	Any	Glycine	Gly, G
	U	Any	Valine	Val, V
	A	A or G	Stop	**Ter, X**
		U or C	Tyrosine	Tyr, Y
	C	Any	Serine	Ser, S
U	G	A	**Stop**	**Ter, X**
		G	Tryptophan	Trp, W
		U or C	Cysteine	Cys, C
	U	A or G	Leucine	Leu, L
		U or C	Phenylalanine	Phe, F

genetic code is **degenerate**, meaning many amino acids are coded by more than one specific triplet. Codons that code the same amino acid are called *synonyms*. An example would be that AGA as well as AGG code for arginine (see later in the chapter, **tRNA Wobble**).

Translation starts with an AUG codon that codes for methionine, called the **start codon**. Therefore, each newly synthesized peptide begins with the amino acid methionine. Usually it is the first AUG in the mature mRNA molecule as seen from the 5′ end. This AUG also determines the reading frame for the remainder of the mRNA molecule. The reading is retained beyond the limits of the original exons because the introns have already been spliced out. The ends of only some exons coincide with the end of a codon. Loss of an exon in the mRNA causes a shift of the reading frame unless the number of nucleotides in the exon can be divided by three.

Important

The genetic code is . . .
Unambiguous—each codon corresponds to a specific amino acid.
- Degenerate—most amino acids are coded by more than one codon.
- Without comma and not overlapping (with the exception of some viruses).
- Universal—the genetic code is the same in most organisms.

Translation

Translation: The mechanism of protein synthesis in the ribosomes that translates the language of nucleic acids into the language of polypeptides.

The mRNAs, tRNAs loaded with amino acids, and ribosomes are the protagonists of the exceedingly complex procedure that involves far more than 100 macromolecules.

Protein synthesis involves three stages: initiation, elongation, and termination. All occur at the **ribosomes**, cytoplasmic particles formed from different proteins and specific RNA molecules, denoted rRNA. They are enzymes that catalyze the mRNA-dependent formation of peptide bonds. Active ribosomes line up at the translating mRNA (like "beads on a string"), with sometimes more than 50 ribosomes working in a row (**polysomes**).

Each individual ribosome consists of two subunits that, when inactive, are separated from one another. The size of each subunit is determined by the sedimentation coefficient "S" (named after the chemist The Svedberg who received the 1926 Nobel Prize in chemistry for his research on colloids and proteins using the ultracentrifuge). The eukaryotic ribosomes consist of a small **40S subunit** (with one 18S rRNA and 33 different proteins) and a large **60S subunit** with three 28S, 5.8S and 5S rRNAs as well as 50 different proteins) (■ Fig. 2.7). 5S rRNA is represented by multiple copies of a gene located on chromosome 1 (~200 to 300 true genes and many dispersed pseudogenes); the others are encoded by multiple copies of a gene on the short arms of all acrocentric chromosomes; the large transcript is cleaved into three separate rRNA molecules. rRNA transcription is carried out in the nucleolus. Eukaryotic cells also have two mitochondrial rRNA molecules encoded by mitochondrial DNA.

■ **Figure 2.7. Model of a Ribosome.**

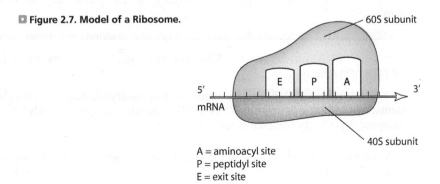

A = aminoacyl site
P = peptidyl site
E = exit site

Initiation. Translation begins with the formation of a "preinitiation complex" that consists of the ribosome's 40S subunit, the initiator tRNA^{Met}, GTP, and several initiation factors. This complex recognizes a mature mRNA at its 5′ end and binds and explores the mRNA in the direction 5′ to 3′, until it encounters a start codon (AUG). At this point the ribosome's 60S subunit binds, the initiation factors detach, and translation begins.

Elongation. The initiator tRNA^{Met} initially occupies the P (peptidyl) site of the ribosome. Elongation begins with the binding of the next tRNA to the second binding site of the ribosome, the so-called A (aminoacyl) site. This is followed by peptide binding between the methionine of the initiator tRNA and the amino acid of the second tRNA. The resulting dipeptidyl RNA then moves from the A to the P site, and the initiator tRNA molecule moves to the E (exit) site before leaving the ribosome. A new aminoacyl tRNA attaches to the free A site to start a new elongation cycle. Elongation factors promote the course of these elongation cycles.

Termination. As soon as a stop codon is reached on the mRNA, the complete polypeptide detaches from the tRNA and the ribosome dissociates into its two subunits.

tRNA Wobble. The codon of the mRNA is recognized by the anticodon of the tRNA. Despite the fact that there are only some 30 different tRNA molecules in cytoplasm (in mitochondria there are only 22), all 64 codons can be recognized. Why is that? Each base of the codon pairs with a complementary base of the anticodon. While the first two bases must pair precisely in the usual way, the steric conditions for the third base are less stringent. Codons that differ in the third position may bind the same tRNA and thus code for the same amino acid. For half of the codons the third base is insignificant, while the remaining codons only distinguish between purines (A and G) and pyrimidines (C and U). The only exceptions are the start codon AUG and one of the three stop codons, UGA, which are specific. It is said that the third position *wobbles*. The degeneracy of the genetic code can therefore be partially explained by the inaccurate pairing of the third base of the codon with the first base of the anticodon. Sometimes synonymous codons differ in the efficiency with which the corresponding amino acid is integrated into the growing polypeptide chain, causing variable effects of apparently silent mutations on gene function.

■■■ **Diphtheria, a Deadly Disease Caused by Faulty Translation**
Diphtheria, a vaccine-preventable disease, was once a frequent cause of death in children. Since the introduction of active immunization, the disease has become rare and today only affects individuals with insufficient immunization. The causative *Corynebacterium diphtheria* produces a toxin that is fatal for nonvaccinated individuals in an amount of a few milligrams. After invading a cell, diphtheria toxin breaks into two fragments, A and B. The A fragment causes ADP-ribosylation and thereby inactivation of the elongation factor EF2, which is required for translocation of tRNAS from the A site to the P site of the ribosome. By stopping translation and protein synthesis, a single A fragment of the toxin can kill one cell.

2.6   RNA

Riboproteins: Complexes of proteins and RNA molecules that carry out various functions in the cell.

Ribozymes: RNA molecules that catalyze enzymatic reactions in cellular metabolism.

Noncoding RNA: Various types of RNA molecules that do not carry sequence information for protein synthesis.

RNA interference (RNAi): A natural mechanism of eukaryotic cells by which short RNA fragments, denoted small interfering RNA (siRNA), identify and cleave mRNAs if the respective sequence is perfectly complementary.

RNA differs from DNA because of the use of ribose instead of deoxyribose as the backbone sugar and the use of uracil (U) instead of thymine (T) as one of the pyrimidine bases. RNA generally exists as a single-stranded molecule but functions as a complementary binding partner for DNA or RNA molecules using the same base-pairing mechanism as double-stranded DNA. Originally the function of RNA was thought to be mostly limited to its role in transcription and translation: **messenger RNA** transports the genetic information from the nucleus to the ribosomes, which contain **ribosomal RNA** and catalyze translation with the assistance of **transfer RNA** as adapter molecules for the amino acids.

This view has changed fundamentally, particularly during the last decade when numerous other functions of RNA molecules have been recognized. Apart from the "classic" RNAs that mediate protein synthesis, there are many types of noncoding RNAs with various functions, particularly in the regulation of gene expression. The first monogenic disease caused by loss of function of an RNA gene, Prader-Willi syndrome (see Section 4.3), has been detected, but we are far from understanding the true extent of the role of ncRNAs in health and disease.

Ribozymes

Catalyzation of biochemical reactions was long thought to be the exclusive domain of proteins, until in the early 1980s Thomas Cech and Sidney Altman showed that RNA can fold into complex shapes and carry out enzymatic functions (they received the 1989 Nobel Prize in chemistry for this discovery). RNA enzymes, called ribozymes, accelerate biochemical reactions, emerge unchanged from them, and can go through several such cycles. Although apparently few RNA molecules remain that function as ribozymes, it has been suggested that prior to the development of proteins in the beginning of evolution all enzymatic reactions were carried out by RNA molecules. It is now recognized that the ribosome is a true ribozyme as there are no ribosomal proteins close to the reaction site for polypeptide synthesis (see Section 2.5).

RNA as a Guide Molecule

Many RNAs together with proteins form part of a ribonucleoprotein (RNP) complex that is responsible for identifying a substrate while the actual (e.g., catalytic) function is accomplished by proteins. For example, **small nuclear RNA** (snRNA, 100 to 300 nt long) manages the splicing of pre-mRNA in the spliceosomes of the nucleus. **Small nucleolar RNA** (snoRNA, 50 to 200 nt long) is found in the nucleolus and after merging with specific proteins is responsible for specific modifications of rRNAs, snRNAs, and tRNAs. A specific region of snoRNA, 10 to 20 nt long, guides the enzymatic active proteins to the complementary RNA targets. Other important RNA molecules are **SRP-RNA**, a component of the signal recognition particle (SRP) that directs ribosomes that produce specific secreted proteins (with an endoplasmic reticulum signal sequence) to the membrane of the endoplasmic reticulum, and **Xist-RNA**, a 17-kb segment of the *XIST* gene on chromosome Xq13, which together with several proteins forms a DNA methyltransferase that initiates X chromosome inactivation.

RNA Interference

RNA interference (RNAi) is a natural mechanism of eukaryotic cells that plays a major role in the degradation of foreign genetic material in the cell (e.g., in viral infections). It also has a major role in regulating the cell's own genes. Gene expression can be regulated at several stages: at the chromatin stage, after transcription, or at transcription. The principle of RNA interference was discovered in 1998 in studies involving the tapeworm *Caenorhabditis elegans*; Andrew Fire and Craig Mello received the 2006 Nobel Prize in medicine for this discovery.

Double-stranded RNA is cut into short RNA fragments (**siRNA** [*small interfering* RNA] or **miRNA** [*micro*-RNA]) of a length of 21 to 23 nt by a nuclease called DICER. One siRNA is incorporated into a multiprotein complex known as **RNA-induced silencing complex (RISC)** that identifies and cleaves mRNAs if its sequence is perfectly complementary to the siRNA. It is an effective mechanism for removal of unwanted mRNA species. In some cases, the binding of siRNA might not initiate cleavage and degradation, but rather prevents translation of the respective mRNA for the duration of binding. Under some circumstances, siRNAs associate into complexes other than RISC that silence gene transcription in the nucleus.

In some organisms (not in humans) an RNA-dependent RNA polymerase can use the double strand of siRNA and bound mRNA as a template, leading to a new double-stranded RNA (dsRNA) that is once again recognized and separated by DICER (a self-potentiating cycle).

In the past few years RNAi has become an important tool for molecular biology. Through the introduction of synthetic dsRNA into cells, it is possible to effectively "switch off" specific target genes by preventing translation. The potential use of RNAi to target the elimination of disease-associated genes in vivo is awaited with great hope.

2.7   Chromosomes

With the exception of the germ cell (sperm or egg cells), all cells of the human organism contain **23 pairs of (46 total) chromosomes** (*chroma* [Gr.], "color," "color particle"). One chromosome of each pair comes from the mother, the other from the father. Each egg cell and each sperm contains a **haploid** (*haploos* [Gr.], "simple") set of 23 chromosomes (1n). A merger of these two haploid chromosome complements in the fertilized egg cell creates a **diploid** (diploos [Gr.], "double") set of 46 chromosomes (2n). Twenty-two pairs of **autosomes** do not differ between male and female. They are numbered according to size in descending order: the largest is chromosome 1; the smallest, however, is not chromosome 22, as originally thought, but chromosome 21. The **sex chromosomes** are denoted X and Y. Males have a single X and a single Y chromosome. Females have two X chromosomes. According to the position of the centromere, the chromosomes are designated as metacentric (central centromere), submetacentric, or acrocentric (terminal centromere).

Centromere: The element of a chromosome that serves as an anchor point for the spindle apparatus during cell division; it contains repetitive α-satellite DNA sequences and divides the chromosomes into a short arm, **p** (for "petite"), and a long arm, **q** (the letter that follows p in the alphabet).

Metacentric chromosomes: The centromere is positioned in the middle of the chromosome.

Submetacentric chromosomes: The centromere is positioned between the middle and the end of the chromosome.

Acrocentric chromosomes: The centromere is positioned at the end of the chromosome, separating a normal long arm from a short arm that contains only multiple (many hundred) copies of rRNA genes (chromosomal satellites).

Telomere: The ends of the chromosomes that consist of numerous tandem repeats of 5'-TTAGGG-3' sequences.

Genes are arranged in a more or less linear fashion along both strands of the DNA double helix of each chromosome. The two partners of each pair of chromosomes (**homologous chromosomes**) normally carry the same genes in the same progression. Sequence homology enables binding and recombination at meiosis, which is not only essential for the generation of a haploid set of chromosomes but also an important factor in the diversification of the species. Throughout the entire genome, however, there are millions of sequence variants that differentiate the two homologous chromosome complements and that, in their entirety, are responsible for the genetic differences between people (see Section 2.3 and Chapter 3).

DNA Packaging

The haploid human genome contains approximately 3×10^9 base pairs of DNA. Since 3,000 base pairs of pure DNA are 1 μm long, the total length of the haploid human genome is 1 meter. Thus, 2 meters of DNA per body cell needs to be packaged efficiently, compactly, and without knots into the nucleus that has a diameter of 10 μm. This is achieved with the help of **histones**, specific evolutionarily conserved proteins that are similar in all eukaryotes. There are two major types of histones: core histones (which come in four different classes: H2A, H2B, H3, and H4) and linker histones (class H1). Each class has a considerable number of subtypes encoded by individual genes that are arranged in clusters throughout the genome. Because of their function in organizing chromosomal structure, histones contribute to virtually all chromosomal processes, such as gene regulation, chromosome condensation, recombination, and replication.

Histones: Specific evolutionarily conserved proteins that are used to package the DNA strand in a chromosome.

Nucleosome: The basic packaging unit in a chromosome that consists of 8 core histones and 146 base pairs of DNA.

Chromatin: The combination of DNA and (histone and nonhistone) proteins that makes up a chromosome.

Euchromatin: Relatively loosely packed chromatin that represents transcriptionally active DNA or may be recognized as light bands during chromosome analysis (G-banding).

Heterochromatin: Highly condensed chromatin that represents transcriptionally inactive (often repetitive) DNA or may be recognized as dark bands during chromosome analysis (G-banding).

The basic packaging unit of a chromosome in all eukaryotes is the **nucleosome**. The outside of the DNA double strand is wound around eight core histones (two each of H2A, H2B, H3, and H4) in a defined spatial arrangement. Per the nucleosome the DNA completes 1.75 full twists, which correspond to 146 base pairs or a packaging ratio (the degree of compaction of the double helix) of 1:6. Neighboring nucleosomes are connected by 60 bp of spacer DNA, aided by histone H1, which has a key role in the coiling and packaging of chromatin and also helps to seal the DNA strand at the surface of the nucleosome. Under the electron microscope the individual nucleosomes with their respective linkage regions look like pearls on a chain. The individual pearls are approximately 10 nm in size.

The next level of packaging is a super helix with a diameter of 25 to 30 nm formed by nucleosomes and histone H1. It represents the **chromatin fiber** of interphase chromatin and achieves a packaging ratio of 1:36. A packaging ratio of about 1:10,000 is achieved during condensation of the chromosomes for cell division through the attachment of loops of the chromatin fiber, each containing 20 to 100 kb of DNA, to a central **scaffold**. This contains various nonhistone proteins including a remarkable enzyme called *topoisomerase II* that can pass one DNA double helix through another by cutting a gap and sealing it. The loop—scaffold complex is further twisted in metaphase chromosomes, finally resulting in a highly coiled chromatid with a diameter of approximately 1,000 nm.

Euchromatin and Heterochromatin

Only in metaphase is the entire chromosome in a highly condensed state. During all other phases of the cell cycle it is possible to distinguish varying degrees of condensation. A large portion of the chromosomes appear as euchromatin that contains rather loosely packed chromatid fibers and represents transcriptionally active DNA. Other segments, called heterochromatin, remain in a relatively high state of condensation during the entire cell cycle; they also show late replication during the S phase of the cell cycle. Much heterochromatin exists near the centromeres of the chromosomes or in the region of the telomeres of the acrocentric chromosomes. The DNA of heterochromatin cannot be transcribed because it is packed too tightly to allow the transcription mechanism sufficient access to the DNA strand. Heterochromatin contains few genes but a large portion of the highly repetitive areas of the human DNA.

A special form of heterochromatin is found in the inactivated X chromosome of women. Large parts (80% to 85%) of the genes of this chromosome are not expressed and remain condensed as heterochromatin in somatic cells throughout life. In oocytes, however, heterochromatin turns into euchromatin as soon as the cell progresses from the dictyotene stage during the first meiotic division.

Centromeres and Telomeres

Centromeres and telomeres of the human chromosome contain a large number of repetitive DNA sequences and are conserved during evolution. About 5% of the repetitive sequences of the human DNA are located in the area of the **centromeres**, primarily α-satellite DNA that binds structural proteins that form the kinetochore, the anchor point for the spindle apparatus during cell division.

Telomeres (*telos* [Gr.], "end") consist of numerous tandem repeats of 5′-TTAGGG-3′ sequences. Since the replication of DNA can only proceed in the 5′ to 3′ direction, a small segment of nucleotides on one of the two DNA strands (the one whose 5′ end is part of the telomere) remains unreplicated by DNA polymerase. TTAGGG repeats at the telomere can be resynthesized by the enzyme **telomerase**, which is a reverse transcriptase that contains its own RNA template 5′-CCCUAAA-3′ and therefore can bind nucleotides independently of a DNA strand at the free 3′ end. Humans express telomerase mostly in germ cells. Fully differentiated cells no longer show telomerase activity and therefore their telomeres are shortened by roughly 50 nt per cell cycle. Complete loss of the telomere triggers cell death, and the progressive shortening of telomeres thus contributes to aging and to cellular degeneration. By contrast, many tumor cells have telomerase activity, resulting in no cellular senescence and thus they are less susceptible to programmed cell death (apoptosis).

2.8   Special Features of the Sex Chromosomes

The evolutionary diversion of the sex chromosomes X and Y probably started 150 to 200 million years ago when a transcription factor gene on what was at that time a pair of autosomes developed a new variant with gender-determining properties. When present, this allele (today represented by the SRY gene on the Y chromosomes) triggered the gonads to obtain a male constitution, while the corresponding allele on the X chromosome (SOX3) had no primary role in gonadal development. Over time, parts of the chromosome that contained the *SRY* precursor (i.e., the precursor of the modern Y chromosome) started to degrade because they were not essential for life. Only a few genes remained functional, most of these having acquired a male gender-specific function that ensured their existence. One problem that arose from this development was the fact that female cells have two copies of X chromosomal genes, whereas male genes have only one. To counteract a deleterious gene dosage effect, the mechanism of X inactivation evolved, which allows silencing or late expression of the genes on one of the two X chromosomes. The end result is a large X chromosome with about 1,000 genes and a small Y chromosome that in humans only contains 45 unique coding genes, largely related to X chromosomal genes. Females have two copies of the X chromosome, one of which is mostly inactivated. Presence of the Y chromosome (or rather, the SRY gene) determines that the individual will become male. Individuals with one X chromosome develop a female phenotype (Turner syndrome), while people with two X and one Y develop as males (Klinefelter syndrome). The number of X chromosomes is inconsequential for sexual differentiation, as is their numeric ratio to the autosomes. The Y chromosome is the dominant factor for the development of testes. In its absence, the primordium develops as female.

Today most parts of the X and Y chromosomes are nonhomologous, with the exception of two larger regions located at the distal end of the short arms (2,600 kb) and at the distal end of the long arms (320 kb), the so-called pseudoautosomal regions (PARs). Genetic markers of these segments are inherited irrespective of sex. **PAR 1** is the larger of the two at the distal end of chromosome Yp or Xp, **PAR 2** is at the distal end of chromosome Yq or Xq.

Pseudoautosomal regions: The distal ends of the X and Y chromosomes that contain homologous gene sequences, pair in meiosis, and experience obligatory crossing over.

The Y Chromosome

The human Y chromosome is approximately 60 Mb long and on its long arm has lengthy segments of repetitive, noncoding DNA. Many of the functional Y chromosomal genes (outside the PAR) play an important role in sexual differentiation, the development of sexual characteristics, and spermatogenesis; there is also a large number of apparently nonfunctional genes or pseudogenes.

Y and Sexual Differentiation. The **chromosomal** sex of the embryo is genetically determined at the time of fertilization. The gonads begin as sexually indifferent genital ridges and do not develop the morphological characteristics for the male or female sex until the seventh week after conception. As mentioned previously, the presence of a Y chromosome dictates how the indifferent rudiments of the sexual organs evolve. For a long time, it was unclear which gene of the Y chromosome was the deciding **testis-determining factor** (TDF). Answers to this question were provided in men with a karyotype of 46,XX, who were phenotypically normal males (XX male syndrome). Cytogenetic and molecular genetic tests showed that most of these men had an unbalanced translocation that caused the genetic material to be translocated from the region directly proximal to PAR-1 of the Y chromosome to the X chromosome. Additional studies identified the gene *SRY (sex-determining region on Y)* in this region as the long-sought *TDF*.

The *SRY* directly affects the differentiation of the gonads: its presence induces male development; its absence, female development. During embryonic development, *SRY* is expressed for a short time in the cells of the genital ridges, immediately before testicular differentiation occurs. It codes for a DNA-binding protein, a transcription factor that as initiator of a gene cascade determines the further development of the indifferent rudiments of the sexual organs. The majority of these other genes are located on the autosomes.

Y and Spermatogenesis. Interstitial deletions in the long arm of the Y chromosome are responsible for 10% of all cases of nonobstructive azoospermia. This discovery led early on to the assumption that one or several genes for azoospermia (denoted **azoospermia factors** or **AZFs**) are located on the Y chromosome. Four different regions whose microdeletion is associated with azoospermia can be distinguished: AZFa, AZFb, AZFc, and AZFd. Detailed research of these gene loci led to the identification of various genes that are important for spermatogenesis, such as the *DAZ* genes (*d*eleted in *az*oospermia) in the AZFc region that code for RNA-binding proteins (i.e., not transcription factors) and are only expressed in the premeiotic germ cells of the testes. It can easily be understood that the microdeletions aided by *DAZ* are de novo deletions. If the father had had this deletion, he would have been infertile and unable to procreate.

The X Chromosome

The X chromosome is a large, submetacentric chromosome with approximately 1,000 genes. As already mentioned, females have two X chromosomes, males only one. The principle by which this dosage difference is compensated was first postulated by the geneticist Mary Lyon in 1961 and is called the Lyon hypothesis.

Lyon hypothesis: In somatic cells of female mammals, only one X chromosome is transcriptionally active. Additional X chromosomes are randomly inactivated during early embryogenesis; once established, the X-inactivation pattern will be passed on to daughter cells during mitosis.

X inactivation most likely begins shortly after fertilization and is complete after approximately 1 week (ca. 100-cell stage). X inactivation in this phase is **random**. It is equally likely that the maternal (X^m) or the paternal X chromosome (X^p) is inactivated. As soon as the X inactivation of a cell is completed, all cells originating from it will have the same inactive X chromosome. Every female with karyotype 46,XX therefore has a functional **mosaic** of cells with an active maternal X chromosome and cells with an active paternal X chromosome. Inactivated X chromosomes are visible by light microscopy as heterochromatic "sex chromatin" or **Barr bodies** in the interphase nucleus. Like all types of heterochromatin, the inactive X chromosome shows late replication during the S phase of the cell cycle.

Quite Simply: All except One (except in Polyploidy). In most circumstances all X chromosomes except one are inactivated. Therefore, a man with the karyotype 46,XY does not have any Barr bodies. A man with 47,XXY has one Barr body, just like a woman with 46,XX. A woman with 45,X (Turner syndrome) has no Barr bodies. A woman with 47,XXX has two, and a woman with 48,XXXX has three Barr bodies. A notable exception to this rule is tetraploidy (e.g., 92,XXXX), in which two active X chromosomes remain, or triploidy, with either one or two Barr bodies. X inactivation thus seems to depend partly on the number of autosomes, but how exactly this is regulated is still unclear.

The molecular mechanism underlying X activation is better understood. It is based on the same principles that are used throughout the genome for transcriptional control and formation of heterochromatin i.e., methylation of cytosine residues at CpG dinucleotides in the DNA, particularly at gene promoters, and modification (e.g., hypoacetylation) of histones (see also Section 2.4). Silencing of one X chromosome is triggered by the RNA transcript of the *XIST gene (X-inactive specific transcript),* which is active on the X_i chromosome that is going to be inactivated. The *XIST* gene is located in the **X-inactivation center (Xic)** on the long arm of the X chromosome (Xq13). The inactive X chromosome is covered with Xist RNA. Initially, this is reversible and genes become reactivated if Xist is lost. However, subsequent DNA methylation makes X inactivation irreversible even in the absence of Xist, which is thus not required for maintenance of the silent state.

If the X inactivation was complete and would affect all genes on the X chromosome, neither patients with karyotype 45,X nor patients with 47,XXY would present a clinical phenotype. In reality, all genes of the PARs (among them the *SHOX* gene, which is important for growth) as well as many other genes (possibly up to 20% of all genes on the X chromosome) escape X inactivation. The genes in the two pseudoautosomal regions have homologous regions on the Y chromosome and need no compensation of gene dosage. For the other genes that escape X inactivation, dosage differences may not be functionally relevant (such as in recessive diseases) or may contribute to the female phenotype.

Because inactivation in the early embryonic stage is random (with reference to the entire organism), the ratio of inactivated maternal X chromosomes to inactivated paternal X chromosomes should be 1:1. This, however, is only a statistical number that follows a Gaussian distribution. Approximately 10% to 15% of all women have an uneven distribution with a definite shift to either side. This phenomenon is called *skewed X inactivation*. Skewing of X inactivation is frequently seen in females carrying a severe mutation or structural anomaly of their X chromosomes. Because inactivation of the "normal" X may have significant consequences for the fitness or even viability of the individual cell, there is skewing (i.e., preferential inactivation of the "abnormal" X). The obvious prerequisite is the presence of the X-inactivation center Xic; large structural anomalies that remove Xic are incompatible with life. Not infrequently Turner syndrome is caused by extensive structural changes of one X chromosome (e.g., ring chromosome X), which gets lost in a proportion of cells. Especially complex are the cases of X chromosomal autosomal translocations because they may cause spreading of X inactivation into autosomal material.

■■■ Skewed X Inactivation

The phenomenon of *skewed X inactivation* explains why the expression of X-linked disorders is variable in heterozygous women. Let us consider the example of Duchenne muscular dystrophy caused by mutations in the DMD gene on chromosome Xp21.2 (Chapter 31.4). Most heterozygous females are asymptomatic in childhood. Nevertheless, they usually show elevated blood concentrations of the muscle enzyme creatine kinase (CK) because of the damage to muscle cells that express the mutant copy of the gene, and as adults they are at risk for cardiomyopathy. Clinical features of DMD in a young female should lead one to suspect an underlying chromosomal disorder such as Turner syndrome, a chromosomal translocation between X and an autosome, or skewed X inactivation.

> **Important**
>
> It is important to recognize that heterozygosity for a mutation has fundamentally different consequences depending on whether it lies on an autosome or (in the case of women) on the X chromosome. In the case of an autosomal mutation, all cells contain a mixture of normal and mutated (or missing) gene products. In the case of an X-chromosomal mutation, there is functional mosaicism for two different cell lines: one has the normal gene product, whereas the other has the mutated or missing gene product. Clinical consequences in the latter depend on the function of the gene product or the type of mutation.

2.9 Mitosis and Meiosis

There are two kinds of cell division in eukaryotes: mitosis and meiosis. While meiosis (*meiosis* [Gr.], "reduction") occurs in the germ cells, mitosis (*mitos* [Gr.], "thread," "loop") is the normal cell division of somatic cells. In mitosis each of the two daughter cells is identical to the mother cell from which they derive. The chromosome complement of the daughter cells resulting from mitosis has 46 chromosomes and is therefore diploid (2n). By contrast, meiosis involves a **reduction division**. It results in four haploid gametes (n) with 23 chromosomes each in males, and one haploid gamete and three polar bodies in females.

Chromatid: One of the two identical copies of DNA, attached at the centromeres, making up a duplicated chromosome during mitosis.

Sister chromosomes: During mitosis the two identical DNA copies after their separation at the centromeres.

2.9.1 Mitosis

The chromosomes of a normal cell not in the state of division are uncoiled (interphase) and not visible under the light microscope. Before the cell enters mitosis, it doubles its genetic material through replication during the S phase (synthesis phase). At the end of the S phase the cell contains 46 chromosomes (2n) with two chromatids each (4C). Mitosis lasts approximately 60 minutes. It is a continuous process of five different consecutive phases: prophase, prometaphase, metaphase, anaphase, and telophase (◻ Fig. 2.8).

Prophase (*pro* [Gr.], "before"). This phase is characterized by the onset of chromosomal condensation, initially recognized in the light microscope by a rough chromatin structure of the nucleus. The entire cellular microtubule system breaks down. The centrosomes travel in the direction of the two cell poles.

Prometaphase. The cell enters prometaphase as soon as the nuclear envelope disassembles. Through progressive condensation the chromosomes become fully visible. The centrosomes reach the opposite cell poles, while their microtubules form the so-called mitosis spindle. The chromosomes begin to travel toward the center of the cell ("congression").

Metaphase (*meta* [Gr.], "central," "between"). In the metaphase, the chromosomes have reached their maximum condensation. The two strands of each duplicated chromosome (chromatids) become visible. The chromosomes align exactly in the center between the two spindle poles (equatorial or metaphase plate).

Figure 2.8. Mitosis. (From Löffler et al., 2007.)

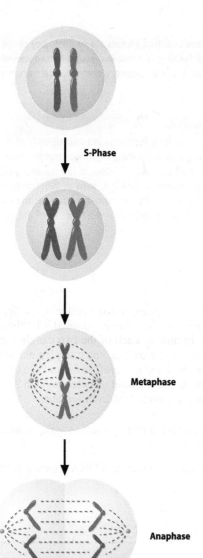

S-Phase

Metaphase

Anaphase

Cytokinesis

Anaphase (*ana* [Gr.], "up," "upward"). It begins as soon as the sister chromatids at the centromere begin to separate and move away from one another toward the opposite cell poles.

Telophase (*telos* [Gr.], "goal"). The separated sister chromatids have reached the region of the centrosomes. The chromatids begin to uncoil. A new cell membrane is formed.

Following telophase, there is **cytokinesis** when actual cell division takes place. It occurs in the middle between the two nuclei of the daughter cells (equatorial division).

At the end of mitosis, there are two equally large daughter cells with 46 chromosomes each. Each of these 46 chromosomes consists of one chromosomal strand.

> **Important**
>
> **The Phases of Mitosis**
> - **Pro**phase: **Pro**log, the chromosomes become **pro**minent (visible).
> - **M**etaphase: The chromosomes are at **m**aximal condensation and aligned in the **m**iddle (equator).
> - **A**naphase: There is pull **at** the chromosomes, and they move **a**way from one another.
> - **Telo**phase: **Telo**s means end—just like **telo**meres are the ends of the chromosomes!

2.9.2 Meiosis

The aim of meiosis is the production of haploid gametes (oocytes or spermatozoa) (1n). This is necessary so that during the fusion of the two gametes an oocyte with a diploid chromosome complement (2n) is created, to generate new life. Meiosis occurs in two consecutive cell divisions. The **first meiotic division** results in the creation of two daughter cells each with a haploid chromosome complement yet still containing double chromatids (1n, 2C). The **second meiotic division** basically is a mitosis without the synthesis phase and during which the two sister chromatids are separated (◻ Fig. 2.9).

Meiosis I

The first meiotic division is an extremely complicated process of reduction division. It is also the phase in which genetic recombination occurs through crossover between homologous chromosomes. The particular challenge for meiosis I is to get one homologous chromosome (with both chromatids) of the 23 chromosome pairs into each of the daughter cells. For that purpose the homologous chromosomes (the four homologous chromatids) are paired to one another at the synaptonemal complex; they remain connected until the division spindle makes contact with each chromosome.

Prophase I. Prophase I is divided into five stages: leptotene, zygotene, pachytene, diplotene, and diakinesis. Pachytene is the stage of the meiotic crossover. During the diplotene stage the homologous chromosomes are separated yet remain attached at the crossover points, the so-called chiasmata. The average number of chiasmata per human spermatozoon is 50 (i.e., multiple for each **bivalent** [chromosome pair]).

Subsequent Phases. The remaining stages of meiosis I correspond to those of mitotic division. They are called prometaphase I, metaphase I, anaphase I, and telophase I. During anaphase the two sister chromosomes of each bivalent are pulled to the opposite cell poles. This process is called **disjunction. Nondisjunction** occurs when both sister chromosomes of a bivalent enter a common daughter cell. Nondisjunction during maternal oogenesis is, for example, the most common cause of Down Syndrome (trisomy 21).

> **Important**
>
> The prospective ova remain in the prophase of the first meiosis, more specifically in the stage of diakinesis (which is then called *dictyotene*), from the early embryonic stage up until the ovulation of the respective ovum. Meiosis I is completed during ovulation; at that point meiosis II is initiated and lasts until fertilization. Meiosis I in women, therefore, lasts up to 40 to 50 years. The long arrest in prophase I most probably increases the likelihood of nondisjunction in oocytes of older mothers and in consequence the increasing incidence of chromosomal disorders associated with "advanced maternal age" (see Chapter 19).

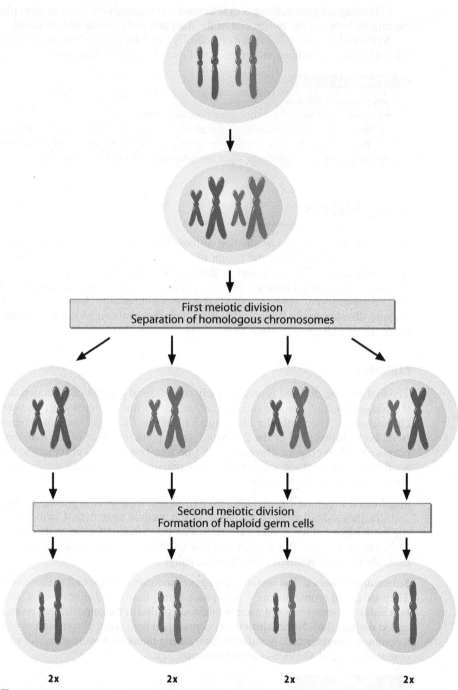

🔵 **Figure 2.9. Meiosis.** (From Löffler et al., 2007.)

Meiosis II

Meiosis II occurs after a short interphase without S phase. Just as in mitosis, the two sister chromatids of the individual chromosomes are separated (1n, 2C → 1n, 1C). As in mitosis, the phases are prophase II, prometaphase II, metaphase II, anaphase II, and telophase II.

> **Important**
>
> During meiosis I and II each female germ cell generates four daughter cells, each with the chromosome complement 23,X. Only one of these daughter cells develops into a mature egg. The other three, the so-called *polar bodies*, contain very little cytoplasm and degenerate. One male germ cell generates four mature spermatozoa, two with the chromosome complement 23,X and two with 23,Y.

> **Important**
>
> In terms of biological evolution meiosis is of twofold importance:
> - It guarantees a reliable distribution of the 23 chromosome pairs into two germ cells. How homologous chromosomes (those from the grandfather and those from the grandmother) are distributed among daughter cells is strictly random (corresponding to the Law of Independent Assortment, the Second Mendelian law). This guarantees continually new chromosomal combinations and evolutionary variety.
> - Crossover between homologous chromosomes during meiosis I generates an exchange of genetic material (recombination). This contributes to additional chromosomal variety, sometimes leading to rearranged genes.

3 Mutations and Genetic Variability

LEARNING OBJECTIVES

1 Define the terms *mutation, polymorphism,* and *genetic variant,* and explain the conceptual differences.

2 Name and define five terms that are used for the description of numerical chromosome anomalies.

3 Explain the different clinical consequences of balanced and unbalanced structural chromosome anomalies.

4 Name and define five different types of point mutations with regard to their functional effects.

5 Define *anticipation* and demonstrate its clinical significance using myotonic dystrophy as a clinical example.

3.1 Mutation or Polymorphism?

Genetic changes are frequent. New alleles arise at an estimated rate of approximately 70 per diploid human genome per generation. Most of these genetic changes are functionally irrelevant, but some may have minor effects on the phenotype or, occasionally, may be of such serious consequence that the conception will result in a miscarriage rather than a live birth.

Complex Problems—Simple Answers? The variants in the human genetic material are as manifold as their consequences. One of the big challenges in molecular genetic diagnostics is the correct interpretation of novel variants in a patient's genetic sequence, especially in cases of point mutations where a different amino acid is predicted to occur in the coded protein ("coding nonsynonymous"), or where there is (seemingly) no influence on the protein sequence. Is it a serious "mutation" or a silent variant? The human genome is too complex to permit simple answers. Mutations in the promoter regions, in splice sites, within introns, or in the untranslated regions may (or may not) lead to changes in gene expression or the posttranslational modification of gene products. In comparing a random piece of human DNA, one finds that two individuals (or rather the homologous chromosomes of the diploid genome) differ in their sequence at every 1,000th base. Therefore, a sequence of 3 billion base pairs would have 3 million base-pair differences between two individuals! When limiting the comparison to coding sequences, 1 in 2,500 bases varies between two individuals (due to the fact that these variants are more likely to have functional effects and to be subject to selection).

A Question of Frequency? In determining the functional effects of a particular genetic variant, it is useful to consider its frequency within a population. A rare variant found in a person (or several persons) with a specific clinical abnormality but not in control individuals is more likely to be disease causing than a variant that is frequently found in the general population. Nevertheless, a novel variant identified in a patient may be clinically irrelevant even if it has never been observed in hundreds of other persons. Determining the effect of "unclassified variants", also called variants of uncertain significance or varicents of unknown significance (VUS) is a particular challenge in the dominantly inherited cancer predisposition syndromes such as inherited breast and ovarian cancer (Chapter 32.3). More than 1,000 disease-causing mutations in the *BRCA1* and *BRCA2* genes have been identified so far, but there are also many VUSs whose pathogenetic relevance is uncertain. This can present a challenge in genetic counseling since it cannot be ruled out that they are disease causing. Nevertheless, predictive mutation analysis would not be offered to a family based on the detection of such a VUS.

Attempting a Definition. Mutation or polymorphism? These two terms are used inconsistently even by geneticists. **Mutation** derives from the Latin *mutatio,* which means "alteration." It can mean both the *occurrence* of a change in the genetic information and the resultant change itself.

The term is primarily unrelated to the functional effect of a genetic alteration, even though in general practice it is mostly used for rare disease-causing variants. Sequence alterations without functional effects are often called polymorphisms, but again this definition, based on functional criteria, may be problematic in some instances. How can one be sure that a specific sequence variant has no functional effect? What about frequent variants that do have functional relevance yet rarely or never trigger a disease or serve as common risk factors for a disease? The blood groups of the ABO system, for example, are due to "mutations," but most people would not use this term to describe carriers of blood group O.

Most geneticists recommend that the term **polymorphism** be defined according to frequency. Polymorphisms are genetic variants where the rarer allele in a population occurs with a **frequency of at least 1%**, independent of the functional or pathogenetic relevance of this alteration. There is nothing wrong with using the term mutation colloquially for rare DNA alterations that cause disease, but one should be aware of the gray zones of such a definition. When in doubt, it is advisable to use the neutral term **variant** for all deviations from the wild-type sequence (the standard "normal sequence").

Polymorphism: A genetic variant where the rarer allele in a population occurs with a frequency of at least 1%, independent of the functional or pathogenetic relevance of this alteration.

Single nucleotide polymorphism (SNP): A polymorphism where the alleles vary within one single nucleotide base.

Mutation: The occurrence of a change in the genomic sequence, or the resultant change itself. The term is generally used for disease-causing genetic variants.

Allele: One of two or more variants of a gene; the term may be used in connection with various denominators such as a particular DNA sequence (e.g., polymorphism), a combination of genetic markers (haplotype), functional characteristics (wild type vs. disease causing), or parental origin (maternal or paternal).

■■■Allele

Allele is another term that is often used imprecisely. It derives from the Greek word *allelon*, which means "belonging together." It designates a specific version or variant of a gene or a chromosome segment that is different from another allele (or several other alleles). This can be in reference to a mere DNA sequence at the same locus, but the term can also refer to a combination of genetic markers (haplotype) or to functional aspects (normal allele vs. disease allele).

Homologous chromosomes contain corresponding gene copies. If a person is homozygous for a particular gene sequence in all its characteristics and base positions, then this person has two copies of the same allele of this gene. Stated differently, this person carries the same allele on both chromosomes, and therefore is homozygous for that allele. At the same time, it is okay to refer to the alleles as maternal and paternal in this situation, since the origin of the chromosomal strand may be a valid distinguishing feature even if it is the same allele with regard to the DNA sequence. The use of the term *allele* thus depends on the distinguishing feature that one likes to emphasize.

Single Nucleotide Polymorphisms

More than 90% of all variations in human DNA involve exchanges of single nucleotide bases. These are called *single nucleotide polymorphisms* (SNPs). By definition, these are loci of the human genome where the alleles vary within one single nucleotide base, and where the rarer allele occurs with a frequency of at least 1% in the population (as stated previously). SNPs are found in coding as well as noncoding regions of the human genome. In the coding regions they are called cSNPs. In the noncoding regions, as a rule, one such polymorphism occurs at every 1,000th nucleotide of the human genome. Most of the known SNPs differentiate humans from primates and are found worldwide in people of all populations.

In the course of the Human Genome Project, SNPs became a central tool for genetic analyses, ranging from the genetics of complex diseases to pharmacogenetics and population genetics.

Because of their low mutation rate (compared to other polymorphisms), great stability, and high frequency in the entire genome, SNPs are especially suited for association analyses in the identification of complex diseases. They can also easily be used for familial segregation analyses.

3.2   Types of Mutations

Genetic disorders can be caused by numerous types of mutations. Generally speaking, there are three groups:
- Numerical chromosome abnormalities
- Structural chromosome abnormalities
- Gene mutations that alter the function of individual genes

Chromosome abnormalities occur as congenital abnormalities in all or most body cells, or as somatically acquired clonal abnormalities that play an important pathogenetic role (e.g., in the formation or progression of various tumors). Our perspective on what we consider "chromosomal abnormalities" has changed considerably over the past 5 to 10 years. Originally, chromosomal anomalies were those that could be detected by light microscopy. The development of molecular cytogenetic techniques enabled the detection of submicroscopic deletions that encompass many genes and have typical characteristics of "chromosomal disorders," even though specific features may be due to haploinsufficiency of specific genes. The recent advent of array technology (Chapter 15.3) allows for the detection of smaller and smaller copy number variants (CNVs), thereby bridging and blurring the gap between "chromosomal" and "monogenic" conditions. We now know that most individuals (65% to 85% of the population) harbor a CNV of at least 100 kb of DNA. Much larger (exceeding 500 kb) variants occur in 5% to 10% of individuals, while at least 1% of the population carries a CNV exceeding 1 Mb. While some of these CNVs are clearly pathogenic, others may represent risk modifiers for common diseases or may be completely benign.

Numerical chromosome abnormalities stem from errors that occur during the segregation of intact chromosomes in meiosis or mitosis. They are always clinically evident, and as a rule, they are de novo (i.e., not inherited). By contrast, **structural chromosome abnormalities** can be balanced (without loss or gain of genetic material), in which case they are typically not evident clinically. Structural chromosome abnormalities can be passed on from generation to generation. Among structural chromosome abnormalities are duplications, deletions, inversions, and translocations. Larger chromosome abnormalities are demonstrable by light microscopic chromosome analysis (cytogenetically, typical resolution is down to approximately 4 Mb); smaller deletions and duplications are demonstrable by molecular cytogenetic or DNA analytical methods. **Gene mutations** can occur in many different forms and are identified through a multitude of molecular genetic methods. Gene mutations occur within the process of DNA replication, either spontaneously or through specific physical or chemical agents (mutagens). The vast majority of gene mutations are identified and corrected by efficient mechanisms for DNA repair. **Constitutional** mutations are found in all cells of the body and are present in the zygote, while **somatic** mutations are present in only a proportion of cells and arise after fertilization.

Frequency of Individual Mutation Types

Numerical chromosome abnormalities represent some of the most frequent genetic disorders. Overall, 10% of all spermatozoa and 25% of all oocytes are estimated to be aneuploid. The average frequency of numerical chromosome abnormalities in newborns is 1 in 400. This, however, is only the tip of the iceberg, since most chromosomal abnormalities affect fetal development so severely that they result in spontaneous miscarriage. Approximately one-sixth of clinically recognized pregnancies are spontaneously aborted. Approximately 50% of all spontaneous abortions in the first trimester are caused by chromosomal anomalies. These figures do not include the large number of pregnancies that went unnoticed because the loss of the embryo occurred soon after conception. Chromosome abnormalities occur in somatic cells as a result of faulty mitotic cell division. Especially frequent are aneuploid cells in malignant tumors.

Structural chromosome abnormalities are less frequent than numerical abnormalities; they are estimated to occur at a rate of 1 chromosomal rearrangement per 1,700 cell divisions. Among structural abnormalities, deletions are the most frequently observed, followed by insertions and duplications. This is partly due to the fact that deletions used to be more readily identifiable by molecular cytogenetics (fluorescence in situ hybridization [FISH] analysis) than duplications; also, the clinical consequences of a missing chromosome region (monosomy) are usually more severe than those of a duplication (trisomy), which means that deletion patients are more likely to come to our clinical attention as compared to duplication patients.

As far as **gene mutations** are concerned, we are also just seeing the tip of the iceberg. The vast majority of replication errors are promptly recognized by the human cell's excellent DNA repair mechanism, excised from the DNA, and repaired. DNA polymerase has this *proofreading* function. It initially recognizes the faulty strand of the newly synthesized DNA double helix, excises the wrong base, replaces it with the correct complementary nucleotide base, and takes care of re-ligating the fragments. DNA polymerase works so efficiently that despite a speed of 20 base pairs per second, only 1 in 10 million bases is inserted incorrectly. Of the initial replication errors, 99.9% are identified and repaired, so that the total mutation rate due to replication errors amounts to 1 in 10^{10} base pairs. In theory, this means that less than 1 replication error remains as a de novo mutation for the 6×10^9 base pairs of the diploid human genome per cell division. To have a significant impact, this mutation would have to be clinically relevant, either as a somatic mutation (e.g., in cancer cells) or as a germline mutation with implications for the following generation. The effect of exogenous agents, such as cigarette smoking, is not part of this calculation. Among the known gene mutations, *missense* mutations are the most frequent, followed by *nonsense* mutations and splice mutations.

3.3 Numerical Chromosome Abnormalities

Changes in the total number of chromosomes (aneuploidy) are called numerical chromosome abnormalities. They arise from faulty segregation (**nondisjunction**) of the chromosomes in meiosis or mitosis. Meiotic failure of a pair of chromosomes to disjoin occurs either in the first meiotic division (i.e., in 75% of cases two homologous chromosomes move together to one cell pole instead of to opposing cell poles) or in the second meiotic division (i.e., in 25% of cases two sister chromatids of a homologous chromosome reach the same cell pole). Examinations of aneuploid fetuses have shown that in greater than 90% of cases the aneuploidy resulted from meiotic nondisjunction in the mother. The risk of numerical chromosome abnormalities is largely dependent on maternal age. While the risk of giving birth to a child with an abnormal chromosome count is less than 0.2% for mothers up to age 30 years, it increases to greater than 0.5% at 35 years, and to 1% at 38 years. At the time of delivery, a 45-year-old mother has a risk of 1 in 20 for the newborn to have a chromosomal abnormality—which also translates to a 95% chance of the child having a normal chromosomal complement. It should be remembered that more chromosome abnormalities are diagnosed at the time a chorionic villus biopsy or amniocentesis is performed, since many aneuploidies result in miscarriages or fetal death as late as the second or even third trimester.

Faulty segregation during mitosis only occurs in a portion of the cells of an organism. This creates a mosaic of normal cells and cells with chromosome abnormalities, called a **somatic mosaic** if the germ line is not affected. Nondisjunction of chromosomes during the generation of germ cells or in meiosis, however, results in chromosome abnormalities that affect all cells of the offspring.

Not only individual chromosomes but also entire chromosome complements can occur in abnormal numbers. This is called polyploidy. Triploid (3n) and tetraploid (4n) chromosome complements have been observed during prenatal chromosome analyses. Some children with triploidy are born alive but usually die within the first few days. The most frequent cause of triploidy is fertilization of an oocyte by two spermatozoa (dispermy). Less frequent are oocytes or spermatozoa with a diploid chromosome complement. Tetraploidies always have the karyotype 92,XXXX or 92,XXYY, which suggests that they originate in normal zygotes that subsequently went through an incomplete division during the first meiotic division.

Only three numerical chromosome abnormalities involving **autosomes** are viable after birth: trisomies 13 (see p. 187), 18 (see p. 185), and 21 (see p. 180). Exceptions are partial trisomies or mosaics of trisomic and normal cell lines. Monosomies of autosomal chromosomes result in a very early spontaneous miscarriage, often before the pregnancy is identified. Numerical abnormalities of the human **sex chromosomes** cause relatively mild phenotypes, unlike numerical abnormalities of the autosomes (see pp. 189). The human cell utilizes mostly the genetic information of one X chromosome and, therefore, can largely compensate for the loss of a Y chromosome or the second X chromosome, as well as additional X chromosomes (by way of X inactivation, as described in Chapter 2.8). As a result, numerical sex chromosome abnormalities in newborns rarely lead to severe physical changes and, in most instances, do not cause substantial intellectual disability. Monosomy X is the only viable monosomy in humans.

Euploidy: A normal diploid chromosome complement (2n) of 46 chromosomes (46,XX or 46,XY).

Aneuploidy: The number of chromosomes varies from that of a normal diploid chromosome sequence (e.g., 47,XY,+21).

Polyploidy: Multiples of the haploid chromosome complement of greater than 2n.

Triploidy: Triple chromosome complement (3n) (e.g., 69,XXX).
— Digynic triploidy: The origin of the additional set of chromosomes is maternal. This results in a partial mole.
— Diandric triploidy: The origin of the additional set of chromosomes is paternal.

Tetraploidy: A quadruple chromosome complement.

Trisomy: Three copies of a chromosome.

Monosomy: One copy of a chromosome.

Triploidy and Tetraploidy

In triploidy (3n) each chromosome occurs threefold, meaning a total of 69 chromosomes. Tetraploidies (4n) have a quadruple chromosome complement, or a total of 92 chromosomes.

Triploidy accounts for approximately 20% of all chromosome abnormalities identified in spontaneous miscarriages. Clinical features depend on whether the origin of the additional set of chromosomes is paternal or maternal. If the extra chromosome complement is of maternal origin, the condition is called digynic triploidy. It results from the fertilization of a diploid ovum by a haploid sperm. The placenta is small and fibrotic, while the fetus shows significant growth retardation and a relatively large head (◘ Fig. 3.1). In up to 70% of cases, the additional chromosome complement derives from the father (diandric triploidy). The fertilization of a haploid ovum by two sperm (double fertilization) is by far the most common pathological mechanism. Much more rare is the incidence of triploidy caused by the fertilization of one ovum with one diploid sperm. Diandric triploidy results in a **partial mole** (from Latin *mola*, "millstone/abnormal embryo") with a large cystic placenta, while the normal-size fetus is microcephalic. If the maternal chromosome complement in paternal diploidy is entirely absent, there results a **complete hydatidiform mole** with a vesicular hypertrophied placenta without fetal elements (e.g., risk of malignant degeneration). Triploid infants are rarely born alive, and their chances of survival are extremely poor. The longest reported survival period is 5 months.

Tetraploidies occur in approximately 5% of all chromosomally abnormal spontaneous abortions. In all cases, the chromosome complement is either 92,XXXX or 92,XXYY. In pathogenetic terms this indicates that tetraploidy is an early division abnormality of the zygote.

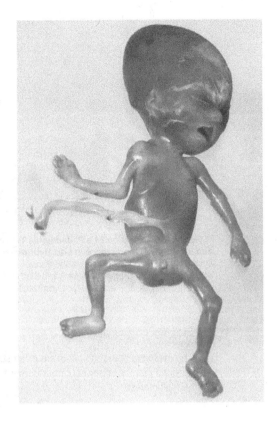

Figure 3.1. Digynic Triploidy. In digynic triploidy the extra chromosome complement stems from the mother, and the fetus is markedly growth retarded and relatively macroencephalic. The placenta is typically small and fibrotic.

3.4 Structural Chromosome Abnormalities

Structural chromosome abnormalities have a cumulative frequency of 1 out of every 375 newborns. They are caused by chromosome breakage with subsequent abnormal realignment. This frequently happens spontaneously. Chromosome breakage can also be caused by ionizing radiation, viral infections, and various chemicals (especially alkylating agents).

Balanced structural abnormalities involve no loss or gain in chromosomes despite the recombination; the entire genetic material is normal. Such aberrations typically have no clinical relevance unless they interrupt a gene with dominant loss of function or cause gain of function through fusion of two unrelated segments. **Unbalanced** chromosome abnormalities involve a gain or loss of chromosome segments and are clinically relevant. Structurally altered chromosomes are denoted according to the origin of their centromere; they are called **derivative chromosomes**.

■■■ **Fusion Proteins**

Fusion proteins are generated by the fusion of two different genes into a single transcribed gene, either by unequal crossing over between homologous chromosomes or by chromosomal translocation.

The classic example for a fusion protein resulting from chromosomal translocation is BCR/ABL at t(9;22), known as Philadelphia chromosome (■ Fig. 3.2) in chronic myeloid leukemia (CML). The *BCR* (*breakpoint cluster region*) gene is located on chromosome 22 and is constitutively active. In contrast, the protooncogene *ABL* on chromosome 9 codes for a tyrosine kinase involved in growth regulation and has a well regulated expression pattern. Translocation t(9;22) results in a fusion gene with loss of expression regulation, leading to increased tyrosine kinase activity and increased cell proliferation. A Philadelphia chromosome occurs in more than 90% of CML (classic CML).

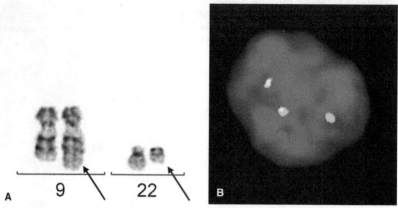

◻ Figure 3.2. Detection of a Philadelphia Translocation t(9;22) by Means of Classical Chromosome Analysis and Interphase Fluorescence In Situ Hybridization (FISH) Analysis. The derivative chromosomes are indicated by arrows **(A)**. FISH analysis **(B)** shows the translocation via two fusion signals (red + green = yellow) of probes for the ABL gene on chromosome 9q34 (red) and the *breakpoint cluster region* (BCR) on chromosome 22q11 (green). (Figures courtesy of H.-D. Hager and A. Jauch, Institute for Human Genetics, University of Heidelberg.)

> **Important**
>
> Chromosomal rearrangements are often stable over numerous cell divisions (mitoses and meioses), provided that the abnormal chromosomes have normal structural characteristics (one centromere and two telomeres).

Deletion

A **deletion** occurs when a chromosome breaks at two sites and the segment between them gets lost. Depending on the size and breakage site, varying numbers of genes can be lost. In rare cases the deletions are large enough to be visible under the light microscope: a loss of 2 to 4 million base pairs (2 to 4 Mb) of DNA is necessary for the deletion to be visible by high-resolution prometaphase banding. Smaller deletions have traditionally been identified by molecular cytogenetic (FISH) analyses, although they are now routinely detected with chromosome oligonucleotide arrays. These are called microdeletions, while the resulting pathologies are called **microdeletion syndromes**. Examples are discussed in Chapter 19.2.

> **Contiguous gene syndrome:** The presence of several distinct (dominant-inherited) monogenic disorders, caused by a deletion affecting several neighboring genes, in one patient.

Duplication

Duplication means that a chromosome segment appears in two (often sequentially inserted) copies on a single homolog. Most of the time, this is caused by a nonhomologous recombination in the first meiotic division.

Inversion

Inversion occurs when a chromosome segment between two breaks is rotated 180 degrees before reinsertion. The gene copy number remains the same; clinical symptoms may arise if there is an additional deletion or duplication, if the breaks occur within the coding region of a gene, or if the regulation of a gene is altered. Like other balanced chromosomal aberrations, inversions may cause infertility, recurrent miscarriages, or an unbalanced chromosome complement in a child. **Pericentric inversions** include the centromere (i.e., one breakpoint is on the short arm and one on the long arm of the chromosome) and are distinguishable from **paracentric inversions**, which do not include the centromere.

Isochromosome

An **isochromosome** is a derivative chromosome with two homologous arms after the centromere divided transversely rather than longitudinally. An isochromosome can be thought of as a "mirror image" of either the short arm or the long arm of a given chromosome.

Ring Chromosome

Ring chromosomes occur when a chromosome breaks at both ends and the ends join together. They typically become clinically relevant through the loss of chromosomal material distal to the breaks. Ring chromosome X causes 5% of Turner syndrome cases.

Marker Chromosome

Chromosome analysis in approximately 0.06% of the population reveals small additional chromosomes, so-called "**marker chromosomes**". These might be too small to be character-ized by traditional chromosome analysis. FISH testing or array analysis is usually necessary to identify their origins. Some marker chromosomes are known to be pathogenic, while others seem to have no phenotypical effect at all. They develop as either isochromosomes (through transverse or longitudinal separation at the centromere) or inverted duplications of certain chromosome segments. Known diseases caused by marker chromosomes are Pallister-Killian syndrome (i.e., isochromosome 12p, which is discussed in Chapter 4.4) and cat-eye syndrome (i.e., an inverse duplication of the short arm and a small part—22q11—of the long arm of chromosome 22, which is characterized by iris coloboma, anal atresia, hearing defects [typically total anomalous pulmonary venous return], and other abnormalities, but normal intelligence).

Translocations

Translocation involves the exchange of chromosome segments between two nonhomologous chromosomes. Two major types can be distinguished: **reciprocal translocations** and **Robert-sonian translocations**.

Reciprocal Translocations. These translocations involve the transfer of chromosomal material from one chromosome to another, and vice versa (◻ Fig. 3.3). Since the exchange is reciprocal, the total number of chromosomes remains unchanged, as does the total amount of chromosomal material. Reciprocal translocations are frequent and occur in 1 out of every 600 newborns. Even

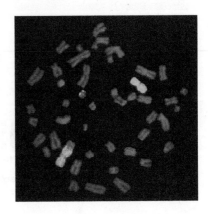

◻ **Figure 3.3. Female Patient with Balanced Translocation of Chromosomes 3 and 13 [46,XX,t(3;13)].** Fluorescence in situ hybridization (FISH) testing with *painting* probes for chromosome 3 (green) and chromosome 13 (red) reveals the reciprocal translocation t(3;13). A large part of the long arm of chromosome 13 is attached to the long arm of chromosome 3, while the small terminal piece of the long arm of chromosome 3 is found near the centromere of chromosome 13. (Courtesy of A. Jauch, Institute for Human Genetics, University of Heidelberg.)

when balanced de novo, reciprocal translocation carries a 6% risk of adverse clinical effect. Symptoms may occur if the breakage destroys the integrity of a gene, causing a dominant monogenic disease. Carriers of reciprocal translocations generate gametes with an unbalanced chromosome complement. Balanced translocations are therefore significant in the differential diagnosis of infertility and/or recurrent spontaneous miscarriage.

The identification of an unbalanced translocation in a child is of special clinical importance, as it frequently is linked to a balanced translocation in one of the parents. Unbalanced translocations usually affect two chromosome segments, of which one is duplicated (trisomic) and the other deleted (monosomic). These segments typically include the respective chromosome ends. For this reason, parental chromosomes should be analyzed in every case of a structural chromosome abnormality that involves the telomere of the respective chromosome. A balanced translocation in one of the parents has significant implications for the calculation of recurrence risk in future pregnancies.

> **Important**
>
> In cases of unbalanced structural chromosome aberrations in a fetus or newborn, the parents should always undergo karyotyping to determine the risk of recurrence.

Robertsonian Translocations. These translocations involve the fusion of two acrocentric chromosomes in the centromeres (centric fusion), with the loss of the respective short arms (◘ Fig. 3.4) and the reduction of the total number of chromosomes to 45. Since the short arms of the acrocentric chromosomes only carry highly repetitive satellite DNA, their loss does not result in a clinical phenotype. The cumulative incidence of Robertsonian translocations is 1 out of every 500 newborns. Most frequent are translocations rob(13;14) and rob(14;21), which carry a risk of translocation trisomy 13 or 21 in their offspring. In the case of a robertsonian translocation with fusion of two homologous chromosomes, there is de facto no possibility of having a healthy child; all live births of a parent [e.g., with a rob(21;21)] karyotype have a translocation trisomy 21. Exceptions to this rule are extremely rare.

> **Important**
>
> Acrocentric chromosomes: 13, 14, 15, 21, 22, (Y).

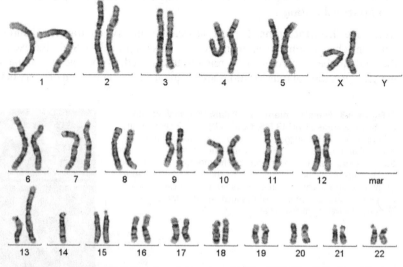

◘ **Figure 3.4. Robertsonian Translocation.** Female karyotype 45,XX,rob(13;14) with fusion of the long arms of chromosomes 13 and 14. (Courtesy of H.-D. Hager, Institute for Human Genetics, University of Heidelberg.)

3.5   Gene Mutations

Monogenic diseases can be caused by many different types of mutations, both with regard to changes in the DNA sequence (e.g., point mutations, trinucleotide repeat expansion, and gene duplication) and with regard to functional changes (e.g., altered expression, disrupted messenger RNA [mRNA] splicing, and alteration in protein structure).

Point mutation: A mutation that affects one single base pair; most frequently refers to a single nucleotide substitution, but the term also describes single nucleotide insertions or deletions.

Missense mutation: A point mutation that causes the substitution of an amino acid with a different amino acid in the protein.

Nonsense mutation: A point mutation that leads to a stop codon.

Splice mutation: A mutation that alters the sequence of an intron–exon transition or another relevant sequence in a way that prohibits or impairs correct splicing.

Frameshift mutation: The deletion or insertion of coding nucleotides in a number not divisible by three, which destroys the reading frame beyond the mutation and leads to a completely wrong protein.

In-frame mutation: The deletion or insertion of coding nucleotides in a number divisible by three, which leaves the reading frame intact.

Null mutation: Any type of mutation that causes complete loss of function of the gene.

Silent mutation: A mutation that has no functional effects.

Hypomorphic mutation: A mutation that causes only partial loss of function of the gene.

Gain-of-function mutation: A mutation that causes increased or novel function of the gene.

Point Mutations

The most frequent type of mutation with monogenic diseases involves point mutations, which are alterations that affect one single base pair. One differentiates between three different types of point mutations as follows:
- Substitution (base exchange), by far the most frequent type
- Insertion (one additional nucleotide)
- Deletion (loss of a nucleotide)

Substitutions include transitions and transversions, depending on whether they occur by simple modification of the correct base (transition, e.g., in CpG mutations see below) or whether they involve a change of the base type (transversion). Transitions are more frequent than transversions.

Transition: The substitution of a purine (A, G) for a purine, or of a pyrimidine (C, T) for a pyrimidine.

Transversion: The substitution of a purine for a pyrimidine or vice versa.

■■■ CpG Mutations
Cytosines in CpG dinucleotides (cytosine followed by guanine, where p stands for the phosphate bond between C and G) are frequently methylated. Deamination of methylcytosine results in uracil and, ultimately, in the substitution of cytosine for thymine in the DNA sequence. "CpG mutations" CG→TG or the complementary CG→CA are the most frequent point mutations in the genome. CpG mutations frequently show independent

recurrence in different individuals (e.g., when the "same" recessive disease mutation is traced to more than one "founder") or represent common somatic mutations (e.g., in tumors). The high frequency of C→T or G→A conversions is one of the reasons why cytosine and guanine occur less frequently in the genome than thymine and adenine. Exceptions are the coding sequences that often have a high proportion of C and G due to conserved codon usage.

Missense Mutations and Nonsense Mutations

The functional effects of **missense mutations** can be manifold: they might not be functionally relevant at all, they may render the protein nonfunctional, they may affect binding sites with other proteins, they may impair the protein's ability to be functionally modified (e.g., by phosphorylation), or they may affect splicing of the pre-mRNA, leading to a completely different effect on protein structure and function. Quite often, missense mutations render the protein less stable or are recognized by the cell's quality-control mechanisms, resulting in degradation of the protein and subsequent loss of gene function. Missense mutations are the most frequent mutations detected in diagnostic laboratories, but they are also among the most difficult to interpret. It is not usually possible to determine the functional effects of novel missense mutations with certainty, even when adequate computer programs are used for further analyses. International quality assessment schemes have shown that the incorrect interpretation of missense mutations is among the most frequent errors encountered in molecular genetic diagnostics.

Nonsense mutations result in premature termination of the polypeptide chain and, usually, in a complete loss of function unless their effect is mitigated by variant splicing. Provided they are not located on the last exon or shortly before the last intron of a gene, they additionally lead to *nonsense-mediated decay*, the premature degeneration of mRNA (Chapter 2.4).

Splice Mutations

Some mutations alter the sequences of intron–exon transitions or other relevant sequences in a way that prohibits or impairs the **correct joining of exons or the removal of introns from the pre-mRNA transcript**. Mutations, particularly of the first two or the last two nucleotides of an intron, almost always affect splicing, but this can also be expected for mutations of the last nucleotide of an exon or the fifth nucleotide of an intron. As a rule, splice mutations lead either to the **skipping of entire exons** or to the use of **alternative splice sites** and the inclusion of extended or shortened exons into the protein. The reading frame of the mature mRNA will be destroyed if the number of nucleotides inserted or deleted cannot be divided by three. Splice mutations usually cause a major change of the protein structure; they are typically null mutations. Some variants within a gene (usually within an intron) may affect the **probability** of correct or incorrect splicing. An interesting example is the 5T variant at the splice acceptor site of intron 8 of the *CFTR* gene (■ Fig. 3.5).

	Transition intron 8 – exon 9	Frequency of TG11, TG12, and TG13 in the presence of the 5t variant		
		General population	Men with CBAVD*	Mild cystic fibrosis
TG11-5T	...tgatgtgtgtgtgtgtgtgtgtgtgtttttaacagGGA..	77 %	10 %	–
TG12-5T	...tgatgtgtgtgtgtgtgtgtgtgtgtttttaacagGGA..	21 %	76 %	56 %
TG13-5T	...tgatgtgtgtgtgtgtgtgtgtgtgtgtttttaacagGGA..	2 %	12 %	44 %

*in compound heterozygosity with a severe CFTR mutation on the other allele. Data from Groman et al. (2004) Am J Hum Genet 74:176-179.

■ **Figure 3.5. The 5T Intron Variant of the *CFTR* Gene.**

More than 1,000 different mutations in the *CFTR* gene have been identified as causes for the autosomal reces-sive disease cystic fibrosis (Chapter 22.1). Most mutations are rare, but there is a DNA stretch at the end of intron 8 that is polymorphic with variable functional effects. A stretch of 11, 12, or 13 TG repeats is followed by a stretch of 5 to 9 thymidines (5T, 7T, 9T). Exon 9 starts five nucleotides later. The so-called 5T variant (allele frequency 4% to 5% in individuals of European descent) causes reduced splicing efficiency, particularly when it is preceded by 12 or (even worse) 13 TG repeats. Individuals who are compound heterozygous for a null mutation on one *CFTR* allele and the 13TG-5T variant on the other allele often have a mild form of cystic fibrosis or, in males, infertility due to congenital bilateral absence of the vas deferens (CBAVD). Similarly, presence of the 5T variant can turn a functionally mild mutation into a severe mutation if it is located on the same chromosomal strand (in cis).

Smaller Deletions and Insertions

The functional effect of small deletions or insertions depends primarily on whether they are located within the coding region of a gene and, if so, whether the number of missing or additional nucleotides is a multiple of three. The deletion or insertion of multiples of three causes the dele-tion or insertion of amino acids in the translated protein but does not affect the reading frame beyond the mutation. The deletion or insertion is said to be **in frame.** Gain or loss of nucleotides in a number not divisible by three constitutes a frameshift mutation, which destroys the entire reading frame beyond the mutation and leads to the continued integration of incorrect amino acids, generating a completely abnormal protein. Most frameshift mutations eventually lead to a stop codon that causes premature termination of translation and often nonsense-mediated decay of the mRNA. Small deletions are not infrequent causes of monogenic disorders; they are more frequent than insertions.

Important

Let us, for example, look at the sentence "ONE CAN NOT SEE THE SUN FOR THE FOG"
- A missense mutation changes one nucleotide (one letter) and consequently one amino acid (one word), for example, ONE CAN NOT SEE THE SUN FOR THE DOG. That creates a different meaning, but the sentence is still readable.
- A nonsense mutation results in a breakup of the text: ONE CAN NOT SEE THE **XXX**.
- An in-frame mutation (e.g., deletion of three letters) may or may not affect the meaning of the sentence: ONE CAN NOT SEE THE SUN FOR FOG.
- A frameshift mutation (e.g., deletion of one letter) changes the reading frame and makes the sentence unreadable: ONE CAN OTS EET HES UNF ORT HEF OG.

A classic example for the different effects of frameshift versus in-frame mutations is the X-linked muscular dystrophy types Duchenne and Becker (Chapter 31.4). These disorders are caused by numerous different mutations of the *dystrophin* gene, which involve large deletions of several exons in more than 60% of cases, but can also involve insertions or point mutations. Mutations that result in a shift of the reading frame almost always cause the more severe form of the dis-order, Duchenne muscular dystrophy. However, mutations without a shift in the reading frame (including in-frame deletions of several exons) often result in a protein with residual function and, consequently, a milder form of the disorder, Becker muscular dystrophy.

Large Genomic Rearrangements

Large deletions or duplications that affect the function of individual genes may not be observed by standard polymerase chain reaction (PCR)-based sequencing. For example, deletions that remove several exons or the entire gene obviously also remove the binding sites for standard PCR primers, leading to loss of amplification that is not recognized unless specific quantitative methods (e.g., multiplex ligation probe amplification [MLPA] or high-resolution oligonucleotide arrays) are employed. Large deletions or insertions almost always result in null mutations that completely remove the function of the gene.

Duplications of individual exons or entire genes have had an important impact on the evolution of the human genome. Many of the functionally important domains of various proteins (e.g., tyrosine kinase domains or immunoglobulin-like domains) are thought to have resulted from the duplication of individual exons. Pseudogenes (Chapter 2.2) usually represent duplicated genes that have been rendered nonfunctional through the accumulation of mutations. In some cases duplications are also the cause of genetic disorders. A classic example is **hereditary motor-sensory neuropathy (HMSN) type 1a** (Charcot-Marie-Tooth disease), which is caused by the duplication of a 1.5-Mb segment encompassing the *PMP22 (peripheral myelin protein 22)* gene on chromosome 17p. The duplication occurs following nonallelic homologous recombination during meiosis I, leaving one gamete with a duplication of the respective region and one with the reciprocal deletion. The deletion results in the typically milder peripheral neuropathy known as hereditary neuropathy with liability to pressure palsies (HNPP).

Functional Consequences of Gene Mutations

From a clinical standpoint, all mutations can be classified according to their functional effect. Mutations that cause a complete loss of function of the protein are called **null mutations.** In the coding regions many point mutations have no functional effects, especially if they involve the third base of a codon; these are called silent mutations.

Mutations may cause disease through various pathomechanisms, systematically described in 1934 by Hermann J. Müller, who was awarded the Nobel Prize in 1946 for his discovery that mutations can be induced by x-rays:

- Mutations that cause complete loss of function or reduced function (hypomorphic mutations). There are various possible mechanisms, including:
  - Loss of a functionally important domain, such as the catalytic site of an enzyme.
  - Loss of the ability to bind relevant other proteins; for example, some mutations in the factor VIII gene cause hemophilia A by altering the thrombin cleavage site of the protein, thereby preventing thrombin-mediated cleavage and activation of factor VIII to factor VIIIa.
  - Changes of the secondary and tertiary structure that lead to instability and premature degradation.
- Mutations that cause an increase in normal gene function (i.e., gain-of-function mutations), for example, through gene duplication, increased gene expression, or changes in a protein domain that results in increased functionality.
- Mutations that act in a dominant negative fashion by interfering with a normal protein in a multimer.
- Mutations that cause a novel function (i.e., neomorphic mutations), either by altered protein effects or expression of a protein in a different organ.

Mutations that Affect Translation. Most gene mutations result in an altered polypeptide sequence of the gene product and, as such, have a functional effect at the level of translation. Mutations in this group include missense mutations (i.e., insertion of a variant amino acid), frameshift mutations (i.e., change in the reading frame), and nonsense mutations (i.e., premature stop codon and termination of translation). Mutations within a start codon (ATG) prevent mRNA from being translated into the correct polypeptide sequence, while mutations in the stop codon lead to abnormal continuation of translation.

Mutations that Affect Gene Expression. Numerous mutations in promoter regions of human genes have been identified. In most cases they result in impaired binding of transcription factors and, thus, cause reduced transcription of the corresponding gene. This has been reported, for example, for mutations in the TATA box of the β-globin gene. The same is true for insertions between promoter and transcription start. Gene expression may be considerably reduced when the promoter is at an increased distance from its gene. The effect of SNPs in promoter regions and their influence on gene expression has been extensively studied. An example would be the frequent G→A variant at position −6 before the transcription start of the angiotensin gene, which stimulates transcription and is considered a risk factor for the development of essential hypertension.

Mutations in Untranslated Regions. Disease-causing mutations can also occur in untranslated regions (UTRs) of a gene. Mutations in the 5′ UTR of a gene may result in a change of gene expression or posttranscriptional mRNA modification. Mutations in the 3′ UTR of a gene may affect mRNA polyadenylation or mRNA stability, may interfere with the export from the nucleus into the cytosol, or may change translation efficiency. One of many examples is the g.20210G>A mutation in the 3′ UTR of the prothrombin gene, which causes more efficient transcription termination and is associated with increased plasma levels of prothrombin and an increased risk of venous thrombosis.

3.6 Dynamic Mutations, Trinucleotide Repeats

Until the beginning of the 1990s, it was assumed that disease-causing mutations, once present, are stable and never change and that they are transmitted intact from generation to generation. The discovery in 1991 that two diseases, fragile X syndrome and spinobulbar muscular atrophy (Kennedy disease), were caused by the extension of trinucleotide repeats led to a completely new understanding of the dynamics and inheritance of certain genetic disorders.

Trinucleotide repeats are in the class of minisatellites in the human genome and are composed of multiple repetitions of three nucleotides (e.g., CAGCAGCAG…CAG or CCGC-CGCCG…CCG), which normally occur in groups of 5 to 30 repeats. An essential feature of disease-associated repeats is their instability: if there are more than a certain number of repeats in the sequence, transmission through gametogenesis may be associated with **expansion** of the repeat. Expansion beyond a certain level may lead to various pathogenetic effects. Several diseases involve so-called **premutations,** which themselves are not usually disease causing but are associated with a significant risk of expansion to a disease-causing **full mutation** in a child. Trinucleotide repeats can change over subsequent generations, and thus the term **dynamic mutation** is used to describe them. Dynamic mutations often cause a variety of clinical features in affected persons of the same family, with younger generations being more severely affected. Apart from trinucleotide diseases, there are also disorders caused by an expansion of dinucleotide and tetranucleotide repeats.

Most trinucleotide diseases are inherited in an autosomal dominant manner. Three main categories of trinucleotide repeat disorders are characterized by distinct pathophysiological mechanisms.

1. **Polyglutamine diseases** have CAG trinucleotides in the coding sequence. CAG encodes for the amino acid glutamine, and expansion of the repeat causes integration of an increasing number of glutamine residues into a polyglutamine tract within the respective protein. Once the number of glutamines exceeds a certain threshold, the physical properties of the protein change, leading to intracellular aggregation and finally cell death. An important disease of this group is Huntington disease, a neurodegenerative disease in adulthood (Chapter 31.1.1). There are also a number of polyalanine diseases that have the same pathomechanism but are caused by GCN repeats.

2. Some disorders are caused by **transcriptional silencing** due to expansion of a repeat sequence in the 5′ untranslated region of a gene. In fragile X syndrome (Chapter 31.2.2), expansion of a CGG repeat beyond 200 copies causes hypermethylation and prohibits transcription of the gene.

3. In a large number of repeat disorders, cellular dysfunction is caused by impaired post-translational processing of the pre-mRNA or **adverse effects of the elongated mRNA.** In myotonic dystrophy (see below), for example, an increasing number of CUG trinucleotides in the 3′ UTR of the *DMPK* mRNA interferes with various RNA-binding proteins, causing a range of symptoms due to aberrant splicing and malfunctioning of other genes. Interestingly, the fragile X–associated tremor and ataxia syndrome (FXTAS) observed in fragile X syndrome premutation carriers is also caused by adverse effects of the abnormal mRNA.

Pathogenic expansions in noncoding repeats are generally much larger (up to several thousand repeats) than those of polyglutamine diseases (◻ Table 3.1).

■ **Table 3.1.** Important Trinucleotide Diseases

Disease	Inheritance	Repeat	Localization of the Repeat	Normal Allele (Number of Repeats)	Full Mutation (Number of Repeats)
Huntington disease (chorea)	Autosomal dominant	CAG	Coding region (polyglutamine tract)	26 or fewer	40 and more
Spinocerebellar ataxias (various subtypes)	Autosomal dominant	CAG	Coding region (polyglutamine tract)	Differs according to subtype	Differs according to subtype
Fragile X syndrome	X chromosomal	CGG	5′ UTR	5–40	200 to several thousand
Myotonic dystrophy	Autosomal dominant	CTG	3′ UTR	5–34	50 to several thousand
Friedreich ataxia	Autosomal recessive	GAA	Intronic	5–33	66 to several thousand

---

Important

Important diseases with trinucleotide expansion and associated mnemonics:
- Huntington chore**A** (C**A**G)$_n$
- Fra**G**ile X syndrome (C**G**G)$_n$
- Myo**T**onic dystrophy (C**T**G)$_n$

Anticipation: The phenomenon that the symptoms become more severe or start at an earlier age as a disease is passed on to the next generation.

Anticipation is an important feature of trinucleotide repeat diseases. This is due to repeat expansion and is most obvious in disorders where symptoms are caused by adverse effects of elongated mRNA. For example, myotonic dystrophy patients with 50 to 100 repeats mostly have a mild form of the disease (e.g., cataracts or mild muscle weakness), whereas carriers of the more severe congenital form often have more than 2,000 repeats. In Huntington disease there is an association between increased repeat numbers and earlier onset of symptoms. No anticipation is found with regard to full mutations causing fragile X syndrome, as differences in repeat length no longer have any clinical relevance once the gene is hypermethylated (i.e., more than 200 repeats).

Father ≠ Mother. It is noteworthy that the likelihood of repeat expansion differs between spermatogenesis and oogenesis. In the case of Huntington disease, repeat expansion occurs mostly through spermatogenesis, while a fragile X premutation only develops into a full mutation through oogenesis. In the case of myotonic dystrophy, this is more complex. Small fragments with fewer than 100 repeats typically expand when transmitted through spermatogenesis, while expansion of large fragments may occur through oogenesis. Therefore, the mother of a child with congenital myotonic dystrophy will have signs (e.g., percussion myotonia) and symptoms (e.g., muscle "cramping") of myotonic dystrophy, although frequently the actual diagnosis is not made until the birth of a child with congenital myotonic dystrophy.

Myotonic Dystrophy

There are two types of myotonic dystrophy, type 1 (DM1) and type 2 (DM2), that are caused by the same pathomechanism but have repeat expansions in different genes. The term *myotonic dystrophy* without indication of the type is used exclusively for DM1.

The history of myotonic dystrophy probably goes back several hundred thousand years. This disease occurs only in European and Asian populations, not in central Africa, and in all clinical cases the mutation is associated with a common haplotype (marker combination at the locus).

This suggests that the first expansion of a normal allele to a premutation occurred in a very early common ancestor of Caucasian and Asiatic peoples. This probably happened at the time when the later European and Asiatic people had separated from the central African ancestor, but before this group split up in order to explore different regions in Europe and Asia.

Case History

Mr. Taylor is 44 years old. He was recently diagnosed with myotonic dystrophy and wants to know more about the disease. He reports that the first symptoms of a muscular disorder appeared approximately 15 years ago, when he was in his late twenties. The first thing he noticed was that he could not let go of objects. Later he also noticed muscular weakness. The disease affects his job as a butcher, for he has trouble with activities that demand manual dexterity. For a while it has also been difficult for him to walk, especially upon awaking in the mornings. As he ages, he notices that he has very little energy. He has difficulty swallowing and needs fluids to help him swallow his food. He also has trouble chewing, and his speech has begun to slur. He has not experienced constipation or diarrhea. Mr. Taylor is married and has two children, aged 17 and 19, who up to now have not experienced muscular weakness. Yet his 17-year-old daughter is often tired and in the last year experienced difficulty in physical education classes. There is no known history of muscular disorder in the rest of the family. Further questioning, however, revealed that Mr. Taylor's 68-year-old father has a drooping eyelid and a somewhat throaty speech. For some years he has been treated for rapid heartbeat with a baby aspirin and a beta-blocker, and he was recently diagnosed with a beginning cataract. You tell Mr. Taylor about the various manifestations of myotonic dystrophy, making sure to point out that his daughter has a risk of having a child with severe neonatal myotonic dystrophy should she herself be affected.

Epidemiology

Myotonic dystrophy is the only disease with both progressive muscular dystrophy and myotonia. At the same time, it is the most frequent of all muscular dystrophies in adults, and the most frequent of all myotonias. The incidence of the classic adult type is 1 in 8,000.

Clinical Picture

For practical reasons, one differentiates between the four different types of myotonic dystrophy. However, expression of the disease is variable and overlapping, and there is no strict correlation between genotype and phenotype (Table 3.2).

Classic Adult Type. The classic form of myotonic dystrophy is a **multisystem disease**. The cardinal symptom is **myotonia** that manifests itself as difficulties with relaxing a muscle and can be elicited

Table 3.2. Correlation between Clinical Presentation and Repeat Size in Myotonic Dystrophy Type I

Type	Age of Onset	Symptoms	$(CTG)_n$ Repeats
Normal allele	—	None	4–34
Premutation	—	None	35–49
Oligosymptomatic	>50 years	May be asymptomatic; cataract, arrhythmias, receding hairline; possibly mild muscular weakness and abnormal EMG (mild myotonia)	50–150
Classic adult	12–50 years	Progressive muscular weakness with myotonia, typical facies, presenile cataract, systemic complications	100–1,000
Childhood	1–12 years	Unremarkable neonatal period, progressive muscular weakness, cognitive deficits	230–1,800
Congenital	Pre-/perinatal	Severe neonatal hypotonia (floppy infant), severe respiratory compromise, clubfoot, developmental delay, intellectual disability	>1,000

EMG, electromyogram.

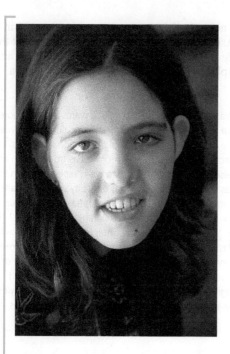

Figure 3.6. Teenager with Myotonic Dystrophy. Individuals with myotonic dystrophy often have a characteristic facial appearance due to long-standing muscular weakness and wasting. The face is long and narrow and the palate is high arched. (Photo courtesy of Rick Guidotti, www.positiveexposure.org.)

by percussing the thenar muscles (i.e., percussion myotonia). The patient's hands may "lock up," for instance, while using a can opener, turning a key in the lock, or holding the steering wheel. Patients often avoid firm handshakes because difficulties in letting go of someone's hand may be embarrassing (i.e., grip myotonia). More concerning for the patient is a progressive **muscular weakness** that initially affects the facial muscles and the muscles of the hands and lower legs. Fatigue and daytime sleepiness may be attributed to "exhaustion." Affected individuals have a typical **myopathic facies** (▫ Fig. 3.6) with a drooping facial expression and bilateral ptosis; it may be impossible for them to firmly close the eyes. Speech may be slurred or throaty, and swallowing may be difficult. Involvement of smooth muscles leads to **gastrointestinal symptoms** including abdominal colic and intestinal pseudo-obstruction. Reduced esophageal motility, in advanced stages of the disease, may lead to aspiration pneumonia, which is among the most frequent causes of death in myotonic dystrophy. As in patients with the oligosymptomatic type of the disease, **cardiac conduction abnormalities** are common; they cause clinically relevant arrhythmias and rarely death in a proportion of patients. All patients with classic myotonic dystrophy show progressive **cataract** in adulthood. In addition, retinopathy may occur. **Endocrine** disorders, such as diabetes mellitus and hypothyroidism, are increased compared to the general population. Fertility is decreased in affected men, who often have testicular atrophy, and in women, who have a higher miscarriage rate. A receding hairline is found in male and female patients.

Oligosymptomatic Type. A cataract radiating from the cortex and cardiac arrhythmias are frequently the only clinical symptoms for this mild form of myotonic dystrophy. The typical receding hairline may be noticed by the trained clinician (▫ Fig. 3.7). Muscular symptoms are usually absent or insignificant, and diagnosis is often not made until a family member is found to have myotonic dystrophy.

Congenital (neonatal) Type. The congenital and most severe type of myotonic dystrophy may become apparent before birth, with poor fetal movement and polyhydramnios due to fetal swallowing difficulties. At birth, these infants are severely **hypotonic** and have myopathic facies, ptosis, and a triangular, open mouth. Congenital contractures and clubfeet are common. Affected neonates show severe, sometimes life-threatening, **respiratory problems** and typically require ventilatory support. Children who survive usually have improved muscle strength over time, and the majority of children can eventually walk with assistance. Most children will have significant learning disabilities, requiring ongoing support. As a rule, all children with congenital myotonic dystrophy have a symptomatic mother, although the diagnosis may not be recognized until after the birth of the affected child.

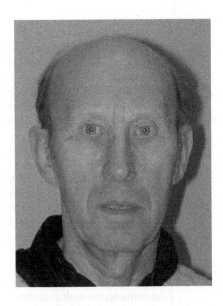

Figure 3.7. Myotonic Dystrophy in Advanced Age. A 67-year-old competitive bowler has cardiac arrhythmias, a beginning cataract, and throaty speech. His face is long and narrow and he has a receding hairline, wasting of the temporalis muscles, and ptosis of the left eye.

In addition to the classic and the congenital types of myotonic dystrophy, there is an intermediate **infantile or childhood type** (Fig. 3.8). After a relatively inconspicuous neonatal period, affected children present with muscular hypotonia, developmental delay, and subsequent learning deficits. Muscle weakness is slowly progressive and later resembles the classical disease type. By the age of 40 years, many of the patients are confined to a wheelchair.

Genetics and Etiology

Myotonic dystrophy is inherited in an **autosomal dominant** manner. It is caused by expansion of a variable **repetitive (CTG)$_n$ sequence** in the 5′ untranslated region (5′ UTR) of the *DMPK* (myotonic dystrophy protein kinase) gene (see Table 3.2). Normal alleles have between 4 and 37 repeats. Occurring in 30% to 40% of cases, (CTG)$_5$ is the most frequent allele. Patients with myotonic dystrophy have more than 50 and up to several thousand repeats. More severely affected patients have a higher number of repeats. Although there is no strict correlation, to enable the physician to predict the severity in any individual patient, a repeat size greater than 1,500 is usually associated with the congenital form of the disease.

Figure 3.8. Myotonic Dystrophy in a 6-Year-Old Boy.

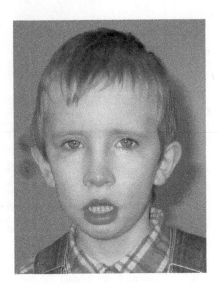

Individuals who have 38 to 49 repeats carry a **premutation,** meaning they will not develop symptoms themselves but have a risk for increased repeat numbers in their offspring. Such premutations, just like the larger disease-causing mutations, are **unstable**. In most cases the repeat number increases, resulting in the phenomenon of **anticipation** (i.e., a more severe clinical picture in the child than in the parent). The risk of significant expansion is higher in males with relatively small expansion size and in females with relatively high expansion size. If a symptomatic woman with 200 to 500 repeats transmits the mutation to her child, the risk of congenital muscular dystrophy is 10% to 30 % in her first child and 40% to 50% if she has had a previous child with congenital muscular dystrophy.

Pathogenesis in myotonic dystrophy is not related to the protein coded by the *DMPK* gene but is due to **abnormal RNA transcript processing**. It is now understood that the long tract with repetitive CUGs in the mRNA leads to sequestration and/or upregulation of RNA-binding proteins and disruption of various RNA processes, ranging from pre-mRNA splicing to protein translation, for a number of different genes. Deficiencies of these genes explain the divergent symptoms in many organ systems.

Diagnosis

The diagnosis of myotonic dystrophy primarily rests on the typical clinical symptoms and signs in conjunction with a conspicuous family history. It should always be confirmed by **molecular genetic analysis** of the trinucleotide repeat using PCR and Southern blotting (□ Fig. 3.9). A normal repeat number excludes the diagnosis of type 1 myotonic dystrophy.

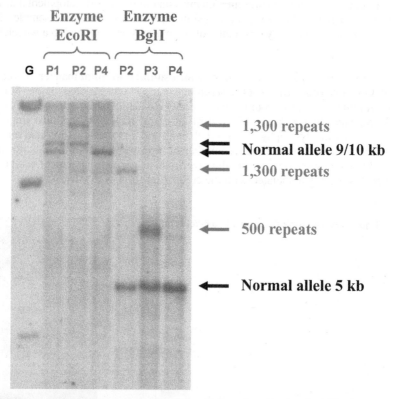

□ **Figure 3.9. The repeat expansion in myotonic dystrophy is analyzed by Southern blotting.** Genomic DNA is digested by restriction enzymes; the fragments are separated by agarose gel electrophoresis and transferred to a nylon membrane. Hybridization with specific probes visualizes bands that contain the repeat sequence and allows exact sizing. The specific fragment normally has a size of 5 kb after digestion with the restriction enzyme BglI, and either 9 or 10 kb after EcoRI digestion. Patient 2 (P2) in the illustration has myotonic dystrophy with approximately 1,300 repeats, while patient 3 (P3) has myotonic dystrophy with approximately 500 repeats. Fragment sizes in patients 1 and 4 (P1, P4) are normal. G, size standard. (Courtesy of B. Janssen, Institute for Human Genetics, Heidelberg.)

Differential Diagnosis

The most relevant differential diagnosis of myotonic dystrophy type 1 is **myotonic dystrophy type 2**, previously described as proximal myotonic myopathy (PROMM). The clinical picture of DM2 is milder than that of DM1, with mild myotonia and predominantly proximal weakness, but **muscle pain** is a distinguishing feature. Onset of symptoms usually occurs in the patient's thirties; no neonatal forms and no developmental retardation have been observed. DM2 is caused by large expansions of a CCTG tetranucleotide repeat in the *ZNF9* gene, which results in sequestration of the same RNA-binding proteins as DM1. Inheritance is autosomal dominant.

Therapy and Management

There is no specific therapy for myotonic dystrophy at this time. Long-term management should include regular neurological, ophthalmological, cardiological, and endocrinological evaluations and management. Cataracts are treated surgically, while diabetes mellitus usually responds to oral hypoglycemic agents or insulin. Arrhythmias sometimes require medications or a pacemaker. Patients with myotonic dystrophy have an increased sensitivity to various drugs given in connection with general anesthesia, and surgery should be carried out either using regional anesthesia or in a tertiary care center.

Prognosis

Life expectancy for patients with oligosymptomatic myotonic dystrophy is generally normal. Patients with classic myotonic dystrophy, however, often die during their middle to late adulthood. Pneumonia or cardiac arrhythmias and sudden cardiac death are the most common primary causes of death. The average life expectancy for patients with the congenital type is approximately 45 years, which is not much lower than for the classic type.

4 Pathomechanisms of Genetic Diseases

LEARNING OBJECTIVES

1 Explain why osteogenesis imperfecta, Huntington chorea, and familial breast cancer are inherited as dominant traits; why cystic fibrosis and phenylketonuria are inherited as recessive traits; and why the terms are not suitable for Fra(X) syndrome and hemophilia.

2 Discuss why sickle cell anemia is relatively common in African Americans.

3 Assess the recurrence risk of Angelman syndrome in a family with regard to the different types of mutations.

4 Discuss the (theoretical) risks for the children of a man with mosaicism for an X-chromosomal disorder.

4.1 From Genotype to Phenotype

It is unlikely that a patient will seek medical advice by saying, "Good morning, doctor. I have a problem with my compound heterozygosity. On one allele of my *CFTR* gene is a classical F508del mutation, on the other the 5T-intron variant—this worries me. Can you please help me?" Medical practice deals with real patients and not with variable copies of pathological gene sequences. So, when does a molecular alteration turn into a "real patient"? How does the genotype become a phenotype? And how can the understanding of this correlation help the doctor in diagnosis and therapy?

The term **genotype** denotes the entire genetic information of an organism or a cell. More specifically, especially with regard to a certain phenotype, the term relates to the genetic information at a specific locus (i.e., the combined DNA sequence information on the two copies of a particular gene). For example, the genotype of an autosomal gene tells whether a genetic variant occurs on both copies of the gene (homozygous) or only on one (heterozygous). It considers the fact that two different variants of a gene can occur on the two homologous chromosomes (in trans) or just on one chromosome (in cis), the latter having occurred through successive mutations or after recombination. The genotype also makes a distinction between homozygosity and hemizygosity. If there is only one copy of a gene, such as most X-chromosomal genes in males, variants in this gene are hemizygous even though in standard molecular genetic tests they look like homozygous variants in autosomal genes.

> **Genotype:** The total genetic information available to an organism or a cell, either as a whole or with regard to a specific function.
>
> **Phenotype:** The physical manifestation of the genetic information.
>
> **Homozygous:** A genetic variant/sequence on both copies of a gene.
>
> **Heterozygous:** A genetic variant/sequence on only one of the two copies of a gene.
>
> **Hemizygous:** A genetic variant on a gene of which there is only a single copy.
>
> **In trans:** Two different genetic variants of a gene that occur on the two homologous chromosomal strands.
>
> **In cis:** Two different variants of a gene that occur beside each other on the same chromosomal strand and not on the homologous chromosomal strand.

A **phenotype** is "what we see," meaning the physical manifestation of the genetic information. It describes what the cell or the organism creates from the genotype. It is important to

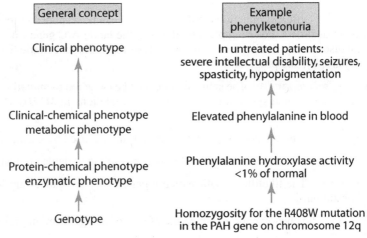

Figure 4.1. From Genotype to Phenotype.

note that the phenotype results from multiple factors, both genetic as well as nongenetic. The phenotype can be defined in different ways, depending on the focus that we choose to take (□ Fig. 4.1).

Patients and physicians usually think and work primarily at the level of the **clinical phenotype**. The patient normally consults a physician because of symptoms that may be perceived as serious and stressful. The physician examines the clinical phenotype, both physically and through diagnostic imaging techniques, and tries to change it through therapeutic intervention. Indeed, nongenetic factors (i.e., "environmental factors"), including treatment, exert their biggest impact on the clinical phenotype.

On a functional level, the **metabolic** or **clinical chemical phenotype**, meaning the concentration of certain key substances in body fluids, is of special diagnostic relevance. Not every clinical phenotype has a measurable clinical chemical correlate; for many genetic disorders there are no measurable biochemical abnormalities. On the other hand, there are genetically caused conditions that have a distinct clinical chemical phenotype yet lack any clinical correlate. Autosomal recessive–inherited histidinemia is a good example of such a "nondisease." There are clear metabolic abnormalities associated with increased histidine concentration in plasma and urine but no clinical symptoms whatsoever.

The same is true for the **molecular phenotype**, which represents the direct gene product and can be examined, for instance, through laboratory methods such as enzyme studies. Protein structure and function is more directly determined by the genotype, and its analysis, if possible, allows a more direct assessment of gene function. Nevertheless, measurable abnormalities in protein structure or function do not automatically imply clinical relevance. Histidinemia, caused by a loss of histidase enzyme activity, once again serves as an example.

Ultimately, the **genotype** is the etiological basis of many human conditions. However, it is not always easy to determine what a particular genetic variant really means for the patient. Geneticists may be specialists for diagnostic tests at the genotype level, but they must also be familiar with the various ways of identifying a genetic disorder on the phenotype level (e.g., clinical, functional, structural, cellular, and molecular levels). Determining which diagnostic approach to choose depends on many factors, and quite often a phenotype-based assay is superior to a gene test. Nevertheless, for many disorders described in this book, it is not possible to measure the activity of enzymes, amounts of protein, substrate accumulation, or other phenotypic parameters in order to reach a firm diagnosis. Only if we understand the relationship between genetic variants and the different levels of phenotypic presentation will we be able to understand the patient's disorder and to interpret the results of genetic tests correctly.

Pleiotropy: Different mutations in the same gene can be responsible for the development of different disorders. For example, mutations in the lamin A/C gene can result in several different disorders, including mandibuloacral dysostosis, Charcot-Marie-Tooth disease, familial lipodystrophy, and progeria.

Genetic heterogeneity: The same disorder can be triggered by mutations in different genes. For example, Lynch syndrome can result from mutations in *MLH1*, *MSH2*, *PMS1*, *PMS2*, or *MSH6*.

Expressivity: The variable phenotypic manifestation caused by a genetic variant.

Variable expressivity: The same mutation can result in variable clinical phenotypes.

Penetrance: The likelihood with which a genetic variant causes any kind of phenotypic manifestation.

Epistasis: The phenomenon in which the effects of one gene are modified by one or several other genes.

Polyphenism: The phenomenon in which the effects of one gene are modified by external factors.

Monogenic: A disease that is caused by mutations in a single gene.

Digenic: A disease that is caused by the combined effect of mutations in two different genes.

Polygenic: A disease that is caused by the combined effect of mutations in multiple genes.

Multifactorial: A disease that is caused by the combined effect of multiple genetic and non-genetic factors.

The identification of genotype–phenotype correlations is one of the main tasks for human genetics, both in research and in clinical practice. Quite often mutations in a gene are associated with different clinical manifestations even within the same family (i.e., variable expressivity) or in some individuals may have no functional effect whatsoever (i.e., **reduced** penetrance). This may be due to the influence of other genetic factors within the organism (i.e., epistasis), due to chance effects in dominant disorders caused by clonal loss of the second (i.e., wild-type) allele (e.g., **loss of heterozygosity** as seen in cancer predisposition syndromes), or due to exogenous factors (i.e., polyphenism). Interestingly, successful treatment that changes the phenotype, such as dietary treatment that prevents intellectual disability in phenylketonuria (PKU) (as discussed in Chapter 24.1.3), could be regarded as a form of polyphenism, but the term is mostly used for the adaptation of animals and plants to different environments. For the development of some clinical phenotypes, the mutation(s) of one single gene is not sufficient. Only if mutations in two or several specific genes interact does the clinical phenotype develop (i.e., digenic or polygenic inheritance). An example is Bardet-Biedl syndrome (see Section 29.3).

4.2 Dominant and Recessive

The founder of modern genetics was the Augustinian monk **Johann Gregor Mendel** (1822–1884), who in 1865 published "Experiments on Plant Hybridization" after cultivating and studying varieties of garden peas at his monastery in Brünn (now the Slovakian town of Brno). He showed that inheritance is based on distinct and separate factors. Today these "factors" are called **genes**. Mendel also coined the terms dominant and recessive by writing, ". . . those characters which are transmitted entire, or almost unchanged in the hybridization, and therefore in themselves constitute the characters of the hybrid, are termed the dominant, and those which become latent in the process, recessive." Understanding the molecular basis of dominance and recessiveness is the basis for understanding the molecular basis of inherited disorders.

There are two different approaches to the terms dominant and recessive. The traditional approach is to look at inheritance patterns in a family and to check whether a phenotype (i.e., a disease) is found, for example, in successive generations, siblings, or male individuals (see Chapter 5). Although this works in many instances, it has major limitations and does not really help in understanding the pathophysiology. Much more enlightening is the question of what happens clinically (i.e., phenotypically) when an individual is heterozygous, a "hybrid" in Mendel's terms. The terms dominant and recessive can only be understood properly as a description of **the functional relationship of two different alleles of the same gene in a (compound) heterozygous organism**. Mendel demonstrated this in the case of pea plants, which bloomed either red or white. If a genetically pure red-blooming plant is pollinated by a genetically pure white-blooming plant (or vice versa), the resulting seed produces only red-blooming plants in the F1 generation. The "red" allele dominates over the "white" allele in the hybrid. The same is true with regard to disease-causing mutations in humans. A pathogenic mutation on one allele (with the wild-type allele on the homologous chromosome) is enough to cause a dominant disorder, while heterozygous carriers of recessive disorder are phenotypically healthy. Recessive disorders only arise if there are mutations on both copies of the respective gene.

It is not quite that simple in most cases, however, and the analysis of what really happens on the molecular or cellular level in dominant and recessive disorders helps one understand the pathogenesis of human disorders.

Dominant: A genetic variant that causes a recognizable phenotype in the heterozygous state, or the phenotype caused by this type of variant.

Recessive: A genetic variant that causes a recognizable phenotype only in the homozygous state, or the phenotype caused by this type of variant.

Semidominance (incomplete dominance): The phenomenon that a genetic variant causes a recognizable phenotype in the heterozygous state and another (usually more severe) phenotype in the homozygous state.

Codominance: The phenomenon that two distinct phenotypes associated with two different genetic variants are both found in a compound heterozygous individual.

Dominant in Every Respect? It is possible that heterozygous carriers of a recessive disease can have relevant phenotypic traits. Heterozygous carriers for PKU have slightly elevated phenylalanine concentrations in their blood and markedly reduced enzymatic activity of phenylalanine hydroxylase in the liver. This is not clinically relevant, but it shows that the normal allele does not completely dominate over the mutated one.

■■■ Heterozygote Advantage

Evolutionary pressure reduces the allele frequency of recessive disease mutations if affected (i.e., homozygous) individuals do not procreate. Why is it, then, that some recessive disorders are very common in various different populations? Why is cystic fibrosis so common in Europeans, with a carrier frequency of up to 5% or more? Why are 9% to 10% of African Americans heterozygous carriers for sickle cell anemia? It appears that, in certain situations, heterozygosity represents a selection advantage over homozygosity for the wild-type allele (i.e., **heterozygote advantage**). The best-known examples of this are the hemoglobinopathies. In Equatorial Africa, where malaria is endemic, the mutation for **sickle cell anemia** (i.e., a mutation in the β-chain of hemoglobin; see Chapter 21.5) has an extremely high allele frequency of 20% to 40%. Epidemiological studies have shown that heterozygous carriers for sickle cell anemia are more resistant toward *Plasmodium falciparum*, the pathogen that causes tropical malaria. Infected erythrocytes of heterozygous individuals are probably destroyed more rapidly, thereby reducing the ability of the plasmodium to multiply in the blood. Homozygotes for normal hemoglobin are more likely to have serious complications of tropical malaria and to die early; in consequence, they are less fertile (have fewer offspring). Although homozygous patients with sickle cell anemia mutation have a serious life-threatening disease that, in the past, precluded them from having children, this effect was counterbalanced in areas with a high incidence of malaria, as reproduction of

carriers of sickle cell mutation is increased by about 15%. If exogenous factors are stable over many generations, the favorable and unfavorable effects of a genetic variant in a population achieve a balance, which is
readjusted only when exogenous effects change. The sickle cell mutation, in this regard, represents a **balanced
polymorphism** in populations with a high prevalence of malaria.

Semidominance or Incomplete Dominance. For most disorders inherited as dominant traits,
homozygosity for a disease-causing mutation results in a much more severe clinical phenotype than heterozygosity. An example is familial hypercholesterolemia (Chapter 24.3), a
genetic disorder resulting from mutations of the low-density lipoprotein (LDL) receptor gene.
Individuals with a heterozygous loss-of-function mutation show elevated LDL cholesterol
levels (greater than 7 to 10 mmol/L) and typically suffer their first myocardial infarction in
midlife. Homozygous carriers have a much higher LDL cholesterol level (10 to 30 mmol/L),
with the onset of symptoms in early childhood and coronary heart disease as early as school
age. Another example is achondroplasia (Chapter 26.2), in which homozygosity for the
disease-causing *FGFR3* mutation causes a severe skeletal dysplasia typically leading to
death in utero or shortly after birth. In these examples, as indeed in most genetic traits, the
phenotype of heterozygotes (Aa) is somewhere in between the phenotypes of wild-type and
mutant homozygotes (AA and aa). The inheritance pattern is called semidominant or incompletely dominant, in contrast to **complete dominance** that is found in very few conditions,
such as Huntington disease (Chapter 31.1.1), in which the phenotype of the heterozygous
and homozygous mutation carriers is more or less identical. It is worth thinking about reasons why a condition may show complete penetrance. For practical purposes, both types of
conditions may be called dominant because the definition rests on the clinical phenotype
in the heterozygote, irrespective of what is observed in the homozygote.

Codominance. There are a few cases in which two alleles of the same gene code for proteins
with different specific functions, both of which may be found simultaneously in (compound)
heterozygous individuals. Such alleles are said to be codominant to each other. The classic
example is the ABO blood group system, in which individuals with genotype AB show phenotypic characteristics of allele A as well as allele B, and there is also a null allele that causes
complete loss of protein function.

■■■ The ABO Blood Group System

The blood groups of the ABO system are determined by the *ABO* gene on chromosome 9q34. With
regard to its function, three different alleles can be distinguished: A, B, and O (■ Fig. 4.2). Both allele A
and allele B code for glycosyltransferases, enzymes that take part in the glycosylation of proteins in the
cell membranes. The respective proteins have different substrate specificities, names, and EC numbers.
Isoform GTA, coded by allele A, catalyzes the transfer of N-acetylgalactose (GalNAc) to the carbohydrate
chain, while GTB, coded by allele B, transfers galactose (Gal). The presence of GTA results in blood group
A, whereas GTB results in blood group B. Individuals who are compound heterozygous for alleles A and B
(who have genotype AB) modify some of their glycoproteins with GalNAc and others with Gal. They have
blood group AB. The third allele, O, contains a frameshift deletion, which completely removes enzyme
function. Individuals homozygous for the O allele have blood group O, while compound heterozygosity for
alleles O and A leads to blood group A, and compound heterozygosity for alleles O and B leads to blood
group B. Alleles/blood groups A and B are thus dominant over allele/blood group O, but are codominant
toward each other. Stated more generally, **function competes with function, and dominates over
absence of function**.

Dominant Negative Effect. Most dominant mutations cause symptoms through reduced
function of the respective protein. The inability of the remaining wild-type allele to fully compensate for the loss of the other allele results in a **haploinsufficient phenotype**. Some mutations, however, generate a structurally altered but stable protein that interferes with the normal
protein coded by the wild-type allele. In this situation the clinical effects are more dramatic
than complete loss of the mutant allele. Such a **dominant negative effect** occurs with many
structural proteins functioning as subunits of a larger protein multimer. A classic example is
osteogenesis imperfecta.

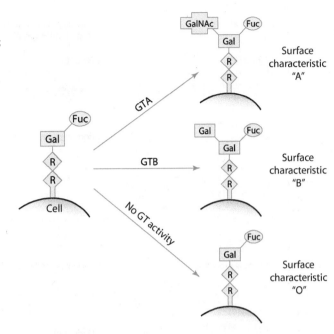

Figure 4.2. ABO Blood Group System. R, residue; Gal, galactose; Fuc, fucose; GalNAc, N-acetylgalactose; GTA, glycosyltransferase A; GTB, glycosyltransferase B.

Dominant Negative Effect in Osteogenesis Imperfecta

Osteogenesis imperfecta (OI), commonly called **brittle bone disease**, is a clinically and genetically heterogeneous disease of connective tissues. It is a disorder of calcified as well as soft connective tissues. Its major symptom is extremely **fragile bones**. The oldest documented case is that of an Egyptian mummy dating to about 1,000 BC.

Osteogenesis imperfecta is caused by the deficiency or abnormal production of **collagen I**. Collagen makes up roughly one-fourth of the human body's protein content. Collagen I occurs in bones, tendons, ligaments, teeth, skin, cornea, sclerae, and the middle and inner ear. It consists of long polypeptides with a high content of the amino acids glycine, proline, and hydroxyproline. Every third position in the polypeptide sequence is occupied by glycine (i.e., Gly-X-Y structure). Three polypeptide chains are aligned and twisted to form a **triple helix**. Procollagen 1 consists of two $\alpha 1$(I)-chains and one $\alpha 2$(I)-chain encoded by different genes (Fig. 4.3A). *COL1A1* is located on chromosome 17 and *COL1A2* is located on chromosome 7.

The clinical effects of mutations in either *COL1A1* or *COL1A2* depend on how much normal protein is produced and whether mutant protein interferes with the function of the normal protein. **Null mutations** that cause complete loss of one of the two copies of either *COL1A1* or *COL1A2* give rise to the relatively mild phenotype of **OI type I**, which results in a 50% reduction of collagen synthesis, but the collagen is of normal quality. This phenomenon corresponding to complete loss of one of two gene copies causes clinical symptoms and is described with the term **haploinsufficiency** (Fig. 4.3B).

Severe neonatal OI (type II), in contrast, is generally caused by **point mutations** that give rise to an abnormal but stable protein that is integrated into the procollagen triple helix along with the normal protein and thus severely disrupts its structure (Fig. 4.3C). In this way, the mutated protein affects the function of a normal protein, and the resulting clinical picture is more severe than in cases of haploinsufficiency for this protein. This phenomenon is called the **dominant negative effect**.

Clinical Case

Mrs. Bender's mother has osteogenesis imperfecta type I, and Mrs. Bender wants to know whether her own children are at risk for developing this condition. Mrs. Bender's mother experienced her first fractures at age 3. Until puberty she had about 10 fractures, mostly of the lower extremities. She became more careful and experienced no more

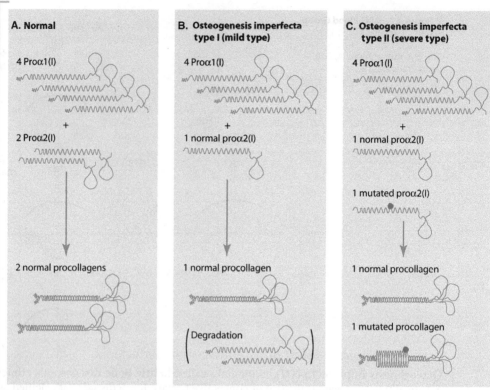

Figure 4.3. A–C. Dominant Negative Effect in Osteogenesis Imperfecta.

fractures. She did not have deformities of the long bones, but her right leg is slightly shorter because of multiple fractures. Mrs. Bender says that her mother is 1.54 m (approximately 5 ft.) tall, is double jointed, and bruises easily. Her sclerae have been a blue-gray color since birth. She has severe periodontitis. Beginning in her thirties, her mother suffered hearing loss, and because of otosclerosis had plastic surgery of the stapes at age 33. Additional diagnoses were osteoporosis and scoliosis of the lumbar vertebrae. Mrs. Bender herself is 26 years old, is 1.67 m (approximately 5 ft. 5 in.) tall, and has never had a fracture. Her sclerae are not discolored and she has normal hearing and normal joint mobility. Although Mrs. Bender was at 50% risk of inheriting this autosomal dominant condition from her mother, as she has no symptoms of OI type I, she does not have the disorder. Of course, this implies that the risk for OI type I in her children is not higher than the risk for the general population.

Epidemiology

The overall incidence of osteogenesis imperfecta in the first year of life is 1 in 20,000. Type I is the most frequent subform, followed by type II and type III. Males and females are equally affected. OI is an important differential diagnosis of nonaccidental trauma during childhood.

Clinical Features

Osteogenesis Imperfecta Type I (■ Fig. 4.4)
- Fractures are rare in newborns, but there is increased bone fragility and an increased fracture rate, sometimes with minor trauma
- No bone deformities, only slightly double jointed
- Slightly smaller than normal
- Blue-gray sclerae (though not a constant feature)
- Normal dentition
- Thin skin, increased risk of hematoma because of fragile blood vessels
- Conductive or mixed hearing impairment through fractures of the ossicles and/or stapes fixation

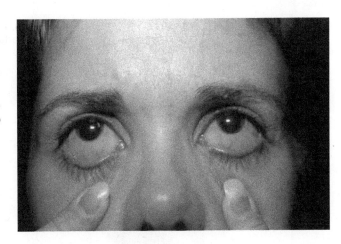

▢ Figure 4.4. Osteogenesis Imperfecta Type I. In osteogenesis imperfecta of any type and more evident in younger persons, the scleral collagen matrix is thinner than normal, allowing scattered light from the deep choroidal melanin to give the normally white sclera a slate-gray (sometimes improperly called "blue") hue. (Courtesy of R. Lewis, Baylor College of Medicine, Houston.)

Osteogenesis Imperfecta Type II (▢ Fig. 4.5)

- Perinatal lethal type
- Disproportionate short stature due to abnormally short, fractured, and bent extremities
- Torso of normal length, but narrow chest because of multiple rib fractures (i.e., "pearl string ribs")

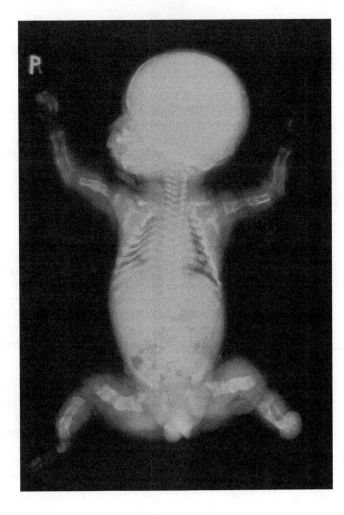

▢ Figure 4.5. Osteogenesis Imperfecta Type II. Multiple fractures of tubular bones and ribs, prenatally lethal. (Courtesy of Hj Müller, Department of Medical Genetics, University Children's Hospital Basel, Switzerland.)

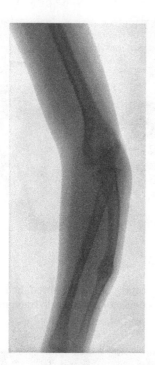

Figure 4.6. Osteogenesis Imperfecta Type III. Deformed, fractured ulna.

- Large head with membranous calvaria (soft and minimally ossified—"caput membranaceum")
- Slate-gray sclerae

Osteogenesis Imperfecta Type III (Fig. 4.6)
- Progressive deformities affecting mobility
- Severely limited growth
- Dentinogenesis imperfecta with blue-gray or yellow-brown translucent teeth

Osteogenesis Imperfecta Type IV
- Moderately severe type
- Short stature, moderate deformities
- Possible fractures during birth

Diagnosis

The clinical diagnosis is supported by radiological tests revealing pathological fractures with good healing tendencies, sometimes with pseudarthrosis. The large tubular bones have "telephone receiver"–like deformations and serial healed rib fractures that resemble rosary beads (type II). In severe cases the skull has membranous calvaria or a typical basilar impression (OI type III), occasionally leading to compression of the brainstem. The diagnosis may be confirmed by mutation analysis or collagen analysis in fibroblasts.

Genetics

The disease is mostly caused by various mutations in either of the *COL1A* genes. The genes are quite large, and sequence analysis is relatively laborious and expensive. Most mutations are unique in a given family (i.e., private mutations). Inheritance of most types of OI is **autosomal dominant**, and the children of affected patients have a 50% risk of also being affected. If unaffected parents have a child with OI, there is a 6% to 7% chance for each subsequent child to also be affected with the same mutation, due to germline mosaicism in one of the parents. Causative mutations in other genes, sometimes with autosomal recessive inheritance, have also been identified.

Therapy and Clinical Management
— Bisphosphonate drug therapy reduces pain and lessens fracture rate.
— Although OI patients are not growth-hormone deficient, treatment with growth hormone may result in increased height for type I and IV patients.
— OI patients should be in a physical therapy program to improve strength and mobility and should be regularly seen by an orthopedist to monitor bone growth, deformity, and bone density.

4.3 Epigenetics and Genomic Imprinting

Not only is genetic information stored in the actual sequence of nuclear (and mitochondrial) DNA (e.g., ATCG), but also for many genes hereditary information is transmitted with a parental-specific **imprint** based on whether the gene was transmitted through spermatogenesis (i.e., from the father) or through oogenesis (i.e., from the mother). This imprint can be thought of as the font of the genome (e.g., *ATCG* vs. **ATCG** vs. ATCG). For these imprinted genes, even though the nucleotide sequence in the maternal and paternal copies is identical, the expression differs depending on the parental imprint. The science of these phenomena is called **epigenetics** (*epi* [Gr.], "above," "at," "near").

Epigenetic factors: Hereditary factors that are independent of the actual DNA sequence.

Imprinting: Inherited inhibition of gene expression by epigenetic factors (either maternal or paternal gene copy). An imprinted gene is not expressed and thus is inactive.

Epigenetic Mechanisms

Epigenetic phenomena, as a rule, are transmitted via changes in the regulation or expression of genes. The most important known mechanisms are methylation of genomic DNA and modification of histones, yet a congenital regulation of gene expression can also be transmitted by way of cytosolic RNA.

Differential **methylation of genomic DNA** is a central mechanism in the regulation of the expression of genes. Of special importance is the methylation of cytosine in CpG (cytosine-phosphorus-guanine) dinucleotides. In the 5' untranslated region (UTR) in front of the start codon, many genes have numerous "CpG islands" with a large number of CpG dinucleotides. Hypermethylation in this region results in transcriptional silencing, meaning the gene can no longer be read. The methylation pattern of DNA and, consequently, the activity pattern of the genes are generally transmitted as a stable trait in mitosis; however, for imprinted or epigenetically sensitive genes, this "trait" is reset in meiosis. A clonal change of the methylation pattern and thus an increase or decrease in expression of important genes is, for example, a major pathomechanism in tumor cells.

As already shown in Section 2.6 (Euchromatin and Heterochromatin), the readability of genes is essentially dependent on the chromatin structure. The condensation level of chromatin and the packaging density of DNA are also regulated through chemical **modifications of histones**, which, in turn, depend on the methylation status of DNA. The reversible acetylation of lysine residues in the N-terminal region of histones, for example, results in loosening of DNA binding and, in this way, enables access of transcription factors. Conversely, there are proteins like MeCP2 (which is mutated in Rett syndrome) that bind to methylated CpG dinucleotides and recruit histone deacetylases, leading to a condensation of the chromatin. Other types of histone modification are phosphorylation of serine residues, methylation of lysine and arginine residues, and ubiquitination and poly-ADP-ribosylation.

Genomic Imprinting

Genomic imprinting is an epigenetic process, first recognized in the 1980s, that differentially modifies (i.e., defines) certain genes or chromosomal segments in the male or female germ line.

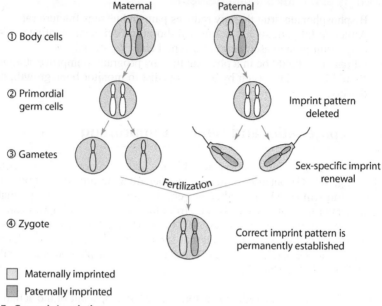

Maternal   Paternal

① Body cells

② Primordial germ cells   Imprint pattern deleted

③ Gametes   Sex-specific imprint renewal

Fertilization

④ Zygote   Correct imprint pattern is permanently established

☐ Maternally imprinted
☐ Paternally imprinted

Figure 4.7. Genomic Imprinting.

As a result, either the paternal or the maternal allele of the gene is inactive in the somatic cells of offspring. A gene is called maternally imprinted if the maternal allele is inactive and not expressed. Conversely, a gene is imprinted paternally if the paternal allele is inactive. The specific parental imprinting pattern within the somatic cells is maintained unchanged throughout all mitotic divisions. Only in the germ line (i.e., the primordial germ cells) is the imprinting pattern reset to reflect the parent of origin. Regional imprinting centers within the relevant chromosomal areas control the epigenetic process. In spermatogenesis, all germ cells receive a male imprinting pattern, while in oocytogenesis, all germ cells receive a female imprint. Thus, after fertilization there exists a balanced and correct imprint of the zygote's entire genome (■ Fig. 4.7).

■■■ Genomic Imprinting—Battle of the Sexes?

Why does genomic imprinting exist? One possible explanation is the **conflict model**: in evolution, the father's genes prevail only if his child survives (possibly to the detriment of the mother, for there are other women), while the mother has to ensure her own survival; after all, she can become pregnant again. Therefore, many paternally expressed genes (imprinted on the maternal allele) should promote the growth of the fetus, while maternally expressed genes should counter this effect and attempt to protect maternal resources. Many imprinted genes support this hypothesis. This imprinting effect also mirrors the clinical differences of embryonal triploidy: in the presence of one paternal and two maternal chromosome complements (digynic triploidy), the placenta is small and fibrous and the embryo's growth is severely retarded, while during diandric triploidy (partial mole), the placenta is cystic-hyperplastic and the embryo of normal size. If all chromosomes of a diploid chromosome complement originate from the paternal germ line, this creates a complete hydatidiform mole (i.e., a hypertrophic placenta without fetal elements and with risk of malignant degeneration).

Genomic imprinting has only been observed in mammals. It is estimated that more than 90 genes of the human genome have parental-specific imprinting; most are located in 1 of 13 known imprinting clusters. All clusters have an imprinting control region (ICR) that is typically 1 to 5 kb in size, is differentially methylated, and regulates imprinting across the entire domain. Clusters contain at least one long noncoding RNA (ncRNA) that is usually expressed from the maternal allele and multiple paternally expressed protein-coding genes; also, there are usually maternally expressed genes and multiple ncRNA genes. Regulation of imprinting is not fully understood but, at least in some cases, involves a long ncRNA that silences the expression of protein-coding genes bidirectionally in cis.

Among the disorders that are linked to genomic imprinting are Prader-Willi syndrome, Angelman syndrome, Beckwith-Wiedemann syndrome, and Silver-Russell syndrome. An imprinting-related disorder may be caused by different mechanisms:

— Typically, there is a **microdeletion** with loss of the nonimprinted (expressed) gene copy. The cell is left with the homologous yet imprinted gene copy, thus prohibiting expression of the gene. Therefore, there is no functional gene copy, and the gene product cannot be synthesized. Usually there are both maternally and paternally imprinted genes in the same region. A microdeletion that encompasses the entire region has completely different clinical consequences depending on whether it is inherited from the mother or the father: a maternally inherited microdeletion causes a deficiency of the paternally imprinted gene(s), and vice versa. Most microdeletions have occurred de novo, and there is only a small recurrence risk for subsequent children in the family. In rare cases an unbalanced chromosomal translocation can be found as the cause of an imprinting-related disorder.

— Disorders related to genomic imprinting can also occur when two homologous chromosomes come from the same parent. This phenomenon is called **uniparental disomy (UPD)**. In maternal UPD the paternal chromosome is missing, and in consequence there is no functional copy of genes that are expressed on only the paternal chromosome. In paternal UPD it is the other way around. An imprinting error through UPD is not transmitted to the next generation since imprinting is started anew (and correctly) in the germ line. Recurrence risk in subsequent children is the same as in the general population unless one of the parents has a chromosomal abnormality (such as a Robertsonian translocation) that predisposes that individual to UPD.

— Occasionally, the loss of function of an imprinted gene is caused by a **mutation in the nonimprinted copy of this gene**. Whether or not a mutation causes disease thus depends on whether the mutation was inherited from the mother or father. This mechanism is especially important because one parent of an affected child could be an asymptomatic mutation carrier. For example, if a woman has inherited a mutation in a paternally imprinted gene from her father, she would be asymptomatic, but a child (son or daughter) who inherits the mutation from her would be affected. The risk of recurrence for subsequent children would thus be 50%.

— In some cases imprinting abnormalities are due to a mutation affecting the imprinting control region, such as a small deletion or abnormal methylation.

— Some disorders are caused by an imbalance between maternally or paternally imprinted genes that have an antagonistic effect (e.g., in the balance of growth promotion and growth retardation). Such an imbalance can be caused by the **duplication of an imprinted gene**, as has been shown for Beckwith-Wiedemann syndrome.

Uniparental Disomy

How is it possible that two homologous chromosomes come from one and the same parent? There are two major mechanisms, both of which involve rescue of a numeric chromosomal abnormality.

— **Trisomy rescue.** Autosomal trisomy in a zygote is not usually compatible with life and leads to early miscarriage. However, if the chromosomal complement number is "normalized" by the loss of one of the trisomic chromosomes, the conceptus is likely to survive to term. Due to the nature of oogenesis, the majority of trisomic conceptuses will have one paternal copy of the chromosome and two maternal copies due to maternal nondisjunction in either meiosis I or meiosis II. In the rescue scenario, if the *paternal* chromosome is the one lost to "rescue" the conceptus, the two remaining chromosomes will be maternal in origin—that is, **maternal uniparental disomy**. So, in one out of three cases, this mechanism leads to UPD. Rarely, nondisjunction occurs in spermatogenesis, and in that case one of the paternal chromosomes would need to be lost to avoid paternal UPD (◘ Fig. 4.8A).

— **Monosomy rescue.** Just like the rescue of trisomy through loss of the additional chromosome, monosomy is occasionally rescued by duplication of the single, available chromosome in one

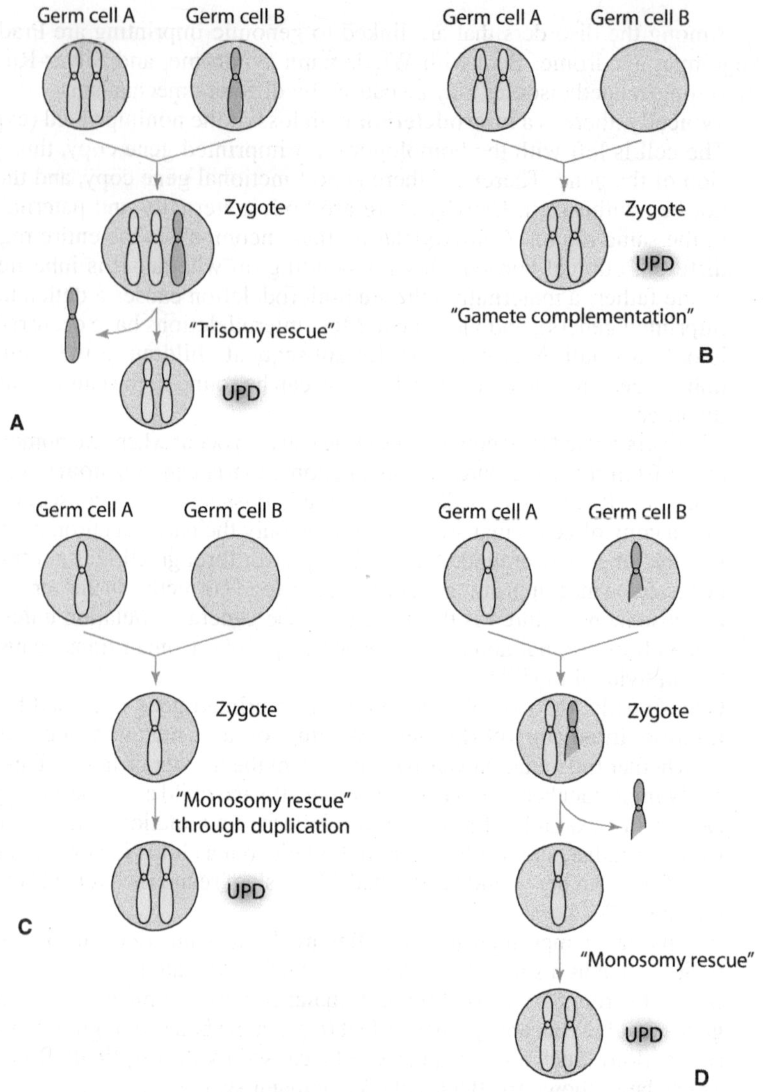

Figure 4.8. Mechanisms Leading to Uniparental Disomy. Green, imprinted maternally; blue, imprinted paternally. UPD, uniparental disomy. See the text for a detailed discussion of the mechanisms.

of the daughter cells. This always results in uniparental disomy (Fig. 4.8C). Monosomy can also be a postzygotic event (e.g., if a structurally abnormal chromosome is "deleted") (Fig. 4.8D).
— In extremely rare cases a disomic germ cell of one parent accidentally fertilizes an egg cell from the other parent that is nullisomic for the same chromosome. The resulting zygote then manifests uniparental disomy for the respective chromosome (Fig. 4.8B).

A Robertsonian translocation is an important risk factor for UPD, since it increases the risk of trisomy or monosomy in the offspring. Care must be taken to exclude UPD if prenatal diagnosis is performed and one of the parents is a carrier of a Robertsonian translocation, even if the chromosomal complement is normal or itself shows a balanced Robertsonian translocation.

Molecular testing of DNA markers on the homologous chromosomes that exhibit UPD allows a more detailed assessment of its origin. All markers are identical if the UPD is derived from

monosomy rescue; this is described as uniparental **isodisomy**. Trisomy due to nondisjunction in meiosis II will also give rise to isodisomy, (in regions that have not undergone recombination). In contrast, nondisjunction in meiosis I will lead to uniparental **heterodisomy** (except for chromosomal regions that have undergone recombination); marker alleles will differ on the homologous chromosomes but will all be derived from the same parent.

Prader-Willi Syndrome and Angelman Syndrome

Prader-Willi syndrome (PWS) and Angelman syndrome (AS) are classic examples that illustrate **genomic imprinting** in humans. Both conditions are due to imprinted genes on the long arm of **chromosome 15**, relatively close to the centromere (15q11-15q13), and may be caused by identical deletions of this region. Of crucial importance is the origin of the mutant allele; lack of the paternal copy gives rise to PWS, while lack of the maternal copy is the cause of AS. This is explained by the fact that some genes in this region are expressed on only the paternal allele, others on only the maternal allele. These genes are silenced (imprinted) on the respective other allele.

It has been known for some time that AS is caused by the deficiency of a **ubiquitin-protein ligase** encoded by the *UBE3A* gene. This gene is paternally imprinted in the brain (i.e., expressed only on the maternal allele). Interestingly, the *UBE3A* gene shows biparental (maternal and paternal) expression in all other organs, which explains why the pathogenic effects in AS are restricted to the brain. The pathogenesis of PWS, in contrast, remained a mystery for a long time, since all protein-coding genes in this region could be excluded as candidates. Recently it was shown that PWS is caused by the loss of a **cluster of small nucleolar RNAs (snoRNAs)** encoded by the non-protein-coding *HBII-85* gene on chromosome 15q11-15q13. Thus, PWS is the first known monogenic disorder caused by the **loss of a noncoding RNA gene**; the function of the snoRNAs remains to be characterized.

> **Important**
>
> Clinically, PWS and AS are totally different disorders, even though they may be caused by identical deletions of the same chromosomal region. They are listed here because of their complementary pathomechanism and not because of differential diagnostic considerations.

Prader-Willi-Syndrome

Case History

A 2½-year-old girl, Katharina, is referred to the genetics clinic for assessment of developmental delay. The mother reports that Katharina was born in the 36th week of pregnancy because of a nonreassuring fetal heart rate. Reduced fetal movements had been noticed previously; amniocentesis had produced normal results. Katharina's birth weight and body length were in the low to normal range. Because of feeding problems and severe muscular hypotonia, Katharina had to be tube fed for 3 weeks. With intensive care at home and weekly visits to the pediatrician, she continually gained weight. Spoon feeding was started at around 6 months. Because of continued hypotonia and developmental delay, Katharina received physical therapy from the age of 3 months onward. She was able to sit at the age of 1 year and stand with support at 2¼ years; she still cannot walk. She babbles but has an active vocabulary of only four to six words. Katharina is a friendly, extroverted child. She had started to eat well during her second year of life, and her weight is now in the upper normal range. However, the parents did not notice an unusual desire to eat. The combination of symptoms is regarded as suggestive of Prader-Willi syndrome. The diagnosis is confirmed by methylation-dependent polymerase chain reaction (PCR) testing, which reveals the absence of the paternal allele at the SNRPN locus. Additional fluorescence in situ hybridization (FISH) tests show a deletion in the PWS critical region. In the subsequent genetic consultation, the parents are educated about the diagnosis, provided information for the PWS national support organization, and referred to a nutritionist for consultation and follow-up regarding the propensity for morbid obesity (and sequelae thereof) should her diet and activity go unchecked. Consideration for growth hormone therapy will be made, as this treatment, in combination with diet and exercise, prevents obesity in PWS.

Epidemiology

Incidence of PWS is approximately 1 in 10,000.

Clinical Features and Progression of the Disease

The clinical symptoms of PWS are age dependent and can be divided into **four developmental phases**:

- In the early months of life, severe **muscular hypotonia** is the predominant clinical feature. Reduced fetal movements may have been noticed before birth. Postnatally, hypotonia results in **severe feeding problems and failure to thrive**, typically requiring tube feeding. In contrast to later obesity, children with PWS are always underweight during their first year of life. **Genital hypoplasia** may be noted at birth, with cryptorchidism and a hypoplastic scrotum in males and hypoplastic labia in females.
- The second phase lasts from ages **1 to 4 years**. During this period, the hypotonia and poor feeding gradually improve. Affected children start to enjoy eating and begin to gain weight, often to the delight of the parents and relatives. Eventually, **hyperphagia** ensues, and without behavioral and dietary intervention children rapidly gain weight. Knowledge of the diagnosis at this stage is very important, because without rigorous restriction of food intake, which may require locking the refrigerator, pantry, and trash, the child will become obese. Affected children also display variable delay of psychomotor development. Typical, minor **facial dysmorphisms** become noticeable, such as a hypotonic facial expression with a tented upper lip, bitemporal narrowing, and almond-shaped eyes (Figs. 4.9 and 4.10). The viscosity of the child's saliva increases, which later results in a higher incidence of caries.

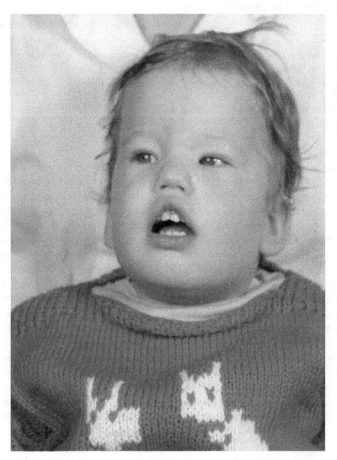

 Figure 4.9. Facial Features of a Young Male with Prader-Willi Syndrome. Note hypotonic facial expressions with a tented upper lip and almond-shaped eyes.

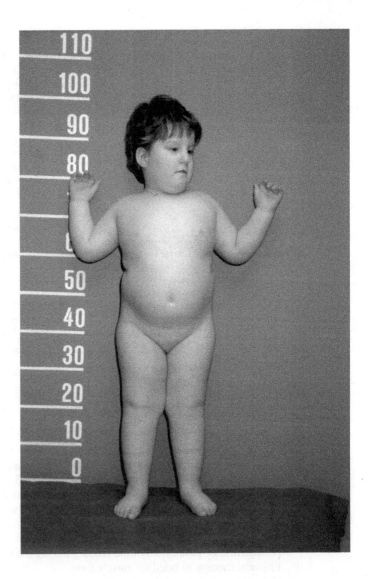

Figure 4.10. Prader-Willi Syndrome in a 3-Year-Old Male. Note truncal obesity and micropenis. The hands are relatively small (acromicria). (Courtesy of G. Tariverdian, Institute of Human Genetics, Heidelberg.)

Individuals who harbor a deletion of chromosome 15q12 often have reduced pigmentation because of haploinsufficiency of the *OCA2* gene that is also located in this region.

- In **childhood and adolescence**, unchecked hyperphagia leads to obesity with truncal distribution of fat. The children have small stature and small hands and feet. Frequently there is precocious puberty, yet **hypogonadotropic hypogonadism** remains. Typical neurobehavioral symptoms of this third phase are mood swings, obsessive scratching, skin picking, and excessive daytime sleepiness often due to nocturnal obstructive sleep apnea. Formal cognitive testing reveals mild to moderate intellectual disability in the vast majority of affected individuals.

- **Adulthood** is seen as the fourth phase. Untreated patients are morbidly obese, have small stature, and display incomplete sexual development. All of this can contribute to a loss of self-worth and increasingly prominent **psychological problems**.

Genetics and Etiology

In approximately 70% of cases, absence of the paternal copy of the *HBII-85* snoRNA gene cluster is caused by a **microdeletion** of chromosome 15q11-15q13 (Fig. 4.11). Approximately

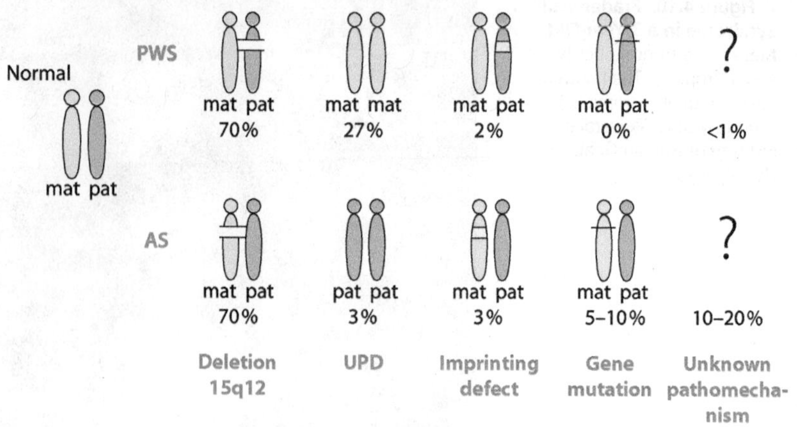

Figure 4.11. Molecular Bases for Prader-Willi Syndrome and Angelman Syndrome. UPD, uniparental disomy. (Modified from Schuffenhauer, 2001).

20% to 30% of cases are caused by UPD, in which both copies of chromosome 15 were inherited from the mother. UPD in PWS is caused by rescue of trisomy 15 that arose during oogenesis through loss of the paternal chromosome 15. In 2% to 5% of cases, PWS is caused by a primary deficiency of the imprinting center responsible for erasure and regeneration of the parental imprint.

> **Important**
>
> **Prader-Willi syndrome: P**aternal **d**eletion; paternal genetic information is missing.

Diagnosis

First-line tests for PWS traditionally assess the methylation status of the chromosomal region 15q11-13 (Fig. 4.12). Normal methylation excludes PWS. If the methylation pattern is exclusively maternal, further tests such as FISH analysis (for deletion), molecular analyses (to identify UPD), or chromosome analyses (for structural anomalies involving chromosome 15) are required.

Therapy

- Nasogastric or gastrostomy tube feeding during the neonatal period and early infancy.
- Physical therapy to build up muscle tone.
- Caloric restriction and diet control.
- Close supervision to minimize food stealing.
- Treatment with **growth hormone** results in a reduction of body fat, an increase in muscle mass, improvements in agility, an increase in mobility, and improvements in language and cognitive skills.
- Consider **testosterone supplement** therapy for PWS boys beginning at the onset of puberty. Girls should receive cycle-simulating hormonal supplement therapy; increased risk of thrombosis should be taken into consideration.

Angelman Syndrome

Case History

Hanna is diagnosed with Angelman syndrome at age 2½ years. The parents report that pregnancy was uncomplicated and delivery was in the 38th week of pregnancy. Hanna's weight and length at birth were in the low normal range. Hyperexcitability was noted at the well-child visit at 1 week of age. Hypotonia, poor weight gain, and developmental delays were noted in early infancy. Hanna did not sit independently until

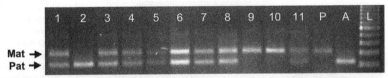

Figure 4.12. Molecular-Genetic Analysis for Prader-Willi Syndrome and Angelman Syndrome. Both disorders are recognized with the same test. An initial bisulfite treatment of the genomic DNA converts each nonmethylated cytosine (C) into uracil, which, during polymerase chain reaction (PCR) amplification, is read and amplified as thymine (T). Next, two different primer pairs are used together to generate specific PCR products for the maternal and paternal alleles. During electrophoresis the upper band corresponds to the maternal and the lower band to the paternal allele. In Prader-Willi syndrome (control P as well as patient 9 and 10), the paternal band is missing; in Angelman syndrome (control A as well as patient 2), the maternal band is missing. L indicates the molecular weight marker.

age 14 months and was not able to walk independently when she presented at age 2½ years. She had no words and could not follow simple commands. Her parents note that she communicated through facial expressions and gestures and that she always seemed happy and content. They also report that her movements are often excessive and undirected and that, at night, she "moves in her bed," but did not notice seizures or convulsion-like movements. On examination, Hanna has no strikingly dysmorphic features, but she is microcephalic and has an open-mouthed posture, laughs frequently, and is unsteady when sitting and standing.

Epidemiology

Angelman syndrome occurs less often than PWS (1:15,000); however, this incidence may be inaccurate, as it depends on the physician's ability to clinically suspect AS and confirm the diagnosis by genetic diagnosis.

Clinical Features and Progression

AS is characterized by severe intellectual disability, ataxia, epilepsy, absent speech, typical behavior (frequent inappropriate laughter), postnatal-onset microcephaly, and prognathia (large jaw) in later childhood and adulthood (Fig. 4.13).

Symptoms of AS in newborns and infants are generally nonspecific, with mild to moderate muscular hypotonia and psychomotor delay. Affected children typically begin to sit at around their first birthday and typically do not begin to walk until 4 to 5 years. The diagnosis of AS is most frequently made in the second or third year of life based on typical neurological anomalies and **absent speech**. Marked **ataxia** in combination with truncal hypotonia and hypertonia of the arms and legs causes a peculiar movement pattern, described as puppet- or robotlike. There is severe intellectual disability, with language acquisition particularly affected. Individuals with AS learn, at most, a few words during their lifetime. Demeanor is said to be "happy" based on frequent, seemingly **inappropriate laughter**.

About 80% of the patients develop overt seizures that often are difficult to control with anticonvulsants. The electroencephalogram (EEG) is almost always pathological and shows characteristic changes with large-amplitude slow waves as well as groups of accentuated frontal spikes and sharp waves. Only over time do the typical traits of the face develop, among them a prominent chin (prognathia), a relatively large mouth with widely spaced teeth, and (postnatal-onset) microcephaly. Similar to patients with PWS, AS patients with haploinsufficiency of the *OCA2* gene manifest hypopigmentation.

Genetics and Etiology

The absence of a maternally inherited normal copy of the *UBE3A* gene is caused by a **microdeletion** in the region 15q12 in approximately 70% of AS cases. About 5% to 10% of patients have a primary *UBE3A* gene mutation on the maternal allele, and 3% to 5% of cases are due to uniparental disomy (both chromosomes 15 derive from the father) or an imprinting center

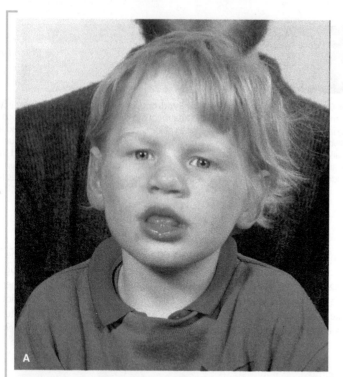

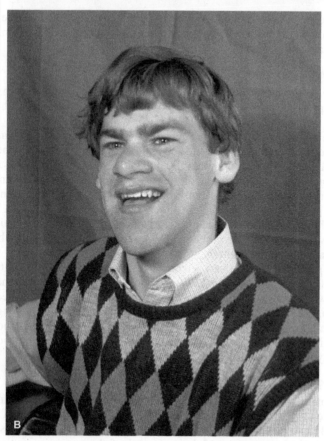

Figure 4.13. Angelman Syndrome. A. Toddlers show only discreet facial dysmorphisms, with deep-set eyes and a relatively large mouth. Many children are blond and have blue eyes, particularly when AS is caused by a large deletion. **B.** With increasing age the face enlarges, the mouth broadens, and marked prognathia becomes apparent. (Courtesy of G. Tariverdian, Institute of Human Genetics, Heidelberg.)

mutation. For 10% to 20% of patients with classic AS, the cause is unknown; it is assumed that abnormal imprinting in some of patients is due to an epigenetic error, which occurs sporadically.

> **Important**
>
> **AngelMan syndrome:** The maternal genetic information is missing.

Diagnosis

Approximately 80% of AS cases are diagnosed with the PWS/AS-specific assay demonstrating the absence of the maternally methylated band in the test described in Figure 4.12. The exact aberration can be determined with a FISH test or UPD analysis. If the methylation pattern is normal but a strong suspicion of AS remains, sequence analysis of the *UBE3A* gene may confirm the diagnosis.

Therapy

— Anticonvulsive treatment
— Physical therapy to strengthen balance and improve gait
— Early training in nonverbal communication (e.g., sign language and nonverbal communication devices)

4.4 Mosaicism

> **Mosaic:** The occurrence of two or more genetically different cell lines within a tissue or within an organism.

It would be a gross simplification to imagine that all 10^{14} cells of the human body carry the same genetic information. In the course of a lifetime (prenatally and postnatally), individual cells of our organism experience countless numbers of smaller or larger mutations (gene mutations as well as chromosomal alterations) that change its genetic constitution. If these mutations are not eliminated by repair mechanisms or cell death, they will be transmitted over many mitotic divisions to all daughter cells and, thereby, form new cell clones with slightly varying genetic information within our organism. Depending on when a mutation arises, mosaicism may be found in the whole body or may be confined to a certain cell type or body segment. A special constellation is present with mosaicism confined to the germ line that has no particular relevance for the person's health but is important with regard to disease risk in the offspring.

Somatic Mosaicism. Most somatic mutations never become clinically relevant, although some may be recognized by harmless phenotypic changes, such as variation in skin pigmentation occurring in a segmental or patterned distribution. Other mutations have important physiological or pathogenic effects. For example, the ability of the body to produce a large number of specialized cells that recognize specific antigens would not be possible without somatic mutation and recombination events. On the other hand, all tumors in the body represent mosaicisms since their abnormal growth is due to altered genetic information (see Chapter 7).

Somatic mosaicism is also found in many disorders that are inherited as autosomal dominant traits. If a disease-causing mutation is inherited from one of the parents or arises in the germ line of one of the parents, all cells of the body will contain the mutation, and the person will have the usual form of the disorder. Sometimes, however, mutations arise from a postzygotic event during (early) embryonic development and are found only in a proportion of the body's cells. From the size and distribution of these abnormalities, one can determine when and where during embryonic development the mutation occurred.

Mosaicism should also always be considered when the skin shows unusual pigmentation abnormalities such as stripes of hyper- or hypopigmentation in the lines of Blaschko or when disease pictures are milder than expected. This is also true for chromosomal mosaicism. For example, some patients with physical features of Down syndrome but only mild intellectual disability have mosaic trisomy 21 with trisomic and normal (disomic) cell lines for chromosome 21. Numerical autosomal abnormalities that are not usually compatible with life may be found in mosaic form in children with a "chromosomal" type of disease. It is important to note that chromosomal mosaicism may not necessarily be visible in standard chromosome analysis from lymphocytes, and skin biopsy or FISH analysis of buccal mucosa cells may be required for diagnosis. Also, a low level of mosaicism may not be detected by DNA array analysis.

The identification of somatic mosaicism is important for genetic counseling. For example, neurofibromatosis type 1 (NF1; Section 32.6) sometimes occurs segmentally, only affecting one specific body part. The diagnosis can be difficult to prove, since the mutation may not be present in the DNA extracted from blood. Parents of a patient with segmental NF1 are always asymptomatic, as the disease has arisen de novo as a somatic mutation, and there is only the minute population-based risk for recurrence of the disease in future children. The recurrence risk for children of the affected individual is lower than the usual 50% but may still be relevant if the mutation occurred early during embryonic development, before the separation of the germ cells. Affected children would have the full clinical picture of neurofibromatosis.

■■■ Pallister-Killian Syndrome

Pallister-Killian syndrome is a good example of a complex chromosome aberration found only in some of the body cells. It is caused by an isochromosome 12p in addition to the normal chromosome complement, leading to tetrasomy of the short arm of chromosome 12. In most cases, the isochromosome was generated during maternal meiosis and thus present in the zygote but subsequently eliminated in many cells during embryonic development, resulting in mosaicism. In older children with Pallister-Killian syndrome, the isochromosome 12p is not found anymore in lymphocytes, and the confirmation of the diagnosis requires chromosome analysis in cultured skin fibroblasts. Clinically, the children have intellectual disability, typical facial features with a high forehead, reduced bitemporal hair growth, and pigmentation anomalies of the skin.

Germline Mosaicism. Sometimes parents have several children with the same, dominant monogenic disorder, even though neither of the parents is clinically affected (taking into account the possibility of reduced penetrance or variable expressivity). Could this be attributed to two independent de novo mutations? This is unlikely, considering that the spontaneous mutation rate usually ranges from 1 in 10^5 to 1 in 10^6. Molecular analyses in such families usually show that both affected siblings carry the same mutation, but DNA analyses in the parents' peripheral blood produce normal results without any trace of the familial mutation. The simple, but clinically important, explanation is germline mosaicism. Mutations that occur de novo in a family may have arisen relatively early in germ cell development, resulting in a significant number of gametes that carry the mutation. Since, in the female germ line, approximately 30 mitotic cell divisions precede the actual meiosis and, in the male germ line, sometimes several hundred, there are plenty of opportunities for mutations to arise and cause germline mosaicism. Indeed, disease-causing gene mutations initially appear as a mosaic, either as somatic ($\pm$ germ cell) mosaicism with variable clinical features or as pure germ cell mosaicism with a risk for the disease in offspring.

These considerations are important when parents of a child with a de novo dominant disorder inquire about the recurrence risk in future children. An estimated 5% of subsequent siblings of children with de novo osteogenesis imperfecta (see Section 4.2) will also be affected. In isolated cases of Duchenne muscular dystrophy, the recurrence risk for noncarrier females due to germline mosaicism is 8% to 9%. The recurrence risk partly depends on the type of mutation and is obviously higher when several affected children have already been born in the family. If no statistical data are available for a dominant disorder, it is reasonable to estimate the recurrence risk to be 2% to 5%. Prenatal diagnosis may be offered, if appropriate, when the familial mutation is known.

X-Chromosomal Mosaicism. Each female with karyotype 46,XX is a mosaic of two functionally different cell lines. The basis for this mosaic is the phenomenon of X inactivation. As described in detail in Section 2.8, some cells use the paternal X chromosome, and others use the maternal X chromosome, while the respective other X chromosome is inactive. If there is a disease-causing mutation in an X-chromosomal gene (outside the pseudoautosomal region), it will have a functional effect only in some of the cells, while the others will be normal. X-chromosomal heterozygosity, therefore, functionally corresponds to somatic mosaicism of a dominant mutation and not to autosomal heterozygosity for a (dominant or recessive) mutation. As for autosomes, X chromosomes can undergo de novo somatic mutations, which can lead to a true X chromosomal somatic mosaicism in males or females. This often leads to milder manifestations of an X-linked disorder in males and has been observed in many X-linked conditions.

■■■ Incontinentia Pigmenti (Bloch-Sulzberger Syndrome)

Incontinentia pigmenti (IP) illustrates that every woman with a normal female chromosomal complement is a mosaic of two functionally different cell lines. IP is X-linked and is caused by mutations in the *IKBKG* (NEMO) gene. The gene product, *NF-κB essential modulator*, has an important role in the NF-κB pathway, which not only is involved in the production of chemokines and cytokines but also protects the cell from apoptosis. At

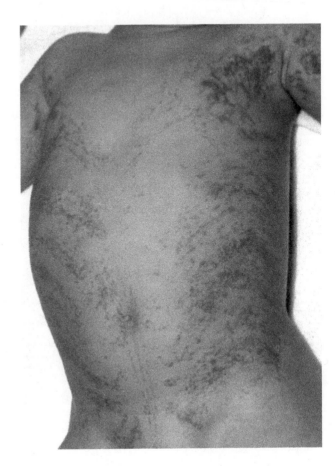

Figure 4.14. Incontinentia Pigmenti. Note the brown-striped hyperpigmentations.

birth, females with incontinentia pigmenti show **striped and meander-shaped skin erosions** and ulcers, representing areas that have been populated by cells that express the mutant copy of the *IKBKG* gene. The erosions normally heal well and evolve to patches of pigmented hyperkeratosis, hyperpigmentation (◻ Fig. 4.14), and finally hypopigmentation, before typically resolving by midadulthood. Since cells that express the mutant copy of the *IKBKG* gene undergo premature apoptosis via the NF-κB pathway, they gradually disappear. Eventually, the body almost exclusively uses cells that express the normal copy of the *IKBKG* gene, a phenomenon described as skewed X inactivation. Most *IKBKG* mutations are **intrauterine lethal in hemizygous males**; exceptions are males with hypomorphic mutations, males with karyotype 47,XXY, or those whose incontinentia pigmenti that originates from a somatic mutation.

5 Modes of Inheritance

LEARNING OBJECTIVES

1 Name the characteristic features of autosomal dominant inheritance, and give five common conditions as an example.

2 Explain the terms *penetrance* and *expressivity* using *BRCA1* hereditary breast and ovarian cancer as a clinical example.

3 Discuss the characteristic features of mitochondrial inheritance, and explain why most mitochondrial disorders do not follow this mode of inheritance.

4 Compose a genetic counseling letter for a family whose first child (female) is affected with pyloric stenosis, integrating your knowledge about gender-dependent threshold effects.

Mendelian Laws of Inheritance

Gregor Mendel described the basic tenets of inheritance through his studies of peas in the 19th century. Although chromosomes and genes were yet to be discovered, Mendel's Laws of Heredity are now applied to human traits and disease, many of which follow **mendelian inheritance**.

The Law of Segregation: The two copies of an individual's genes (the two homologous chromosomes) separate during meiosis such that each gamete has only one copy of each chromosome and one copy of each gene.

The Law of Independent Assortment: Genes that are not linked (i.e., not too close together on the chromosome) are inherited independently of each other, because the maternal and paternal chromosomes exchange genetic material (homologous recombination) during meiosis I. This process ensures genetic diversity in each subsequent generation.

5.1 Autosomal Dominant Inheritance

> **Important**
>
> **Typical Characteristics of Autosomal Dominant Inheritance**
> - Successive generations are affected (vertical transmission).
> - Males and females are affected with equal frequency and severity.
> - The disease is transmitted to subsequent generations by females as well as males (Figs. 5.1 and 5.2).
> - Male-to-male transmission of trait occurs.

Recurrence Risk. As discussed in detail in Section 4.2, a disorder/mutation is called dominant if heterozygosity for a genetic variant causes a clear pathological phenotype. The normal (wild-type) allele, on its own, is not sufficient to secure normal function. Half of the germ cells generated by an individual who is heterozygous for a disease-causing mutation will harbor this mutation, while the other 50% of germ cells will harbor the normal wild-type allele. Statistically, half of the offspring receive the mutated allele and will also be affected by the disorder. If the partner of the affected person happens to have the same disorder (which is generally unlikely, yet is seen frequently in some disorders such as achondroplasia, Section 26.2), 25% of the offspring will be homozygous (or compound heterozygous) mutation carriers. The clinical consequences depend on the disorder and are, in most cases, considerably more severe than with heterozygous affected individuals (Section 4.2).

Penetrance and Expressivity. As already mentioned in Chapter 4, there is not always a direct connection between the genotype and the manifest phenotype. The term **penetrance** is used to describe the probability with which a carrier of a "dominant mutation" will actually show signs of the disorder. For example, not all women who carry a *BRCA1* gene mutation will develop

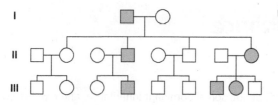

Figure 5.1. Typical Pedigree of an Autosomal Dominant Disorder.

■ ● = Affected

breast or ovarian cancer, and therefore the penetrance is said to be **incomplete**. Incomplete penetrance may explain the occurrence of a dominant disorder in a grandparent and a grand-child, with apparent skipping of one generation. It should be noted that penetrance of some disorders is closely linked to age. An example is Huntington disease (Section 31.1.1), where mutation carriers are normally free of symptoms at a young age but will, with certainty, become symptomatic before they reach old age (complete yet age-dependent penetrance).

The term **expressivity** refers to the variability of a genetic disorder leading to the spectrum of symptoms in a particular patient. Most dominant disorders show variable expressivity, meaning that the clinical presentation varies between different mutation carriers even within the same family. The clinical picture may be influenced by other (usually unknown) genetic factors (a phenomenon called *epistasis*), by gene–environment interactions, or by chance events. For example, whether a *BRCA1* gene mutation carrier will develop breast or ovarian cancer may be, to a large degree, due to chance additional mutation events. In most dominant disorders, it is not possible to predict the exact clinical presentation in an affected child.

De novo Mutations. Many autosomal dominant disorders occur sporadically, which means that healthy parents have an affected child. This occurs when the mutation is de novo (new) in the affected child. In some conditions, all affected individuals have de novo mutations, because the disorder is incompatible with life and there are no affected persons who could have an affected child; one example is osteogenesis imperfecta type II (caused by mutations in the gene encoding type I collagen), which is lethal perinatally. Other conditions do not interfere with reproductive fitness and are frequently inherited from a parent; an example is osteogenesis imperfecta type I, the "mild" form of collagen I deficiency (Section 4.2). It is important to keep in mind that de novo mutations may arise at any stage during germ cell development (more frequently in the male than in the female germ line) and that, because of germline mosaicism (Section 4.4), later siblings of an affected child with a de novo mutation may inherit the same mutation even though it is not found in the blood of either parent. De novo mutations are not observed in trinucleotide repeat disorders (such as fragile X syndrome); nonaffected ancestors may, however, harbor an unstable repeat and, while not clinically affected, are predisposed to transmit an expanded allele. These individuals are known as **premutation carriers**.

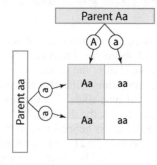

Figure 5.2. Inheritance Pattern of an Autosomal Dominant Disorder.

□ = Affected

A = Dominant allele
a = Recessive allele

○ = Germ cells

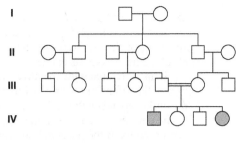

Figure 5.3. Typical Pedigree of an Autosomal Recessive Disorder.

■ ⬤ = Affected

□━◯ = Consanguinity

■■■ **Examples of Disorders with Autosomal Dominant Inheritance**
━ most familial cancer predisposition syndromes (e.g., familial breast and colon cancer, retinoblastoma)
━ most trinucleotide repeat disorders (e.g., Huntington disease, myotonic dystrophy)
━ familial hypercholesterolemia
━ achondroplasia
━ most forms of osteogenesis imperfecta
━ neurofibromatosis type 1 and type 2
━ Marfan syndrome.

5.2 Autosomal Recessive Inheritance

Important

Typical Characteristics of Autosomal Recessive Inheritance
━ Horizontal pattern in a pedigree; the disorder occurs only in one generation, not in successive generations. Several children of one couple are affected.
━ The disorder affects males and females with equal frequency and severity.
━ The disorder is transmitted by phenotypically healthy parents to affected offspring. The parents are heterozygous (carriers) for a disease-causing mutation.
━ The disorder occurs in higher frequency in the offspring of consanguineous couples (e.g., first-cousin marriage) (☐ Figs. 5.3 and 5.4).

Recurrence Risk. A heterozygous carrier for a recessive mutation has a 50% probability of transmitting this mutation to a child. If both partners are heterozygous carriers for the same autosomal recessive disease, the risk for transmission to offspring is as follows: 25% of the offspring of the couple will be homozygous (or compound heterozygous) for the disease-causing

Figure 5.4. Inheritance Pattern of an Autosomal Recessive Disorder.

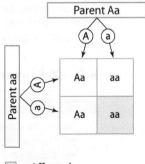

☐ = Affected

A = Dominant allele
a = Recessive allele

◯ = Germ cells

allele and thus be affected by the disorder, 50% of the offspring will be healthy heterozygous carriers just as their parents, and 25% will be homozygous for the wild-type allele. When speaking of the children of carrier parents, two-thirds of the healthy siblings of an affected child are heterozygous carriers.

If an individual with an autosomal recessive disorder has children, a disease-causing mutation will be transmitted to all of them (either of the two mutant alleles). The consequences for the child depend on this individual's partner. If the partner is homozygous for the normal allele of the respective gene (as in the majority of cases), all offspring will be nonaffected heterozygous carriers. If the partner, however, is a carrier (the likelihood is approximately 0.5% to 1% for the more frequent recessive disorders), statistically, half of the offspring will be affected (homozygous or compound heterozygous), and the other half will be carriers. If both partners should have the same recessive disorder (caused by mutations in the same gene), all offspring will be homozygous/compound heterozygous and affected.

Allelic heterogeneity: The phenomenon that different mutations in the same gene (allelic mutations) may cause the same disorder.

Locus heterogeneity: The phenomenon that some clinically defined disorders may be caused by a deficiency of different genes (loci), meaning the absence of different proteins causes the same phenotype.

Genetic Heterogeneity. The possibility of locus heterogeneity is an important phenomenon that needs to be taken into consideration when two persons with the "same" autosomal recessive condition are planning to have children. If the disease in the partners is caused by (homozygous) mutations in different genes, the child will be heterozygous for mutations at both loci but him- or herself will not be affected. This is a common observation in some conditions, such as autosomal recessive deafness.

In rare cases one of the parents of a child with a recessive disorder is not a carrier for the mutation(s) found in the offspring. This can have several causes, including (1) **nonpaternity**, meaning the assumed father is not the biological father; (2) a de novo occurrence of a deletion, which encompasses the gene of interest; (3) uniparental disomy of a chromosome that contains a recessive mutation; and (4) rarely, a de novo mutation of the gene of interest. The most frequent of these is nonpaternity.

■■■ Examples of Disorders with Autosomal Recessive Inheritance
▬ most inborn errors of metabolism (e.g., phenylketonuria, galactosemia, hemochromatosis, Gaucher disease, Tay-Sachs disease
▬ Smith-Lemli-Opitz syndrome)
▬ 21-hydroxylase deficiency (i.e., congenital adrenal hyperplasia)
▬ cystic fibrosis, spinal muscular atrophy
▬ sickle cell disease, β-thalassemia
▬ ataxia telangiectasia.

5.3   X-Chromosomal Inheritance

Important	

Typical Characteristics of X-Chromosomal Inheritance
▬ Males are severely affected; sometimes the disorder in males is incompatible with life.
▬ Clinical symptoms in females are variable depending on the disease mechanism and the individual X-inactivation pattern; females may be asymptomatic carriers.
▬ A heterozygous (carrier) female transmits the disease-causing mutation to 50% of her sons and 50% of her daughters.
▬ A hemizygous (affected) male transmits the disease-causing mutation to all of his daughters and none of his sons (■ Figs. 5.5 and 5.6).

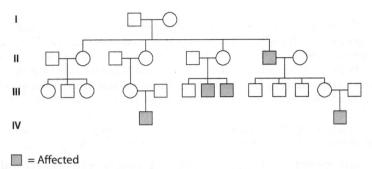

☐ = Affected

☐ **Figure 5.5. Typical Pedigree of an X-Chromosomal Disorder with Asymptomatic Carrier Females.**

As discussed in Section 2.8, males have only one X chromosome and are therefore hemizygous for all X-chromosomal variants outside the pseudoautosomal region. A mutation in a typical X-linked gene is, thus, expressed in all cells of the body. In contrast, females have two X chromosomes and are, thus, either heterozygous or homozygous for X-chromosomal variants. Because of X inactivation in females, only one X chromosome is active in each cell, and a typical X-linked heterozygous mutation is expressed only in a proportion of cells (on average 50%). Thus, the female is a **functional mosaic** for X-chromosomal traits.

The clinical picture of an X-chromosomal disorder depends on the pathogenic mechanism and, in females, is influenced by the variability or compensatory mechanism of X inactivation. A mutation that causes **cell death** will be lethal for male embryos in an early stage of postzygotic development. In females, such a mutation typically causes the loss of all cells that express the mutant copy of the gene, while the other cells may develop normally. A female may show signs of X-chromosomal mosaicism, as in incontinentia pigmenti (Section 4.4), or may be clinically normal with completely skewed X inactivation (Section 2.8). If (as in fragile X syndrome, Section 31.2.2) the mutation **disturbs cellular function** but does not cause cell death, hemizygous males are severely affected while females show variable symptoms, ranging from asymptomatic to severe, depending on the individual X-inactivation pattern. Mothers of boys frequently show skewed X inactivation (favoring the wild-type allele), sometimes explained by ascertainment bias, as females with an unfavorable X-inactivation pattern may be less likely to have children. Different consequences, again, may be expected if a deficiency of an X-chromosomal gene in a cell may be **compensated for by neighboring cells**, as is the case for secreted proteins or some metabolic functions. Hemizygous males will show the typical disease picture (which, in the individual case, may be variable depending on the specific mutation), while heterozygous

☐ **Figure 5.6. Inheritance Pattern of an X-Chromosomal Disorder.**

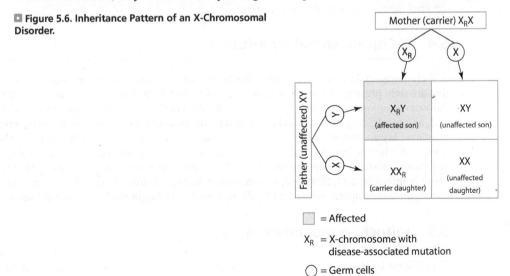

☐ = Affected

X_R = X-chromosome with disease-associated mutation

◯ = Germ cells

females are usually asymptomatic or may show minor disease manifestation due to unfavorable X inactivation. Notable examples are the hemophilias (Section 21.6) and ornithine transcarbamylase deficiency, the most common urea cycle disorder (Section 24.1.3).

Because of the variable clinical presentation in heterozygous females, the terms *recessive* or *dominant* should not be used in relation to X-chromosomal disorders. We would also argue, as Mendel did, that these terms refer to the functional relationship of two different alleles in the heterozygous individual and, thus, cannot apply to X-chromosomal genes of a cell, as only one X chromosome is functionally active in males and females alike. The term *X linked* is sufficient to explain both the peculiarities of disease expression in females and the inheritance patterns within families.

Recurrence Risk. A male patient with an X-chromosomal disorder will transmit his only X chromosome, which contains the mutation, to all of his daughters. All daughters are **obligate heterozygotes** and may be either asymptomatic carriers or have variable (less severe) symptoms of the disorder. On average, 25% of the daughters' children (50% of her sons) will be affected with the disorder of their grandfather, 25% of children (50% of her daughters) will be heterozygous females, while 50% of the children will inherit the normal allele from their mother. All sons of an affected male will have inherited the Y chromosome of their father and, therefore, will not be affected and will not transmit the disorder to their children.

As for many conditions, when evaluating an individual with an X-linked disorder, the family's medical and developmental history may be inconclusive or completely negative for additional persons affected with the disorder. In this instance, the occurrence of a **de novo mutation** must be taken into consideration. Due to the pathophysiology of spermatogenesis, a new mutation is more likely to occur in the male germ line rather than in the female germ line. This implies that the mother of an affected boy can be a carrier for the disease. As for any condition, the individual affected with the condition should be tested first. If a mutation is identified in a male affected with an X-linked disorder, his mother should be tested, even in the absence of signs, symptoms, or positive family history. As **germline mosaicism** can also occur in X-linked disorders, there is a small (~6%) risk of recurrence, even if the mother has a negative DNA analysis; thus, prenatal mutation analysis should be considered.

■■■ Examples of Disorders with X-Chromosomal Inheritance
▬ muscular dystrophy types Duchenne and Becker
▬ hemophilias A and B
▬ Lesch-Nyhan syndrome
▬ ornithine transcarbamylase deficiency
▬ fragile X syndrome
▬ color blindness, and incontinentia pigmenti.

5.4   Y-Chromosomal Inheritance

A Y-chromosomal inheritance pattern (**holandric inheritance**) should be assumed for all genes that are only present on the Y chromosome or for dominant mutations in genes of the pseudoautosomal region of the Y chromosome. An affected father transmits the disorder to all his sons and, as a result, only men would be affected by the disorder. In reality, this mode of inheritance does not play an important role. Most of the unique Y-chromosomal genes that are not homologous to X-chromosomal genes play a role in male sexual differentiation, the development of sex characteristics, and spermatogenesis. This means that mutations in these genes typically result in infertility and, therefore, are not transmitted to children. Artificial insemination through intracytoplasmic sperm injection (ICSI), however, may begin to change this scenario.

5.5   Mitochondrial Inheritance

In addition to the nuclear genome, eukaryotic cells contain a separate **mitochondrial genome** within the mitochondria, which encodes 13 of the 87 proteins of the mitochondrial

Table 5.1. Differences between the Nuclear and the Mitochondrial Genome

	Nuclear Genome	Mitochondrial Genome
Size	Approximately 3,300,000,000 bp (haploid chromosome complement)	16,569 bp
Structure	46 double strands with two ends (telomeres)	Ring-shaped double strand
Number of genes	Current estimate: 22,300 protein-coding genes; 10,000 RNA genes	37
Gene density	Approximately 1/132,000 bp	1/450 bp
DNA-repair mechanisms	Yes	No
Portion coding DNA	Approximately 3%	Approximately 93%
Transcription	Mostly individual for each gene	Mainly continuous
Introns	In almost all genes	Absent
Recombination	Yes	No
Inheritance	Follows mendelian laws	Exclusively maternal

respiratory chain. Mitochondrial DNA (mtDNA) is a 16,569-bp ring-shaped double strand that resembles bacterial genomes. Indeed, it is hypothesized that mitochondria originated as separate Proteobacteria, which were internalized by the cell as endosymbionts. Replication of the mitochondrial genome is independent of the cell cycle. Most eukaryotic cells contain more than 1,000 mtDNA molecules spread out over hundreds of mitochondria, or rather, the extensive mitochondrial network. A particularly high number of mtDNA copies is found in the mature egg cell that often contains more than 100,000 copies. This means that mtDNA represents up to one-third of the total DNA content of mature egg cells. In contrast—as the sperm are built for speed—the mature sperm cell only has mitochondria to propel it forward and rarely, if ever, do those mitochondria contribute to the mitochondrial genomic complement of the conceptus.

mtDNA contains a total of 37 genes. Of these, 13 code for proteins of the oxidative phosphorylation complex. The remaining 24 genes are transcribed into 22 transfer RNA (tRNA) and 2 ribosomal RNA (rRNA) molecules that are required for protein synthesis within the mitochondria (▢ Table 5.1).

Important

Seventy-seven of the 90 mitochondrial respiratory chain proteins, and all other mitochondrial proteins, are encoded by the nuclear genome. After cytosolic synthesis, these proteins are transported into the mitochondria; they have specific import sequences for this purpose. Most mitochondrial disorders, therefore, are caused by mutations of the nuclear genome and are inherited according to the classic mendelian rules of inheritance.

Characteristics of Mitochondrial Inheritance. The human zygote receives almost all of its mitochondria from the oocyte, because during fertilization only the head of the sperm, without mitochondria, penetrates the egg. The result is that a mother with mutations in mtDNA will transmit this mutation to all of her offspring, while the father with the same mutation in the mitochondrial genome will not transmit this mutation to any of his offspring. Mitochondrial inheritance is, thus, purely **maternal** (▢ Fig. 5.7). Another characteristic of mitochondrial inheritance reflects the fact that the mitochondrial genome, unlike the nuclear genome, does not have a controlled segregation mechanism. mtDNA is replicated independently of the cell cycle, and the individual copies are randomly distributed to the daughter cells during mitosis.

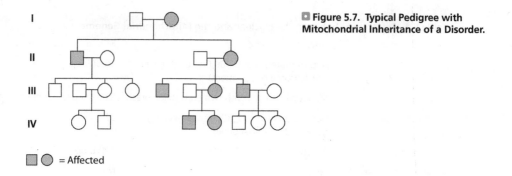

Figure 5.7. Typical Pedigree with Mitochondrial Inheritance of a Disorder.

■● = Affected

> **Heteroplasmy:** An mtDNA variant is found only in a portion of the cell's mitochondria.
>
> **Homoplasmy:** All mtDNA copies have the same sequence (e.g., all mtDNA copies contain a particular mutation).

Frequently, both wild-type and mutant mtDNA sequences at the same locus are found when mitochondrial DNA is studied in a patient, a phenomenon called heteroplasmy (■ Fig. 5.8). Whether a heteroplasmic mitochondrial mutation is actually expressed phenotypically depends on the proportion of the cells' normal mtDNA to mutated mtDNA (**threshold effect**). Reduced penetrance, variable expressivity, and pleiotropy are, therefore, typical features of mitochondrial inheritance. The proportion of normal and mutated mtDNA copies may vary considerably in different organs or in the course of successive cell divisions. Patients with mitochondrially inherited disorders often report that individual symptoms change over time (e.g., cardiac arrhythmias have phases of different severity).

Mitochondrial mutations affect either subunits of the oxidative phosphorylation complex or (in the case of tRNA or rRNA genes) the efficiency of mitochondrial translation and, thus, also the function of the oxidative phosphorylation complex. Mitochondrial mutations always affect the cell's energy metabolism and are especially relevant for tissues that require significant energy, such as the central and peripheral nervous system (including the retina), skeletal muscle, heart muscle, the liver, and kidneys. Typical symptoms of mitochondrial mutations are encephalopathy, ataxia, myopathy, cardiomyopathy, external ophthalmoplegia, retinal degeneration, or renal tubular dysfunction. Even with light physical exercise, affected individuals

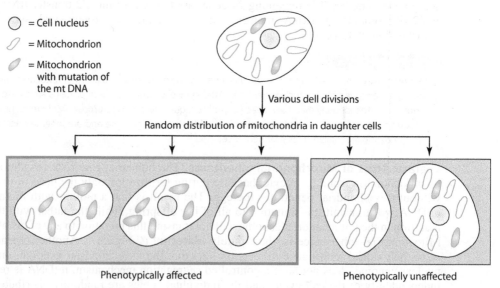

○ = Cell nucleus

⟋ = Mitochondrion

⟋ = Mitochondrion with mutation of the mt DNA

Various dell divisions

Random distribution of mitochondria in daughter cells

Phenotypically affected   Phenotypically unaffected

Figure 5.8. Heteroplasmy.

may have an insufficient oxidative phosphorylation capacity and suffer lactic acidosis. Skeletal muscle histology often shows *ragged red fibers* representing subsarcolemmal accumulation of mitochondria.

Examples of Mitochondrially Inherited Disorders

MELAS Syndrome. The acronym for MELAS syndrome signifies **M**itochondrial **E**ncephal-opathy, **L**actic **A**cidosis, and **S**trokelike episodes. Affected patients initially develop normally yet, over time, experience increasing physical limitations because of progressive myopathy. Typical strokelike episodes (with hemiparesis and hemianopsia) usually start to occur between the ages of 4 and 15 years. Additional symptoms include small stature, migraine, learning difficulties, deafness, and diabetes mellitus. The clinical symptoms vary in affected family members, depending on the degree of heteroplasmy in various tissues. MELAS syndrome is typically caused by m.3243A>G in the mitochondrial *tRNA^{Leu}* gene.

MERRF Syndrome. The acronym for MERRF syndrome signifies **M**yoclonic **E**pilepsy with **R**agged **R**ed **F**ibers. After normal early development, the disorder typically presents symptoms in childhood, with myoclonus progressing into generalized epilepsy, ataxia, weakness, and finally dementia. Additional symptoms include short stature, hearing loss, optic atrophy, and cardiomyopathy. MERRF syndrome is typically caused by the m.8344G>A in the mitochondrial *tRNA^{Lys}* gene.

Another mtDNA disease is **NARP syndrome** (**N**europathy, **A**taxia, and **R**etinitis **P**ig-mentosa), mostly caused by m.8993T>G or T>C in the *ATPase* gene. **Chronic progressive external ophthalmoplegia** (CPEO), **Kearns-Sayre syndrome** (CPEO, retinopathy, ptosis, deafness, cardiac arrhythmias, ataxia), and **Pearson syndrome** (anemia, pancytopenia, exocrine pancreatic function disorder, hepatopathy, failure to thrive, often a precursor of Kearns-Sayre syndrome) are typically caused by large deletions of mtDNA. This list shows that the spectrum of symptoms caused by mtDNA mutations may be overlapping. A mitochondrial disorder should be considered if several members of a family have an unspecific, multisystem disorder with involvement particularly of the nervous system and the skeletal muscles. Even migraine can be a minimal symptom of such a disorder.

Leber Hereditary Optic Neuropathy. An exception among the mtDNA disorders is Leber hereditary optic neuropathy (LHON). It is not a multisystem disorder but only affects the optic nerve. Typical presentation is acute, painless loss of vision, striking "out of the blue." Initially, this is monocular; however, within weeks to months, it also affects the second eye. There may be partial recovery, but the disorder usually progresses to severe optic atrophy. For unknown reasons, males are more frequently affected; the age of onset is early adulthood but may range from 8 to 60 years. LHON is caused by mutations in mtDNA genes coding proteins of complex I of the respiratory chain; common mutations are m.11778G>A, m.3460G>A, and m.14484T>C (90% of cases). Penetrance is low: two-thirds to three-fourths of male and 90% of female mutation carriers remain asymptomatic throughout life.

5.6   Multifactorial Inheritance

In the final analysis, all disorders are caused by the interplay between genetic and nongenetic factors. This means that the classic separation into purely genetic, purely exogenous, and so-called multifactorial disorders is entirely not valid. Even the clinical phenotype of many "monogenic" disorders may be influenced decisively by exogenous factors—otherwise, treatment would not work. As discussed in Section 24.1.3, this can be readily demonstrated in the case of phenylketo-nuria (PKU), a monogenic disorder in which the clinical phenotype is fundamentally influenced by an exogenous factor (i.e., reduced intake of phenylalanine). While untreated individuals with classic PKU develop a severe intellectual disability, a person with PKU who has been treated with an optimal diet is, clinically, not different from a "healthy" person. Some patients with PKU, therefore, say that they are not sick but that they need to adhere to a special diet in order not to get sick. In this way PKU is similar to a risk factor for a disorder; however, in the absence of treatment the risk of disease is far larger than with classic multifactorial disorders.

▪▪▪ What Is a Genetic Disorder?

The term *disorder* refers to the clinical symptoms of a person, not to his or her genome! A carrier for myotonic dystrophy falls ill when the first symptoms occur; before that he or she is an asymptomatic mutation carrier. Some carriers of dominant disease-causing mutations never fall ill (reduced penetrance). While consulting with patients, one should clarify that detection of a mutation, especially during predictive testing, may only imply an increased risk or probability for the disorder that should be critically evaluated in its overall context. This is another reason why genetic analyses should only be done with care, and the findings should be discussed in a formal genetic consultation.

Multifactorial. Multifactorial are those disorders that do not follow a clear inheritance pattern and whose clinical symptoms are suspected to have been caused by the interplay between several genes (polygenic) and exogenous (environmental) factors. Therefore, one also calls these **complex disorders**.

To explain the emergence of some multifactorial disorders (as, for example, congenital malformations), one refers to the concept of **threshold effect**. According to this concept, a certain trait becomes phenotypically evident only once the threshold of genetic predisposition is exceeded; when this happens, the effect is complete (i.e., the all-or-nothing principle). In the case of some conditions, the threshold of genetic predisposition seems to differ between males and females (i.e., is **gender dependent**).

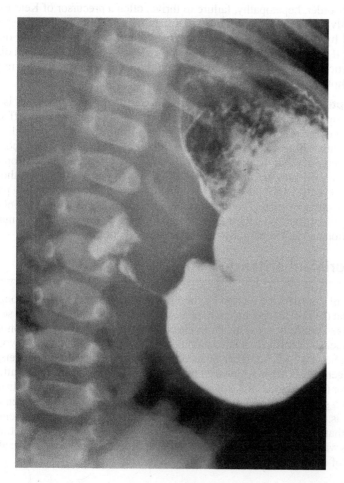

Figure 5.9. Hypertrophic Pyloric Stenosis. A contrast image shows the pylorus as a thin line. (Courtesy of Hj Müller, Department of Medical Genetics, University Children's Hospital Basel, Switzerland.)

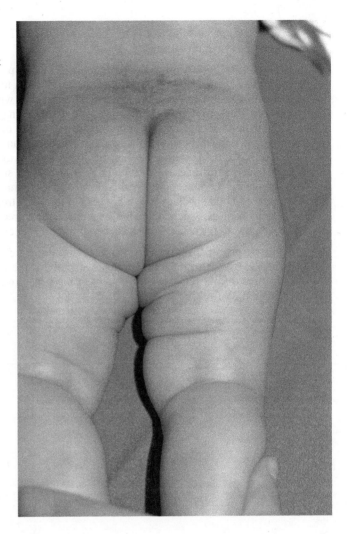

Figure 5.10. Hip Dysplasia in a 6-Month-Old Infant. Note the asymmetrical skin folds in the legs. (Courtesy of Universitäts-Kinderklinik Heidelberg.)

Important

Carter Effect: Multifactorial diseases with a gender-dependent threshold effect have a higher recurrence risk if the index patient is of the less commonly affected sex. This phenomenon was proven by Cedric Carter in his studies on hypertrophic pyloric stenosis, a disease that is more common in males than in females. He showed that its incidence is highest in sons of affected women and lowest in daughters of affected men.

Examples of Multifactorial Disorders with Gender-Dependent Threshold Effects

Hypertrophic Pyloric Stenosis. The disorder **hypertrophic pyloric stenosis** is a postnatal hypertrophy of the circular muscle of the pylorus that results in functional obstruction of the pylorus, projectile vomiting, and failure to thrive (Fig. 5.9). The cumulative frequency of this disease is 1 in 1,000; boys are affected five times more frequently than girls. In most cases, the disorder is diagnosed in infants between 3 and 12 weeks of life. Sometimes the pylorus can be felt as a cylindrical tumor in the upper right quadrant of the abdomen. Water and salt deficiency can result in a hypochloremic alkalosis. The treatment of choice is pyloromyotomy (i.e., Ramstedt procedure).

Congenital Hip Dysplasia. The term **congenital hip dysplasia** includes a range of diagnostic findings, from a slight deformity of the acetabulum to a vertically positioned femur with subluxation to a manifest luxation of the femoral head with hypoplasia of the acetabulum (◻ Fig. 5.10). The early forms are 12 times more frequent in girls than in boys. For manifest luxation, the male-to-female ratio is approximately 1:8. The multifactorial genesis consists of genetic, mechanical, and hormonal causes. The hormonal causes typically manifest as extremely loose connective tissue within the first few days after birth (resulting from the continued presence of maternal estrogen). Of crucial importance for a successful therapy is the earliest possible diagnosis. In some countries, therefore, a sonographic hip screening was introduced as part of the well-child checkup at 4 to 5 weeks of age. The treatment of choice is a soft brace called a Pavlik harness, which maintains the joints in the correct position by keeping the knees apart and bent toward the chest. This is successful in 90% of cases if started in the first months of life.

Hirschsprung Disease. Hirschsprung disease is a deficiency of mobility of the distal colon caused by congenital aganglionosis, usually of the rectum and often sigmoid. The disorder is three to four times more frequent in boys than in girls. A detailed description is found in Section 23.1.

6 Twin Pregnancies

LEARNING OBJECTIVES

1 Give the frequency of different types of twins and discuss predisposing factors.

2 Examination of the placenta and fetal membranes may give clues on whether a twin pregnancy is monozygotic or dizygotic. Discuss the principles and limitations.

3 Discuss twin–twin transfusion syndrome with regard to the type of twinning and clinical presentation.

Multiple gestations are rare but now occur at a greater frequency than in the past due to the effects of infertility treatment. While previously a frequency of 1 out of 85 was observed, today 1 in 40 births worldwide involves twins. Twinning associated with infertility treatment is called **dizygotic**. In the absence of ovulation enhancement therapy, approximately two-thirds of twin pregnancies are dizygotic. Factors associated with dizygotic pregnancies include the ethnic background of the mother, maternal age, reproductive medicine techniques, and as yet undetermined genetic factors (i.e., "Twin pregnancies run in our family"). In contrast, there are no known associated "risk factors" for **monozygotic** twinning.

> Monozygotic twins (MTs): Twins that result from the fertilization of one ovum by one sperm and the subsequent division into two zygotes.

> Dizygotic twins (DTs): Twins that result from simultaneous yet independent maturation, ovulation, and fertilization of two ova.

It is obvious that dizygotic twins share no more genetic information than siblings, whereas monozygotic twins are expected to have the same DNA sequence. However, it is not always clear during a gestation or even at delivery if the twins are monozygotic or dizygotic. If one twin is male and one is female, they are almost certainly dizygotic; rare exceptions exist and involve sex chromosomal abnormalities. The examination of the placenta and fetal membranes is only helpful in determining zygosity when a monochorionic placenta is observed, as only monozygotic twins will have this type of placentation. Any other type of placentation (e.g., two completely separate placentas or a single [fused] placental disc with two separate amniotic sacs) can be observed in either monozygotic *or* dizygotic pregnancies. In those cases DNA analysis is used to determine zygosity, as physical appearance of infants and even small children can be deceiving.

> ■■■ Concordance and Discordance
> Studying phenotypical characteristics of MTs and DTs can, under certain conditions, provide information about which part of the phenotype is genetically determined. If twins have the same phenotypical characteristic, they are concordant; if they differ, they are discordant with regard to this characteristic. If a genetic disorder is determined mainly through genetic factors, concordance will be much higher for MTs than for DTs. In an extreme case, all MTs would be concordant, while the concordance rate of DTs would be the same as that of siblings. If, however, external factors play a major role, the phenotype is independent of the twin status, and there will only be a slight difference in concordance rates between MTs and DTs.

Placental Morphology in Twin Pregnancies. The typing of a twin placenta is done macroscopically as well as histologically. Classification occurs according to the number of chorions and the number of amnions (◘ Fig. 6.1).

| Separate, dichorionic diamniotic | Fused, dichorionic diamniotic | Monochorionic diamniotic | Monochorionic monoamniotic |

Monozygotic or dizygotic twins   **Monozygotic twins**

⬭ = Placenta   ◯ = Chorion   ⬤ = Amnion

▫ **Figure 6.1. The Morphology of Twin Placentas.**

Chorion: The multilayered, outermost fetal membrane, consisting of extraembryonic somatic mesoderm, trophoblast, and, on the maternal side, villi bathed by maternal blood (*chorion* [Gr.]). Part of the chorion becomes the fetal placenta.

Amnion: The thin, avascular inner membrane that envelops the embryo in utero (*amnion* [Gr.], "sheepskin," "skin surrounding the fetus"). Together with the embryonic ectoderm, it forms the amniotic sac.

Early embryonic division (within the first 3 days after fertilization) results in a monozygotic twin pregnancy with dichorionic, diamniotic placentation. This scenario occurs in approximately 25% of all MTs. Division within 4 to 8 days after conception results in a monochorionic diamniotic placenta (74% of all MTs); division occurring between 8 and 12 days after fertilization results in a monochorionic monoamniotic placenta (less than 1% of all MTs). All monochorionic placentas can be traced back to a monozygotic twin pregnancy; dizygotic twins never share a placenta. However, an important caveat to this rule is evidenced when placental discs are fused and appear to be monochorionic.

▪▪▪ Placental Morphology in Twin Pregnancies
— Monozygotic twins often have a common placenta; dizygotic twins almost never share a common placenta (except in the case of a fused placenta).
— Only monozygotic twins share a common amniotic sac.
— Monozygotic twin pregnancy can never be excluded by placental morphology, while dizygotic twin pregnancy can be excluded in all truly monochorionic placentas.

Twin–Twin Transfusion Syndrome

Twin–twin transfusion syndrome (TTTS) is a serious complication of monochorionic twin pregnancies, where one fetus transfuses blood into the other twin. This is caused by placental shunts, especially arteriovenous anastomoses. If TTTS occurs as early as the second trimester, the prognosis is poor. The mortality rate without therapy is 80% to 100% and is caused by anemia and intrauterine growth retardation in the donor and cardiovascular decompensation in the acceptor.

Conjoined Twins

Conjoined twins (sometimes called "Siamese" twins in reference to Chang and Eng Bunker, who were born on May 11, 1811, in Siam [now Thailand]) are monozygotic twins whose failed separation results from the twinning process initiating approximately 13 to 14 days after fertilization. Conjoined twins have exclusively monochorionic/monoamniotic placentation; however, the twins themselves can be joined at the head (cephalopagus), chest (thoracopagus), abdomen (omphalopagus), sacrum (pygopagus), pelvis (ischiopagus), or xiphoid process of the sternum (xiphopagus). The incidence of conjoined twins is approx 1:100,000 births. There are many accounts of conjoined twins either living in a conjoined state or being surgically separated.

Besides conjoined, fully developed twins, there are also cases of asymmetric twinning, where one of the twins is incompletely developed. A conjoined twin that is small, poorly formed, and dependent on the larger twin for survival is called a "parasitic" twin. Parasitic twins are attached at various regions of the body (e.g., highly differentiated dermoid cyst, sacral parasite) and can be removed surgically.

7 Cancer Genetics

LEARNING OBJECTIVES

1 Discuss the statement, "Cancer is a genetic disease."

2 Discuss the functional, molecular, and genetic differences between oncogenes and tumor suppressor genes.

3 Explain why most cancer disposition syndromes are inherited as autosomal dominant traits.

Cancer is second only to cardiovascular disease as the most frequent cause of death in Western, industrialized nations. The "cost" of cancer for the individual, the family, and the nation is substantial and spans many elements, such as direct health care costs, loss of productivity, and costs associated with treatment, research, and development. Most cases of cancer are sporadic; fewer than 10% of all tumors result from a familial disposition. Yet each case, whether sporadic or familial, has a genetic cause. Cancer is a genetic disease.

7.1   Cancer Is a Genetic Disease

The term *cancer* is not a distinct disease but a general term for all malignant neoplasms. A proliferating cell mass is **malignant** when it grows independently of control mechanisms, being capable of transcending tissue boundaries, growing invasively, and metastasizing. Some types of malignant tumors (e.g., basal cell carcinoma) have a very low metastatic potential and may grow and infiltrate surrounding tissue without metastasizing for many years. There are three major groups of cancers: **carcinomas**, which develop from epithelial tissue (e.g., skin, intestinal epithelium, bronchial epithelium, and the epithelium of the glandular ducts such as the mammary glands or pancreas); **sarcomas**, which originate from mesenchymal tissue (e.g., connective tissue, bones, muscles); and the malignant diseases of the hematological and lymphatic systems (**leukemias** and **lymphomas**, respectively).

Most types of cancer develop through the progressive accumulation of various mutations within a cell. These genetic changes are typically acquired somatically, although some can be transmitted through the germ line and are present at birth in every body cell. The genes responsible for cancer development can be classified into two major groups: protooncogenes and tumor suppressor genes.

Protooncogenes: Genes that, through (dominant) activating mutations, can be turned into oncogenes. Oncogenes facilitate malignant transformation by synthesis of structurally altered or defective proteins.

Tumor suppressor genes: Genes that are relevant for the regulation of growth, repair, and cell survival, with malignant transformation supported through (recessive) loss-of-function mutations on both copies of the gene. They typically include DNA repair genes that are responsible for detecting and repairing genetic damage within a cell.

Malignant transformation: The change from controlled to uncontrolled growth of a cell that is caused by mutations in oncogenes or tumor suppressor genes.

The coordinated interplay between growth-promoting and growth-controlling genes is required for maintaining the functional health of individual cells and tissue groups. Cancer development reflects the breakdown of this carefully balanced system. It is never a single mutation that causes cancer; rather, cancer is the result of the accumulation of several genetic and chromosomal changes. Only after a critical number of genetic changes have occurred does the initially controlled growth

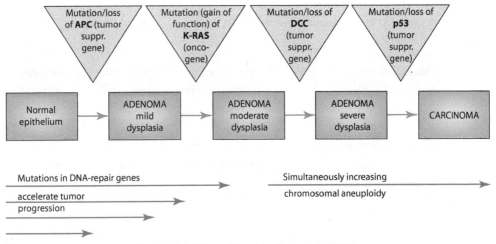

Figure 7.1. Tumor Progression Model. (Adapted from Vogelstein et al. 1996.)

become an uncontrolled, malignant growth (malignant transformation). The most extensive studies on this topic have been done for colorectal cancer. Bert Vogelstein and his colleagues described the **tumor progression model** (adenoma carcinoma sequence). Using this model, they were able to explain the impact of a succession of different gene defects on tumor development. It is remarkable how the accumulation of genetic defects in oncogenes and/or tumor suppressor genes correlates with morphological parameters. Tumor progression, from normal tissue to adenoma and carcinoma of the colon, takes approximately 10 years (◻ Fig. 7.1).

A Question of Balance. Uncontrolled growth is a common characteristic of all tumors, whether they are benign or malignant. Malignant tumors, however, also have the ability to grow invasively and metastasize. Uncontrolled growth of a tumor results from disruptions in intracellular, as well as intercellular, processing of information. Therefore, cancer does not necessarily result from increased cell proliferation. Rather, it is a question of balance between cell division and growth, on one side, and apoptosis (programmed cell death), on the other. It is crucial for embryonic development, as well as adult organisms, that the different signaling pathways are accurately coordinated and regulated. There is an inverse relationship between the degree of differentiation and the extent of a cell's proliferation. A malignant tumor tends to be less differentiated than its tissue of origin.

7.2 Oncogenes

From Protooncogenes to Oncogenes. Oncogenes develop from protooncogenes through so-called "**hypermorphic**" mutations that result in a **gain of function**. Such mutations are mostly missense mutations that cause permanent activation or altered function of the gene product (qualitative changes). Protooncogenes can also be duplicated or multiplied (**amplification**), resulting in increased gene copy numbers and thus more gene products in the cell (quantitative changes). Also, translocations can turn a protooncogene into an oncogene by generating a **fusion gene** with novel function and/or placing it under the control of a new, constitutively active promoter, which might trigger abnormal expression with regard to organ system or developmental stage.

Intracellular Dominance. Typical protooncogenes are involved in pathways that regulate cellular growth, cell proliferation, and the cell cycle. This includes receptor tyrosine kinases, growth factors and their receptors, components of intracellular signaling cascades, and proteins that regulate the cell cycle. Oncogenes are dominant at the cellular level, which means that

■ Table 7.1. Chromosomal Translocations as Causes of Malignant Diseases

Neoplasia	Translocation	Frequency	Fusion Gene or Oncogene Involved
CML (chronic myeloic leukemia)	t(9;22)(q34;q11)	90%–95%	BCR-ABL
ALL (acute lymphatic leukemia)	t(9;22)(q34;q11)	10%–15%	BCR-ABL
Burkitt lymphoma	t(8;14)(q24;q32) t(8;22)(q24;q11)	80% 15%	MYC
CLL (chronic lymphatic leukemia)	t(11;14)(q13;q32)	10%–30%	BCL-1
Follicular lymphoma	t(14;18)(q32;q21)	>90%	BCL-2

Adapted from Nussbaum et al. 2002.

activation or overexpression of one single allele is sufficient to result in a change of the cell's phenotype.

Two examples of oncogenes are the receptor tyrosine kinases *RET* and *MET*. **RET** is the receptor for growth factors of the glial cell line–derived growth factor (GDNF) family. *Activating* mutations in the *RET* gene are responsible for the development of MEN2, one of the multiple endocrine neoplasias (Section 32.5). It is interesting to note that *inactivating* mutations of the same gene can be a cause for Hirschsprung disease (Section 23.1). **MET** is the receptor for hepatic growth factor (HGF). Mutations in the *MET* gene can result in familial papillary renal carcinoma.

Among the most frequent oncogenic changes are mutations of genes of the **RAS family** (e.g., *H-RAS*, *K-RAS*, and *N-RAS*). *RAS* genes code for guanosine triphosphate (GTP) binding proteins that have a crucial regulating function for several important signaling cascades in the cell. *K-RAS* mutations occur in approximately 90% of all pancreatic carcinomas and in 50% of all colon cancers; mutations of *N-RAS* occur in roughly 30% of all cases of AML.

The classical example of a chromosomal translocation resulting in activation of a protooncogene is the translocation between chromosomes 9 and 22 that results in the so-called **Philadelphia chromosome**, t(9;22)(q34;q11). On a molecular level, the translocation causes a fusion of the *BCR* and *ABL* genes, leading to a fusion protein, BCR-ABL, and constitutional activation of the ABL tyrosine kinase (see Section 3.4 and Fig. 3.2).

Translocations of protooncogenes into chromosomal regions that are under the control of promoters for genes of the immunoglobulin chains (chromosomes 14, 22, and 2) result in uncontrolled, constitutive expression, as seen for the *MYC* protooncogene in Burkitt lymphoma (■ Table 7.1).

7.3   Tumor Suppressor Genes

Intracellular Recessiveness. Most familial cancer predisposition syndromes result from mutations in tumor suppressor genes in which **loss of function** favors development of a tumor. The products of these genes inhibit cellular growth, proliferation, or cell cycle progression (gatekeeper genes). Also, they can ensure genetic stability, for example, through DNA repair (caretaker genes). In contrast to oncogenes, which are activated by mutations on a single allele, a tumor-promoting phenotype associated with tumor suppressor genes is triggered if there are inactivating mutations in both alleles. These mutations are, therefore, recessive on a cellular level. Especially frequent are null mutations that cause complete absence of a functional product, such as small frameshift deletions or nonsense mutations that cause aborted protein synthesis. Missense mutations are also commonly encountered; however, if those have not been characterized before, it may be difficult to determine their true functional impact and, consequently, they are labeled "variants of unknown significance" (or "unclassified variants").

Variant of unknown significance (VUS): A genetic variant identified in a patient with a particular disease or a suspected disease predisposition that may or may not be of functional importance. This type of variant is frequently encountered, for example, in mutation testing for cancer predisposition syndromes; as the clinical impact of the variant is uncertain, it cannot be used for predictive testing.

■■■ Two-Hit Hypothesis

In 1971, Alfred Knudson observed that 50% of the offspring of patients with bilateral retinoblastoma develop retinoblastomas themselves, while only 10% to 15% of unilateral retinoblastomas appear to be heritable. He postulated that all cases of bilateral retinoblastoma should be considered heritable. Children with familial retinoblastoma more frequently develop the disease in both eyes or simultaneously at multiple sites while also developing it earlier than children with single unilateral tumors. These observations led Knudson to establish the two-hit hypothesis of cancer development. He postulated that children with bilateral tumors have inherited a constitutional mutation as a predisposition for development of the retinoblastoma. This single mutation is not enough to trigger the disease; a *second hit*, meaning a second somatic mutation, is required. Patients with sporadic retinoblastoma did not inherit a mutation and require two independent somatic mutations affecting the same cell. In both cases two hits are required for tumor development; in congenital retinoblastoma one of the mutations is already present in all cells. Because, statistically, a somatic mutation is likely to occur in at least one relevant cell, the disease occurs almost inevitably and much earlier in constitutional mutation carriers than in noncarriers. Frequently, secondary tumors can develop independently (e.g., osteosarcoma and leukemia).

Two-hit hypothesis of cancer development: Cancer development involves two successive mutations that affect the two alleles of a tumor suppressor gene. In familial cancer disposition syndromes, a mutation on one allele is inherited, and only one additional hit is required for cancer development.

The two-hit hypothesis applies to all known tumor suppressor genes. Mutations are required on both alleles to convert a normal cell into a tumor cell. In constitutional tumor predisposition syndromes, one mutated allele derives from the parental germ line so that offspring will have only one wild-type allele in all of their body cells (*first hit*). Each additional inactivating mutation of the second (wild-type) allele causes loss of function of the respective gene product within the affected cell (*second hit*) (■ Fig. 7.2).

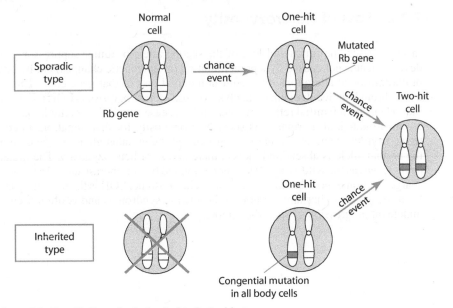

■ Figure 7.2. Two-Hit Hypothesis Applied to Retinoblastoma.

Recessive Equals Dominant. Although inactivation of tumor suppressor genes reflects a recessive mechanism at the cellular level, the associated cancer predispositions are inherited as (autosomal) dominant disorders. This paradox is easily understood if one calculates that the human body contains approximately 10^{14} cells, and the average mutation rate per gene and generation is 1 in 10^6. Even though the specific target organ has much fewer cells, it is just a matter of time for at least one mutation event (one hit) to occur in at least one cell. Normally this event does not have a functional effect, but an effect will occur if the cell already contains an inherited mutation on the other allele. Cancer development is, thus, a question of probability. Patients with an autosomal dominant tumor predisposition syndrome who never experienced a second hit in the relevant organ in their lifetime, therefore, would not develop any tumor. This is reflected by incomplete penetrance of the respective disease. The seeming paradox of a dominant disorder with a recessive pathomechanism at the cellular level applies to all conditions where abnormal functioning of a single cell is sufficient for the development of clinical symptoms.

■■■ **Epigenetic Processes**

A modification of the two-hit hypothesis became necessary when it was realized that the *second hit* in the second allele did not necessarily have to involve a DNA change. Epigenetic processes, such as DNA hypermethylation, can also account for the inactivation of an allele of a tumor suppressor gene. Since the methylation status of a gene remains the same throughout all mitotic cell divisions, the effect resembles that of a true alteration of the DNA sequence.

7.3.1 DNA Repair Genes

The inactivation of DNA repair genes does not immediately trigger abnormal cellular growth or differentiation. However, it causes failure to identify and repair mutations in the entire genome, which may result in a 100-fold to 1,000-fold increase in the mutation rate. This has an impact on protooncogenes as well as other tumor suppressor genes or gatekeeper genes. Since the accumulation of mutations is a decisive factor in tumor progression, inactivation of DNA repair genes significantly accelerates malignant transformation. One example of a hereditary tumor predisposition caused by mutations of DNA repair genes is Lynch syndrome, due to mutations in DNA mismatch repair genes such as *MSH2* or *MLH1* (Section 32.4). Other genetic disorders of DNA repair are discussed in Section 32.7.

7.3.2 Loss of Heterozygosity

In many cases, the functional loss of the second allele of tumor suppressor genes in cancer development is not caused by a point mutation (or epigenetic changes) but by larger deletions or chromosomal alterations that result in the total loss of that gene copy. This can be recognized through molecular genetic analysis of *loss of heterozygosity* (LOH). For example, when individuals with familial retinoblastoma and a disease-causing point mutation in the *RB1* gene are investigated, all normal cells show heterozygosity for that mutation. In contrast, tumor tissue from the same individual will only reveal the mutated allele. In the case of a deletion, the normal allele is absent and, hence, there is loss of heterozygosity. The mutation is really *hemizygous*, as the wild-type allele is not amplified by polymerase chain reaction (PCR) due to a large deletion or possibly loss of the entire chromosome. LOH is the most frequent mechanism for a second hit in heritable tumor predisposition syndromes and is often seen as part of the malignant progression of sporadic tumors.

8 Aging and Genetics

LEARNING OBJECTIVES

1 Name three mechanisms that contribute to cellular aging processes.

2 Malignant cells frequently express the enzyme telomerase, which is able to prevent shortening of the telomeres during replication. Explain why this is of advantage to a cancer cell.

3 Give two reasons why the mitochondrial genome is particularly vulnerable to mutations.

In a literal sense, a person begins to age the moment he or she is born; however, true aging at the cellular level doesn't commence until early adulthood. The pathophysiology of aging is complex; it is characterized in each cell by a limited number of mitoses and is largely associated with the accumulation of mutations, which lead to death of the cell and, eventually, the organism. In a teleological sense, aging occurs to allow evolutionary changes in a species. Many naturally occurring human disorders exist whereby the aging process is greatly accelerated. Despite the elucidation of many of these conditions at a genetic level, the exact regulation of the aging process is, as yet, poorly understood.

8.1 Protein Changes

Life expectancy varies among different species; flies live for about 30 days, rabbits 6 years, and horses 25 years. Even within a species, there is a genetic basis for life expectancy; for example, children of long-living parents usually live significantly longer than average. What is the molecular basis for cellular aging, and in what way is aging determined by our genes? If one examines the tissues of younger individuals and compares them to those of older individuals of the same species, there are significant differences, especially with regard to **posttranslational modification** of proteins. For many mammalian species, it has been shown that, with increasing age, some of the enzymes in their tissues lose a portion of their activity even though immunological methods show that the proteins are still present. It is assumed that chemical processes, such as the generation of free radicals due to oxidative stress, contribute to conformational and consequently functional damage to various structural and nonstructural proteins of the cell.

Free Radicals. Under certain circumstances, oxygen forms highly reactive compounds (e.g., superoxide anions, hydroxyl peroxide radicals, and hydroxyl radicals). These free radicals react with certain amino acids, including histidine, arginine, lysine, and proline, as well as with the sulfhydryl groups of methionine. The changes in the normal polypeptide chains, such as an enzyme, can lead to a conformational change that results in inactivation of the enzyme's catalytic function. Experiments with drosophila have shown that overexpression of catalase and superoxide dismutase, enzymes that trap free radicals and convert them back into H_2O and O_2, can significantly extend the life span.

Glycosylation of Proteins. There is evidence that glycosylation of proteins, meaning the spontaneous, nonenzymatic reaction of the proteins with glucose, significantly contributes to aging. During glycosylation, the aldehyde of glucose reacts with a free amino group of a protein. Subsequent reactions, which may involve free radicals, result in complex final products, so-called **advanced glycation end products (AGEs)**. The content of AGEs rises with age depending on the blood glucose level. AGEs are able to cross-link other proteins and change their physical as well as biological characteristics. It is assumed that AGEs are involved in the development of atherosclerosis, cataracts, and peripheral neuropathies. AGEs, and their reaction products, are recognized by macrophages and, in this way, promote the secretion of inflammatory cytokines and tumor necrosis factor.

Nutrition as an Aging Factor. Can alteration of nutrition and lifestyle prolong life expectancy? A large study on rhesus macaques shows that animals that are fed a low-calorie diet live significantly longer than animals that are fed normal diets. Lower fasting insulin levels, lower fasting glucose levels, higher insulin sensitivity, and lower low-density lipoprotein (LDL)-cholesterol levels are associated with lower atherogenesis in the dietary-restricted animals. This correlates with previous studies in mice, which used biochemical analyses to show that the levels of glycated proteins in the caloric-restricted mice were significantly lower than those in the control group. It was also shown that caloric restriction has a positive influence on the defense mechanisms against free radicals. This may be an indication that free radicals, as well as glycated proteins, contribute to the aging process or even complement each other, synergistically.

8.2   DNA Changes

Studies of human DNA reveal that **somatic mutations** accumulate, and **chromosomal instability** is more likely as an organism ages. Presently, it is not known whether these aberrations are the *result of* or the *cause for* the aging process.

Telomere Shortening

Some especially striking age-related changes of the nuclear genome occur at the telomeres of the chromosomes. These regions are characterized by multiple tandem repeats of a specific sequence, 5'-TTAGGG-3', stretching over many thousand nucleotides (approximately 9 kb). Telomeres have an important function in **stabilizing the chromosome structure** by "capping" the chromosomal ends and preventing interaction with other chromosomes that could lead to rearrangements or chromosomal fusion. They have been compared to aglets at the end of shoelaces that keep them from fraying.

Since approximately 50 nucleotides at the end of each chromosome are lost during each cell division cycle (Section 2.7), the telomeres become progressively shorter during a person's lifetime. When too short, they lose their function as protective chromosomal "caps," and the cell enters **growth arrest and apoptosis**. This mechanism appears to prevent genomic instability and development of cancer in aged human cells by limiting the number of cell divisions. Cell cycle arrest is mediated through cyclin-dependent kinases. While DNA damage can possibly be repaired during cell cycle arrest, lengthening of the telomeres is not possible, since normal body cells do not have telomerase activity. Additional signaling cascades lead to the programmed death (apoptosis) of these cells.

Mitochondrial DNA

Changes in the mitochondrial DNA (mtDNA) are thought to cause some of the phenotypes of an aging organism. The **accumulation of mitochondrial mutations**, including deletions, duplications, and point mutations, has been found in many tissues of older individuals. There are two reasons why the mitochondrial genome is particularly vulnerable to mutations. First, mitochondria lack DNA repair enzymes that maintain a low cumulative mutation burden in the nuclear genome. The mitochondrial genome, therefore, has mutation rates that are 100 to 1,000 times higher than the rate of mutations of the nuclear genome. Second, mtDNA is the preferred target of **free radicals**, because the latter develop during oxidative phosphorylation in the mitochondria themselves. The proximity of mtDNA to the sources of free radicals and the absence of a scaffold of histone molecules render mtDNA far more vulnerable and mutable than nuclear DNA. As with mitochondrial disorders, the accumulation of mtDNA mutations particularly affects tissues with high energy needs and a dependence on oxidative phosphorylation. Reduced mental and physical strength, ataxia, retinal degeneration, hearing loss, cardiac arrhythmias, and myopathy with rapid fatigue are not only typical symptoms of mitochondrial disorders, but also phenomena that manifest themselves in the aging organism, though in varying degrees.

8.3   Human Progeria Syndromes

Human aging is a highly complex and multifactorial process, yet there are monogenic disorders—the so-called progeria syndromes—that are characterized by clinical features of premature aging in young persons.

> Progeria syndromes: Syndromes that recapitulate the phenotype of the aging person in an accelerated manner.

The prototype of this group of diseases is **Werner syndrome** (progeria adultorum), which is an autosomal recessive disorder resulting from mutations of the *WRN* gene. In most cases it manifests itself as the absence of the normal growth spurt in adolescence. At the age of 20 years, most of the patients have gray hair with progressive atrophy and hardening of the skin, premature development of cataracts, osteoporosis, diabetes mellitus, and varying degrees of atherosclerosis. The average life expectancy is 47 years. The most frequent causes of death are myocardial infarction and malignant neoplasms. More than 400 cases of Werner syndrome have been reported in the literature. The gene product of the *WRN* gene belongs to a family of DNA helicases that are required for DNA replication, recombination, chromosome segregation, DNA repair, transcription, or other processes requiring unwinding of DNA. Hindered DNA repair, increased telomere shortening, and increased genomic instability all may contribute to premature senescence in Werner syndrome.

    While Werner syndrome manifests itself in adolescence, children with **Hutchinson-Gilford syndrome** (progeria infantilis) begin to show symptoms of premature aging in their first year of life (◘ Fig. 8.1). The disorder was first described in 1754. Most affected children have distinct

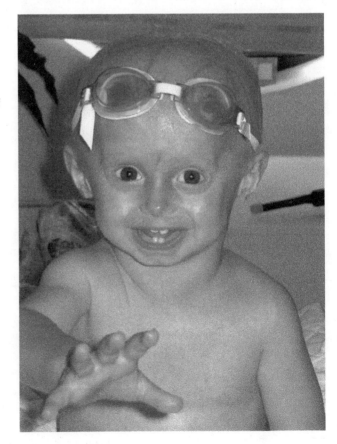

◘ **Figure 8.1. Hutchinson-Gilford Progeria in a 3½-Year-Old Boy.**
Note the sparsity of hair of the scalp and eyebrows, as well as the atrophy of subtemporal fatty tissue, facial hypoplasia with microgenia, and the typically prominent cranial veins. (Courtesy of R. Hennekam, Institute of Child Health, London.)

alopecia by their second birthday. Subcutaneous lipodystrophy makes the children look old at a very young age. Periarticular fibroses result in the stiffening of the joints; there is early osteoporosis with bone fragility. By the time they are 5 years old, patients have generalized atherosclerosis. The average life expectancy is 14 years. Hutchinson-Gilford syndrome is caused by mutations of the *LMNA* gene, which codes for laminin A/C, an essential component of the nuclear membrane. Lamins form microfilaments in the nucleus and are important in maintaining the proper structure of the nuclei. They also influence chromatin structure, regulation of gene expression, and other functions.

9 Pharmacogenetics

For hundreds of years it has been known that medications can have different effects on different people. It has also been known that close relatives often have similar reactions. **Adverse drug reactions** are among the 10 most frequent causes of death. These include dose-dependent, dose-independent, and dose-over-time-dependent (cumulative) effects, as well as withdrawal, paradoxical effects of medications, and resistance to therapy. Many of these unusual effects result from the genetic-biochemical makeup of the individual patient.

9.1 Basics of Pharmacological Metabolism

The **therapeutic window** of a medication is the drug dosage that can treat a disease effectively while staying within the safety range (e.g., giving more desired effects than adverse effects). If the dose is too low or the time span between doses too long, or if bioavailability of the medication is insufficient, the effective dose will not be reached. The same is true if the medication is catabolized too rapidly and/or excreted. If the dose is too high, the time span between doses is too short, or the drug is hardly metabolized and excreted, then the therapeutic window will be exceeded and toxic side effects may occur.

Pharmacokinetics: The representation of the body's action on the drug.

Pharmacodynamics: The effects the drug has on the body, or more exactly, the target tissue.

There may be considerable genetic differences in pharmacokinetics and pharmacodynamics from one patient to another, resulting in extremely different medicinal effectiveness between individuals prescribed the same dose of medication. Processes such as absorption, distribution, biotransformation, metabolism, and excretion are part of **pharmacokinetics**. The distribution and metabolism of a drug can differ greatly between individuals and sometimes depend considerably on genetic factors. Drug levels in the blood are used as an indirect measurement of drug concentrations in the target tissue. **Pharmacodynamics** of a medication describes how the drug molecules bind to the respective receptors and thereby trigger signaling cascades, activate transcription factors, or regulate gene expression. These processes also depend on individual genetic disposition.

Phase I reactions: Modification of a chemical, usually rendering it (more) polar.

Phase II reactions: The attachment of a polar, ionizable group to the respective molecule.

The great majority of drugs are metabolized in phase I and phase II reactions. Phase I reactions can lead either to activation or inactivation of the drug. A large and important group of phase I enzymes are the **P-450 cytochromes**, a class of proteins of which more than 50 have been identified in humans. Cytochromes are monooxygenases that hydroxylate their substrates and create the possibility for conjugation with strong polar agents in a subsequent phase II reaction. Like most phase I enzymes, cytochromes not only play a role in drug metabolism but also have unwanted functional effects. Some of the strongest carcinogens are metabolically activated in vivo by cytochromes of the P-450 system, which change a precursor substance into a chemically reactive form. Other phase I enzymes include various hydroxylases, peroxidases, monoamine oxidases, dioxygenases, reductases, lipoxygenases, cyclooxygenases, and dehydrogenases. After the introduction of a functional group, a polar and ionizable group can then be attached to the respective molecule in a **phase II reaction**. In most cases, this involves conjugation with a strong polar group, typically a glucuronyl group. The introduction of a polar group leads to a molecule devoid of activity with increased water solubility, making it more easily excreted from the body.

9.2   Pharmacogenetics in Clinical Practice

Variability of N-Oxygenation

Trimethylaminuria (fish odor syndrome) is a less known, yet clinically relevant, "pharmacogenetic" metabolic disorder. It is caused by a deficiency of the flavin-containing monooxygenase type 3 (FMO3) that is required for the oxygenation of nitrogen in numerous substances and is inherited as an autosomal recessive trait. FMO3 deficiency affects the metabolism of various drugs, such as tyramine, benzydamine, and nicotine. Clinically, the most relevant symptom is caused by the reduced or absent N-oxygenation of trimethylamine (TMA), a substance that gives old fish its unpleasant odor. TMA N-oxide, the product of the FMO3-mediated reaction, is odorless. In FMO3 deficiency, free TMA accumulates, and large quantities of it are excreted in urine, breath, and sweat, causing a highly unpleasant body odor resembling old fish. Numerous mutations in the *FMO3* gene have been described. A complete loss of FMO3 results in permanent body malodor that is very stressful for affected persons, although often it is not recognized as a disorder. There is also a common hypomorphic allele with reduced, but not absent, FMO3 activity, which occurs at a frequency of 20% in various populations and is homozygous in 3% to 5% of individuals of mid-European descent. Such individuals have "mild" or "intermittent" trimethylaminuria, meaning the unpleasant body odor occurs only in special situations (e.g., after eating fish and certain other food products such as peas, choline, or lecithin-rich substances, or after the administration of carnitine).

Fast and Slow Acetylators

The polymorphism of the **N-acetyl transferase gene** *NAT2* on chromosome 8 is the pharmacogenetic variant par excellence. It was recognized at the beginning of the 1950s, when repeated cases of severe polyneuritis were noted after **isoniazid** was introduced as a new medication for tuberculosis. The cause was soon discovered: some people catabolize the medication slowly and, as a result, develop a toxic overdose reaction. Isoniazid is detoxified by acetylation caused by the hepatic enzyme N-acetyl transferase. With regard to the metabolism of isoniazid or many other substances, people may be classified into two groups: fast and slow acetylators. The difference is caused by hypomorphic variants in the *NAT2* gene that result in a diminished enzyme activity and, thus, slower acetylation. Like most other inborn errors of metabolism, NAT2 deficiency shows autosomal recessive inheritance; slow acetylators are homozygous (or compound heterozygous) for alleles that mediate diminished N-acetyl transferase activity. The frequency of these alleles varies in their ethnic distribution. While fewer than 20% of Asians are slow acetylators, the percentage rises to 50% for African Americans and 65% for Europeans (up to 90% in the Mediterranean). It is unknown why this metabolic variant is so frequent in some populations; it is possible that slow acetylation had once represented an evolutionary advantage.

Clinical Relevance. Fast acetylators need (and tolerate) higher doses of certain medications than slow acetylators. Slow acetylators have an increased risk for developing lupus erythematosus after administration of hydralazine (for hypertension). The antihypertensive drug debrisoquine and the antiarrhythmic drug sparteine are overly active in slow acetylators and may be ineffective in fast acetylators. Routine genetic testing is not yet recommended, since the many possible gene variants and interindividual variability do not permit an accurate prognosis; when relevant, the drug concentrations can be measured directly in the blood.

Malignant Hyperthermia

Malignant hyperthermia is, perhaps, the most dramatic complication of anesthesia and frequently results in death of the patient. Malignant hyperthermia is inherited in an autosomal dominant manner. It is diagnosed more frequently in children (incidence, 1 in 12,000 children) than in adults (incidence, 1 in 100,000 adults), and males are affected more frequently.

Clinical Relevance. Malignant hyperthermia is due to an adverse reaction to inhalation anesthetic agents such as halothane, enflurane, isoflurane, sevoflurane, and desflurane, as well as depolarizing muscle relaxants such as succinylcholine. These agents are routinely administered in anesthesia practice and rarely cause side effects in the general population; however, administration of one of these medications to a patient with a predisposition for malignant hyperthermia may cause a life-threatening reaction with hyperthermia above 42°C, muscular rigidity, and massive elevation of creatine phosphokinase and myoglobin in the blood. Massive myoglobinemia can cause renal failure. Treatment in the acute phase includes intravenous administration of dantrolene, which is continued as long as hyperthermia persists.

Genetics. To date, two genes that predispose an individual to malignant hyperthermia susceptibility (MHS) have been identified, and three additional loci have been mapped. MHS1 is associated with mutations in the gene *RYR1*, which encodes for ryanodine receptor type 1; MHS5 is associated with mutations in the gene *CACNA1S*, which encodes for the skeletal muscle calcium channel. Up to 70% of cases of malignant hyperthermia are caused by mutations in the *RYR1* gene. The type 1 ryanodine receptor is a calcium channel in the sarcoplasmic reticulum of skeletal muscle. *RYR1* mutations can result in the leakage of the channel and an unphysiologically high calcium concentration in myoplasm. Another possible effect of the mutations is that the channel acts independently of the relevant regulatory proteins. Molecular genetic testing for *RYR1* and *CACNA1S* is available on a clinical basis. Mutations in the *RYR1* gene can also cause a nonprogressive myopathy, central core disease.

Pseudocholinesterase Variants

Serum cholinesterase, also called pseudocholinesterase, hydrolyzes cholinesters such as acetylcholine and succinylcholine, which is a depolarizing muscle relaxant that functions at the neuromuscular junction and is frequently used during anesthesia. Succinylcholine consists of two molecules of acetylcholine and is metabolized and inactivated by cholinesterase. Negative reaction to succinylcholine is caused by variants of the *BCHE* (butyrylcholinesterase) gene. As with other conditions relating to enzymatic function, the variants only cause adverse affects when present in a homozygous or compound heterozygous form (autosomal recessive inheritance). Individuals who are homozygous for "variant A" have pseudocholinesterase deficiency, with respective clinical symptoms. Among persons of European descent, the AA genotype occurs in 1 in 3,300 individuals.

Clinical Relevance. The administration of succinylcholine or succinyldicholine (suxamethonium) to affected individuals often results in apnea that last several hours. The affected patient must be supported with extended mechanical ventilation until the drug is eventually metabolized.

9.3   Pharmacogenetic Disorders

Glucose-6-Phosphate-Dehydrogenase Deficiency

Glucose-6-phosphate-dehydrogenase deficiency (G6PDD, favism) is one of the most common genetic disorders, with an estimated 400 million affected individuals worldwide. It is inherited as an **X-linked** condition; mostly males are clinically affected. As with the hemoglobinopathies (sickle cell anemia and thalassemia), the incidence of G6PDD varies considerably by region due to a **partial resistance to malaria** in carriers. G6PD deficiency results in diminished production of reduced glutathione, which protects erythrocytes from oxidative stress. Affected patients have a reduced capacity to detoxify peroxides that, consequently, damage the erythrocyte membrane and cause hemolysis.

Hemizygous or homozygous individuals may develop **severe hemolytic crises in reaction to various external factors** such as oxidative stress triggered by infections, ingestion of fava beans (broad beans), or the administration of certain medications such as quinine, chloroquine, primaquine, sulfonamides, and aspirin. Once the diagnosis is made, crises may be prevented through avoidance of the triggering substance. All affected persons should wear a medical ID bracelet and carry a medical emergency card.

Acute Intermittent Porphyria

Acute intermittent porphyria is an autosomal dominant disorder caused by half-normal activity of porphobilinogen deaminase, the second enzyme of heme biosynthesis. Clinically, it is characterized by **acute episodes of (abdominal) pain, psychiatric symptoms, and tachycardia**. These attacks are triggered by various external factors, including drugs (e.g., cytochrome P-450 enzyme inducers such as barbiturates, pyrazolone, sulfonamides, and halothane), hormones (e.g., progesterone), nutritional factors (e.g., fasting and low cellular glucose), smoking, alcohol, and stress. The diagnosis is typically made in early adulthood (peak age 30 years), and the incidence is estimated to be 1 in 10,000 individuals. Females are more frequently clinically affected than males. Penetrance is low; only 10% to 20% of individuals with a disease-causing mutation in the *HMBS* gene manifest with the disease.

> ■■■ Acute Intermittent Porphyria—A Dominant Metabolic Disorder
>
> Most inborn errors of metabolism show autosomal recessive inheritance since, in most instances, the half-normal activity of an enzyme (caused by a heterozygous mutation) is sufficient for physiological function. In contrast, porphobilinogen deaminase (PBGD), a highly regulated enzyme that functions at the beginning of a biosynthetic pathway, exhibits autosomal dominant inheritance. There are two pathogenetic factors: on one hand, half-normal PBGD activity might be sufficient at baseline, but not when there is increased demand for heme biosynthesis, and on the other hand, there is high toxicity of the respective accumulating substrates (aminolevulinic acid and porphobilinogen). A significant amount of the heme synthesized in the liver is not utilized for hemoglobin but is integrated into numerous enzymes, especially cytochrome P-450 oxidases. Heme synthesis is regulated primarily by its cellular concentration: low heme concentrations result in a strong activation of the first enzyme of this metabolic pathway, δ-aminolevulinic acid synthase. This explains why crises are triggered especially by drugs that induce cytochrome P-450 enzymes. These drugs deplete the cellular concentration of heme, resulting in a strong stimulation of heme biosynthesis that cannot be adequately contained due to the metabolic blockage.

Clinical Relevance. Clinical symptoms can be numerous and misleading. Episodes can manifest as nonspecific, often colicky, abdominal discomfort. Unfortunately, some patients undergo unnecessary abdominal surgery, as signs and symptoms of porphyria can mimic those of acute appendicitis. The neurological and psychiatric symptoms of this condition are protean, are nonspecific, and often pose a diagnostic challenge. These include polyneuropathy with paresis, mood changes, fatigue, and, in severe cases, seizures. Cardiovascular symptoms, such as hypertension or tachycardia, may also occur.

Diagnostics. In 50% of cases, the urine in an acute attack is red or red-brownish, which is enhanced by exposure to air and light. A marked increase in the urinary excretion of porphobilinogen confirms the diagnosis.

Therapy. In an acute crisis, it may be necessary for the patient to receive intensive medical care. Medication associated with causing the disease must be stopped immediately. Heme arginate (as a source of heme) and intravenous glucose infusion can revert activation of heme biosynthesis in the liver. Toxic metabolites may be removed by forced diuresis. The most important therapy, in the long term, is educating the patient about the avoidance of triggers. Affected persons should wear a medical ID bracelet and carry a medical emergency card.

9.4   Pharmacogenomics

Pharmacogenetics: The study of the impact of single genetic variants on drug metabolism.

Pharmacogenomics: The study of drug metabolism in relation to the whole genome or the individual's overall genetic constitution.

Whenever a physician administers a medication to a patient, there is a degree of uncertainty as to how effective the treatment will be and if there will be any unwanted side effects. In most cases, the desired effect is achieved; sometimes the medication has no effect at all, or the effect is excessive or paradoxical. Usually, unexpected drug response is multifactorial rather than monogenic, since it does not result from a single rare mutation but rather from a multitude of functionally important genetic variants. Pharmacogenomics strives for an individualized genetic profile of the patient that can predict the effect of a medication in the respective patient. Such an individualized, genetic-biochemical profile could, theoretically, make it possible to calculate, in advance, the adequate dose and application of a medication. It remains to be seen how rapidly and for which therapies such an approach can be realized.

II

The Clinical Basis of Human Genetics

10   Human Genetics as a Medical Specialty

LEARNING OBJECTIVES

1 List at least three benefits of establishing a diagnosis in an individual with a genetic or developmental condition.

2 Describe the responsibilities of the medical geneticist in a genetic counseling session.

Human genetics has four important functions in medicine:

- **Diagnosis of genetic disorders** through a detailed personal and family history, physical examination, and diagnostic laboratory evaluation
- **Anticipatory guidance and management regarding interdisciplinary care** for individuals with genetic conditions
- **Genetic counseling** regarding prognosis, recurrence risk, and availability of patient advocacy associations
- **Clinical and laboratory-based research** to identify the molecular bases of genetic disorders and disease susceptibility

Human genetics differs from other medical fields because it is not defined clinically as relating to a particular organ system, age, or gender but is instead defined pathophysiologically through specific factors that contribute to the disease. Therefore, an interdisciplinary approach is essential to fully appreciate the intricacies of most genetic disorders. In past decades the medical geneticist diagnosed, treated, and followed individuals with rare heritable conditions or sporadic developmental disorders. However, as the human genome emerges from obscurity, all physicians must have a workable knowledge of human genetics and genomics because they too will be responsible for the diagnosis and treatment of the "genetic patient."

Nevertheless, even in the postgenomic era, the human geneticist is presented with the puzzles of medicine and has a key role in the diagnosis and treatment of relatively common and very rare genetic diseases. The components of these puzzles are nothing more than medical history, familial history, physical examination, and synopsis of findings from specialized examinations; yet, it is the clinical geneticist who has the patience, skill, and insight to fit these pieces into the portrait of the final diagnosis. The challenge for the clinical geneticist is to recognize certain features and patterns found through history and physical examination and to reach a diagnosis, either through recognition of patterns associated with particular syndromes or understanding of the pathophysiology and molecular mechanisms. A detailed and well-structured familial medical history, or pedigree, is extremely important in clinical evaluation and in determining whether or not a disease has a genetic component. Diagnostic workup includes specialized laboratory tests that at times appear technically simple; yet, the correct interpretation and evaluation of these tests demand a high level of expertise. Establishing a diagnosis is important for the obvious reason of commencing specific therapy; but even for those conditions that are not treatable by specific intervention, the diagnosis is imperative for the medical and psychological health of the patient and family. Determining a diagnosis provides the often overlooked benefits of increasing medical surveillance, enabling individualized education plans, developing knowledge of recurrence risk, and enabling patients to network with disease-specific support organizations.

Important

Establishing an etiological diagnosis:
- Is crucial for starting specific pharmacological therapy
- Provides a basis for anticipatory guidance and management of and/or screening for medical, developmental and educational issues
- Allows the determination of accurate recurrence risks in family members
- Imparts a tangible psychological benefit for the patient and family who find closure with the knowledge of a diagnosis and identification of condition-specific support groups

Once a diagnosis is made, the geneticist becomes the conductor for the patient's and often the family's medical **management and care**, which can involve specific treatment (e.g., for metabolic disorders), organ system surveillance (e.g., for cancer syndromes), and coordination of interdisciplinary care. The geneticist also plays the role of educator for many rare disorders, educating the patient, family, and interdisciplinary team of physicians and health care providers. Once these tasks are accomplished for any given patient, the geneticist may take a secondary role in the patient's care.

Genetic counseling is the third important function of the medical geneticist. As mentioned previously, a unique role of the genetic medical specialist is educating the patient and family not only about the medical implications of the diagnosis but also about the educational, social, and reproductive implications. The diagnosis of heritable or developmental conditions carries with it the burden of guilt and uncertainty. While the guilt is not based on scientific fact or even common sense, it is no less real to the individual who harbors it. The uncertainty, however, can be quite real, especially for those rare conditions for which there is little understanding, treatment, or support. The geneticist, through empathetic communication and knowledgeable resources, is charged with ushering patients through this difficult transition from not knowing a diagnosis to knowing that the diagnosis may have prognostic and reproductive implications. How is the disease inherited? What do the genetic findings signify for the patient and his or her family? What is the significance for the affected individual and his or her relatives? What is the recurrence risk for future pregnancies? How did the genetic change occur, and is the patient somehow at fault? How does one cope with knowledge of genetic changes and variants? These questions are of vital significance for the patient and the family and require a competent, professional, and empathetic consultation. Because a genetic counseling session is often long and emotionally charged, and covers complicated material, a geneticist often provides a **counseling report** to the family, which serves as an important reference for them in the future.

One can appreciate that the human geneticist is an investigative physician, effective educator, and empathetic communicator. One can also appreciate that the field of medical genetics and medicine in general would be stagnant if it were not for the efforts of **human genetics research** in the laboratory, at the bedside, and, most importantly, in translation between those two realms. Research is necessary to characterize rare and newly identified syndromes as well as to dissect and define the pathophysiological mechanisms of well-established medical conditions such as hypertension, diabetes, and cancer. We are far from a complete understanding of the genetic bases for health and disease, yet each step toward this goal translates to improved diagnostics, therapy, and prevention.

11   Genetic Counseling

LEARNING OBJECTIVES

1 Define the term *predictive genetic testing* and give an example of a disorder to which this term applies.

2 Discuss the advantages and disadvantages of predictive genetic testing.

3 Discuss the indications and contraindications of molecular genetic testing in children.

4 Define the term *nondirective counseling.*

Genetic counseling has been practiced for thousands of years. For example, the Babylonian Talmud (completed in the 7th century AD) clearly states that a mother is to refrain from circumcising her son if two previous sons had died from (uncontrollable bleeding caused by) a circumcision. Today, the enormous expansion of molecular knowledge makes genetic counseling both more complex and more urgent. Patients as much as doctors need to understand the impact of genetic knowledge on diagnosis and treatment, prognosis, and reproductive decisions.

Communication and Consultation. Clinical genetics deals not only with the purely medical aspects of genetic diseases but also with their social and psychological consequences. It is of great importance that the human geneticist addresses options and strategies for coping with genetic risks and diagnoses of genetic diseases. In contrast to most physicians, the geneticist must focus on the patient as well as the family, including those at risk for having a genetic condition or passing the condition to future generations. Calculating risk (see Chapter 14) plays a major role in this.

A Question of Time. Contrast the time it takes to explain the rationale for treatment of an uncomplicated otitis media to the time it takes to explain the implications of a diagnosis of a heritable neurodevelopmental disorder or familial cancer syndrome. Genetic counseling takes time because the conditions are often complex, affect the person throughout his or her lifetime, and can be passed on from one generation to the next in a family. In the course of a genetic counseling session, the geneticist does his or her best to explain the medical, developmental, and educational implications of the condition, as well as its prognosis and recurrence risk, in a manner that is understandable to a person who is not familiar with medical or scientific concepts or jargon.

The geneticist must anticipate negative reactions from the patient and family such as denial, guilt, and even anger, and empathetically convey that the diagnosis is not a reflection on the person or the family but is a medical condition that they did not cause themselves. An initial genetic counseling session is scheduled for 60 minutes, and many patients and families need one or two additional sessions to have their questions and concerns that arise as a result of their deeper understanding of the diagnosis answered and addressed.

11.1   Aims and Goals of Genetic Counseling

Who? Why? What? Genetic counseling is a medical consultation for individuals who are affected by a genetic disorder (either in themselves or in a child) or who have an increased risk for a genetic disorder. The major focus of the session is to address questions and concerns of the consultand (who can be the patient, parent, or a couple depending on the circumstance) and to provide additional resources to facilitate further understanding of the diagnosis and its implications for the consultand and his or her family. Consultations whose major focus is on diagnosis, on the other hand, basically are not different from any physician's usual diagnostic activities.

> **Important**
>
> **Indications for Human Genetics Counseling**
> - Questions of diagnosis, cause, and prognosis of heritable or developmental disorders
> - Questions of disease risk for family members (primary diagnostic confirmation is often required)
> - Questions of the risk for a genetic disease in an expected or future child
> - Discussions of options of prenatal testing for certain genetic disorders
> - Discussions about and performance of predictive molecular genetic testing (e.g., for cancer disposition syndromes or for late manifesting heritable diseases such as Huntington disease)
> - Questions of management and anticipatory guidance for heritable disorders or disease susceptibility
> - Clarification and advice about:
>   - Infertility or recurrent miscarriages
>   - Advanced maternal or paternal age
>   - Assisted reproductive therapy
>   - Marriage between relatives (consanguinity)
>   - Exposure to teratogens before or during pregnancy

The purpose of the counseling session is to help the consultand to understand the diagnosis in question. Information is an essential component for coping with disease. For that reason, especially with rare genetic disorders of critical significance, it is extremely important to inform the consultand in an intelligible and appropriate way about the disease, its prognosis, and its heritability. Important details should be presented calmly in the most simple terms and using comparisons. Sometimes it is useful to discuss the problem from multiple angles. This might require several counseling sessions.

Another essential component of genetic counseling is the detailed and individualized counseling report addressed to the consultand. This report should summarize the counseling session in plain language; a copy should be sent to the referring physician.

An invaluable resource for physicians and families is a specific advocacy group developed by individuals with a particular genetic disorder. The Genetic Alliance (www.geneticalliance.org) is a nonprofit health advocacy organization that promotes awareness and education for genetic conditions in general and provides links and information regarding specific support groups worldwide.

Genetic Counseling in the Context of Molecular Genetic Testing

The clinical diagnosis of many genetic disorders can now be established (or confirmed) by molecular diagnostic testing, and in many cases a molecular laboratory test supplants or even replaces other, once "gold standard" methods of diagnosis. An example is DNA testing for spinal muscular atrophy that obviates the invasive procedure of a muscle biopsy. Despite the rapid increase in the number of clinically available molecular tests (www.genetests.org in North America, www.orpha.net in Europe) and their integration into routine practice, written consent of the patient or parent is still mandatory in many countries. In any case, it is good clinical practice to inform the patient or parents of the availability of testing and why the molecular study is requested.

Predictive Diagnostics

A situation in which informed consent for genetic testing is often (and should be) required is in the predictive diagnosis for asymptomatic individuals in a family with an adult-onset disorder. The psychological and social implications of the test result may be life altering and sometimes devastating for individuals, particularly if no effective treatment is available. Specific guidelines were first developed by advocacy groups and genetic professional organizations with regard to predictive testing for Huntington disease. These recommendations in principle should also be followed in other conditions such as familial cancer disposition syndromes.

Huntington disease (HD) is an autosomal dominant neurodegenerative disease with age-dependant penetrance. Presymptomatic molecular diagnosis is available and predicts with 100% certainty whether or not the individual will (if he or she survives to adulthood) manifest the disease (see Section 31.1.1). In the case of predictive testing for HD, genetic counseling is required and is often achieved in multiple sessions to educate the consultand and explore the benefits and risks of learning his or her future with regard to manifesting the disease. It is strongly recommended that a predictive diagnosis involve at least a three-step counseling process with the following components:

— Initial counseling session
— Second counseling session with possible blood test
— Third counseling session to report the diagnosis

The **initial counseling session** has two objectives: it serves to clarify whether possible symptoms of the disease are already present and to make sure the patient is responsible and optimally informed about the condition and disease. This includes questions of heritability and diagnostic and therapeutic possibilities, as well as those of familial and social networks. Many individuals have concerns regarding their ability to obtain health, disability, and life insurance if they undergo testing and especially if the testing indicates they will manifest the disease. In the United States, the Genetic Information Nondiscrimination Act (GINA) of 2008 protects individuals against discrimination by health insurers and employers, but this legislation does not yet apply to disability or life insurance.

Because the early manifestations of HD can be subtle, individuals seeking predictive testing should also undergo an evaluation by a neurologist familiar with this diagnosis. In addition, a psychological interview is strongly recommended to assess how the consultand may react to positive (or negative) test results and to facilitate access to psychological help if required after the test. Even a "favorable" test result can cause severe mental stress for an individual at 50% risk. Those who spent a lifetime expecting to fall ill and die from a familial disease may have difficulty readjusting to a future life without the condition, and may also experience "survival guilt" for not having inherited the deleterious mutation while another family member did. Such unexpected (paradoxical) reactions should be discussed before the test is done, and the consultand should be availed of psychotherapy to enable him or her to anticipate and manage these reactions. Many centers require neurological and psychological evaluation to be completed before the molecular test is initiated.

The **second counseling session** should be scheduled after the consultand has had time to decide whether he or she wants to proceed with the test. It allows the consultand time to contact friends or other trusted persons to exchange thoughts about the test. If support groups are available, encourage the consultand to contact them. The second counseling session serves to clarify remaining questions. If the consultand at this point wishes to proceed with the test and if the geneticist and the psychotherapist have no serious objections, the session ends with the drawing of a blood sample and the consultand is informed when to expect the test result.

Communicating the test result or posttest counseling should never be done over the telephone or by mail. Instead, it should be the subject of the **third counseling session**. The consultand should be encouraged to bring a supportive friend or relative, yet some individuals prefer not to be accompanied. Even after the consultand arrives for this session, he or she has the option of electing not to learn the results. How the consultand reacts to a (positive or negative) test result cannot be predicted. This calls for a great deal of empathy on the part of the geneticist, the genetic counselor, and the person accompanying the consultand.

11.2 Molecular Genetic Testing of Children

Children should only undergo molecular-genetic testing if it will be of direct medical benefit to them. Molecular genetic examination of symptomatic children as part of an overall diagnostic concept is indisputable when a congenital disease is suspected; it can sometimes spare the children painful, invasive, or otherwise stressful tests. Predictive testing of children is also meaningful if a positive test result would have immediate preventive or therapeutic consequences (e.g., thyroidectomy in multiple endocrine neoplasia type 2B [MEN 2B] or preventive colonoscopy in children older than 10 years of age in familiar adenomatous polyposis [FAP], or to avoid these invasive measures).

A predictive diagnostic test for a disorder without therapeutic options is contraindicated in children because there may be untoward psychological consequences for the child and his or her parents and family. Likewise, carrier testing for recessive disorders is not done in children. Open communication with the child about the specific condition is important throughout his or her lifetime, and specific information about the availability of molecular testing can be discussed when the child is old enough to understand the implications of this information. Later, when he or she becomes an adult, the person can decide whether or not to proceed with testing.

Indications for molecular genetic testing in childhood include:

— Primary diagnostic testing or confirmation of the diagnosis with a justifiable clinical suspicion. This is most appropriate in the case of a favorable cost-effectiveness ratio, or if there is no better or more cost-effective alternative (e.g., clinical tests, biochemical tests).

— Presymptomatic diagnostic testing if there is a familial implication and if a prevention program for children is available

— Obtaining information about the prognosis, the possible progression, and therapeutic options, insofar as these are relevant in childhood and only if there is a good correlation between genotype and phenotype

— Determining the risk for the family when molecular genetic testing is required or when important information is provided for subsequent examinations (including prenatal tests)

11.3   Nondirective Counseling

The aims of many medical treatments are concurrently evident to the physician and the patient, and the patient generally authorizes the physician to decide the best course of action. Such is the case, for example, with pain relief or emergency treatment after an accident. By contrast, many decisions in genetic counseling are difficult and closely tied to personal values. Genetic counseling aims at providing the patient with enough information to be "a specialist for his or her own disease." Once equipped with the necessary medical information and an understanding of potential risks and benefits, the patient should be able to decide on the correct course of action. The consultand, not the physician, decides whether or not to do predictive testing or prenatal diagnostic testing, or whether or not to terminate a pregnancy. As far as ethical considerations permit, the **autonomy of the patient** should never be questioned. An important aspect of genetic counseling, therefore, is its **nondirectiveness**. Genetic counseling should impart knowledge and competence; the decision of the consultand should not be influenced by the personal opinion or the value judgment of the counselor. Absolute nondirective counseling, however, is impossible because even the selection of various terms reflects the judgment of the counselor (e.g., "grave," "unfortunately," "hopefully," "risk," "chance," "probability"), yet it should remain the objective of the entire counseling process. In this context, the physician can facilitate the consultand's requests yet is still bound by the standards of clinical practice, medical ethics, evidence-based medicine, and the law.

12 The Diagnostic Approach for a Child with Multiple Anomalies or Dysmorphic Features

LEARNING OBJECTIVES

1. Describe the elements of a genetics medical history and physical examination, and apply these to the evaluation of patients.

2. Construct a three-generation pedigree using approved symbols.

3. Become familiar with various resources for genetic conditions, including public and commercially available databases.

4. Following the assessment of physical characteristics and medical and family history, determine which patients would benefit from a clinical genetics evaluation.

A clinical geneticist is often one of the first of several specialists called to evaluate a newborn with multiple congenital anomalies with or without dysmorphic features. Likewise, when two or more systems are involved in the medical history of an individual, the expertise of a clinical geneticist is often sought to help the team arrive at an underlying diagnosis. **Dysmorphology** is the discipline within human genetics that deals with recognizable physical anomalies that are outside the normal spectrum of human morphology or outside what is expected in a family. The objective of any examination for dysmorphisms or multiple anomalies is to identify and interpret the **pattern of structural abnormalities** in order to arrive at a correct diagnosis. The medical literature describes thousands of distinct syndromes, many of which are rare and familiar only to the human geneticist. However, it is important that all physicians recognize when to include a genetic syndrome in the differential diagnosis, obtain specific diagnostic evaluations, and consult a clinical geneticist.

12.1 Medical History

A comprehensive medical history is the key to diagnosing any medical condition. The clinical genetic history consists of a comprehensive synopsis of the patient's own medical history, including pregnancy, the perinatal period, developmental milestones, development of body measurements, etc. Most importantly, it pays special attention to the family history. Genetic disorders are often complex, as they typically affect more than one organ system of the affected person. An **open-ended or semistructured interview technique** is particularly suited for the investigation of human genetic medical history and uses targeted questions to discern the presence or absence of multiple miscarriages, childhood deaths, early-onset cancer, intellectual disability, and psychiatric disorders. Also to be noted are seemingly unrelated symptoms and abnormalities.

Progression and Pathogenesis. The objective of a medical history is to obtain a complete account of the progression of the disease so that the possible factors causing the disease can be identified. This pathophysiological diagnostic aspect of clinical genetics focuses especially on the progression of symptoms. It is important to note not only the existence of a certain clinical phenomenon but also **when** and **how** it developed.

A particular objective of clinical genetics is the diagnosis of children with developmental disorders in or out of the context of a specific or well-known genetic syndrome. Attaining the medical history involves searching for clues that support or refute primary genetic factors of pathogenesis as well as other exogenous factors that could have contributed to the clinical picture. The questioning should focus on exogenous influences that occurred before and during pregnancy (e.g., diseases and infections, medications, trauma, drugs). The following list of the components of a medical history applies primarily to diagnostic questioning in childhood (e.g., the case of a child with etiologically undefined developmental delay and learning disabilities).

A genetic medical history should address the following basic elements:

- Major symptoms and parental concern
- Pregnancy
  - The mother's and father's age at conception
  - Maternal complications (e.g., fever, infection, rashes, bleeding), chronic or acute diseases (e.g., diabetes, preterm labor), hospitalizations
  - Teratogenic exposures (e.g., medications, smoking, alcohol, drugs), special diets, folic acid, vitamins
  - Fetal development (e.g., ultrasonography), amniotic fluid level during pregnancy, onset of first fetal movements (normal: first pregnancy, during week 20; second and subsequent pregnancies, between weeks 16 and 20)
  - Prenatal diagnostics, including indications for testing and the results (e.g., maternal serum screening, ultrasonography, amniocentesis, chorionic villus sampling)
- Perinatal period
  - Gestation age, mode of delivery, complications at birth, Apgar scores
  - Birth weight, length, head circumference
- Neonatal period (activity, muscle tone, feeding)
  - Complications (e.g., prolonged jaundice, convulsions, apnea, fever)
  - Age at discharge from hospital, noting reason for prolonged hospital stay
  - Results of newborn screenings for hearing and metabolic studies
- Development
  - Progression of weight, length, and fronto-occipital circumference (FOC) measurements (does growth parallel the percentile curves?)
  - Milestones of motor development (e.g., head control, sitting, standing, walking, etc.)
  - Expressive language development (e.g., cooing, babbling, first words, first sentences)
  - Receptive language (following one-step, two-step, and complex commands)
  - Communication skills (verbalization vs. manual signing vs. gesturing to make wants known)
  - Bonding and social development
  - Behavior problems (e.g., sleep disturbances, autistic behavior, self-injurious behavior, repetitive movements)
  - Formative and therapeutic measures (e.g., nursery school/school, physiotherapy, exercise therapy, speech therapy)
  - Early childhood intervention (e.g., oral-motor therapy, physical therapy)
- Special diseases, functional disorders
  - Neuromuscular problems (e.g., convulsions, ataxia, weakness)
  - Hearing, vision
  - Organ function disorders (e.g., heart, kidney, gastrointestinal tract)
- Health and test results
  - General physical condition
  - Physicians involved in patient's care
  - Hospitalizations and discharge diagnoses
  - Surgical history
  - Diagnostic imaging (e.g., echocardiogram, magnetic resonance imaging [MRI])
  - Various laboratory tests (e.g., complete blood count [CBC], thyroid function)

12.2   Family Medical History and Pedigree Analysis

A thorough family medical history is an essential component of any genetic consultation. This involves creating a standardized, complete family pedigree over at least three generations, including details on age, relationship, diseases, age at death, causes of death, and

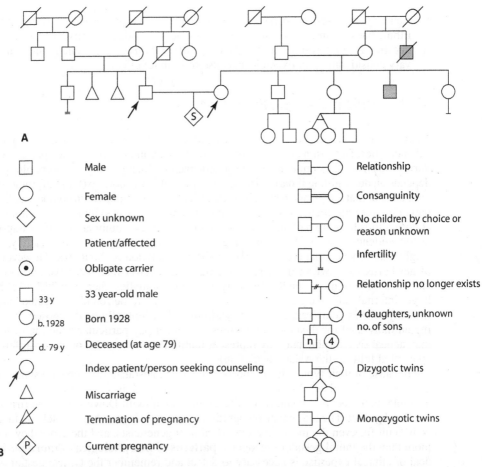

A

☐	Male	☐—○ Relationship
○	Female	☐═○ Consanguinity
◇	Sex unknown	☐⊤○ No children by choice or reason unknown
▨	Patient/affected	☐⊥○ Infertility
⊙	Obligate carrier	☐⫽○ Relationship no longer exists
☐ 33 y	33 year-old male	☐—○ 4 daughters, unknown no. of sons
○ b. 1928	Born 1928	n ④
▨ d. 79 y	Deceased (at age 79)	☐—○ Dizygotic twins
↗○	Index patient/person seeking counseling	
△	Miscarriage	☐—○ Monozygotic twins
⊿	Termination of pregnancy	
◇P	Current pregnancy	

B

□ **Figure 12.1. Creation of a Pedigree. A.** A couple expecting their first child arrives for counseling. Noteworthy in the wife's family history is a diagnosis of Duchenne muscular dystrophy in her brother and in a deceased uncle on the mother's side. The husband's family history includes infertility in a brother; the husband's mother had two miscarriages. **B.** The pedigree is created according to international recommendations. (From Bennett R.L., et al., 2008. PMID 18792771.)

other possibly relevant information. Of special importance are similarly affected siblings, miscarriages, or stillbirths from previous pregnancies, as well as diseases or other health risks among the parents.

International standards should be followed when creating a pedigree (□ Fig. 12.1). It is suggested to start with the indexed patient or the consultand and then proceed on both sides of the family over three generations. The consultands are marked with an arrow. For couples, one usually lists the men (and the paternal family line) on the left and the women (and the maternal line) on the right. Siblings in a family are listed chronologically by birth from left to right. The symbols for affected individuals are shaded.

Important aspects that should be questioned in the course of an assessment of family medical history include:

- Miscarriages, stillbirths, or infant deaths (possibly an indication of an unbalanced chromosomal complement)
- Instances of physical or intellectual disabilities and/or distinctive physical characteristic(s)
- If the couple is childless, is this intentional or unintentional (indication of infertility due to a possible unbalanced chromosomal complement)?
- Similarly affected family member

— Consanguinity—are the parents related to each other (i.e., do they share a common ancestor)?
— Ethnic background of the various family branches (aside from possible consanguinity, this question is of interest because allele frequency within certain ethnic groups can sometimes vary considerably, for example, because of founder effects)

12.3   Clinical Genetic Examination

Perceptiveness Breeds Success. Genetic conditions often manifest clinically with morphological anomalies. Detection and interpretation of these anomalies represent a particular challenge during the physical examination of the genetic patient. Recognizing dysmorphology syndromes depends on determining if particular features are within the normal (familial) range of variation or outside of that range, and hence, **dysmorphic**. It is also important to compare individual body parts directly with their corresponding counterpart to assess symmetry. Often the individual abnormalities have no pathological significance, but their combination offers important diagnostic evidence. The incidence of a single, minor abnormality (e.g., clinodactyly, epicanthus, single transverse palmar crease) in the newborn population is about 30%. However, only 10% of newborns have two or more such anomalies and fewer than 4% have three or more. If a child has three or more small, externally apparent anomalies, there is a 20% likelihood that a larger internal defect (e.g., cardiac or renal anomaly) will be found in targeted examinations. In many of these children, a genetic syndrome will eventually be diagnosed. When evaluating an individual for dysmorphic features, one must pay particular attention to features that may appear dysmorphic but only represent familial characteristics or ethnic differences (e.g., epicanthal folds in the Asian population).

Because of their typical facial morphology (e.g., gestalt), some genetic syndromes can be diagnosed at first glance by an experienced geneticist and, in some cases, a nonphysician. For example, many people would recognize an individual with Down syndrome (trisomy 21) by the facial gestalt. The immediate recognition of rarer syndromes based solely on facial features is difficult for even the most experienced clinical geneticists, and therefore they must rely on more than the initial gestalt to recognize **patterns of morphological abnormalities**. A great deal of clinical expertise is necessary to detect and remember the typical gestalt of rare dysmorphism syndromes.

Time Will Tell? The clinical picture of some congenital disorders can change considerably during the course of a lifetime. An example is neurofibromatosis type 1 (Section 32.6): a newborn with NF1 may have no stigmata of the condition or only a few café au lait macules. The neurofibromas and the pathognomonic Lisch nodules of the iris develop over time and may not be evident until later in childhood or adolescence. In making the diagnosis, it can be helpful to utilize photographic evidence taken over time in the context of, for example, yearly examinations. Genetic dysmorphism syndromes also show changes in facial abnormalities over the course of the child's development; geneticists have termed this phenomenon as "growing into" (or out of) a typical gestalt.

Systematically and with a Tape Measure. Although a gestalt can be a helpful first indication, the clinician must record specific features in the medical record in a systematic manner that is understandable and interpretable to other clinicians caring for the patient. The initial evaluation must include a complete physical examination so that morphological abnormalities are not overlooked. Once an abnormality is seen, a system-based approach to the examination is used to determine if other related features are present. An example of an appropriate time to use this strategy is when abnormal fingernails are noticed during an examination of the hand. This feature directs the physician's attention to other ectodermal-derived structures, such as hair, skin, teeth, and sweat glands. All abnormalities should be described and photographed. Photos are also helpful when quantifying facial measures; in such cases the photograph should include a measuring scale (special attention should be paid to placing it in the same plane as the body part). Of particular importance are the interpupillary distance that could possibly indicate hyper- or hypotelorism as well as the intercanthal distance that, if enlarged, indicates

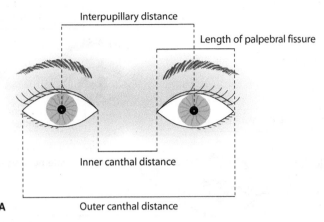

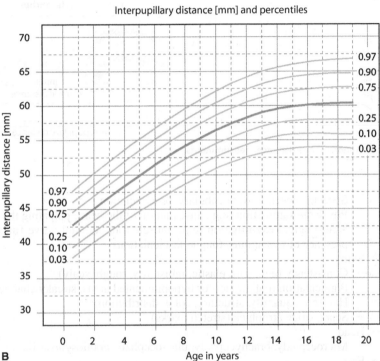

Interpupillary distance

Length of palpebral fissure

Inner canthal distance

A   Outer canthal distance

Interpupillary distance [mm] and percentiles

Interpupillary distance [mm]

0.97
0.90
0.75
0.25
0.10
0.03

B   Age in years

🔲 **Figure 12.2. Distance between the Eyes. A.** Distance measurements between the eyes. **B.** Interpupillary distance in childhood. (From MacLachland C. and Howland H.C., 2002. PMID 12090630.)

a telecanthus (🔲 Figs. 12.2 and 12.3). Percentile curves for the various measurements are available (Fig. 12.2B).

The skin, hair, fingernails, and teeth require special attention (e.g., spots of hyperpigmentation or hypopigmentation in the skin). The latter are readily detectable if the child is examined in a dark room with an ultraviolet (UV) lamp. In young girls, skin changes (such as hyperpigmentation) with a typical distribution along a **dermatome** are indicators of an X-chromosome anomaly that, according to the **Lyon hypothesis**, may be expressed in some dermatomes and not in others.

A clinical-genetic examination should contain the following basic elements:
- General
  - Length (or height), weight, body mass index (BMI), head circumference
  - Behavior, communication, interaction, activity

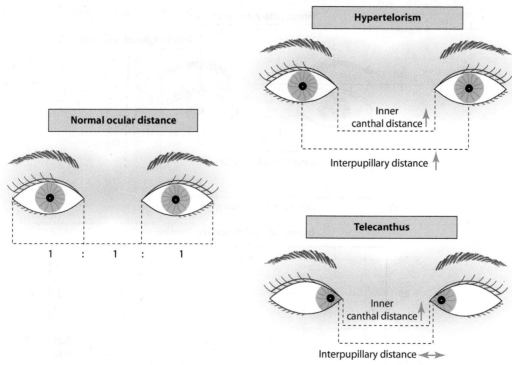

□ Figure 12.3. Abnormal eye-distance measurements.

- — Speech: speech flow, vocabulary, pronunciation
- — Physical examination (e.g., auscultation of the heart, palpating the abdomen)
- — Neurological examination (e.g., muscle tone, cranial nerve function, reflexes, gait, presence of nystagmus, tongue fasciculations)
- — Skin
  - — Consistency (e.g., soft, elastic, moist, dry, rough, scaly)
  - — Pigmentation (e.g., hyper- or hypopigmented areas, streaky changes)
  - — Hair (e.g., quantity, structure, color, distribution)
  - — Scars, striae atrophica (stretch marks)
- — Head
  - — Microcephaly, brachycephaly, plagiocephaly, craniosynostosis
- — Face
  - — Profile (e.g., flat)
  - — Midsection (e.g., hypoplastic)
  - — Jaw/chin (e.g., micrognathia, prognathia, retrognathia)
- — Eyes
  - — Interpupillary and intercanthal distance (e.g., hyper- or hypotelorism, telecanthus)
  - — Eye folds (e.g., epicanthus)
  - — Palpebral fissures (upslanting or downslanting)
  - — Size (e.g., microphthalmia)
  - — Sclera (e.g., blue)
  - — Iris (e.g., color anomalies, heterochromia, coloboma, Lisch nodules, Brushfield spots)
  - — Eyelashes, eyebrows (e.g., fused eyebrows [synophrys], laterally thinned or sparse)
- — Nose
  - — Shape
  - — Root of the nose (e.g., flat, depressed, prominent, broad)
  - — Nares (e.g., anteverted)

- Philtrum
  - Length
  - Structure (e.g., prominent, smooth)
- Mouth
  - Size
  - Lips (e.g., thin, prominent, pigmentary anomalies, pits)
  - Palate (e.g., high arched, frank or submucous cleft, cleft uvula)
  - Teeth (e.g., number, spacing, structure)
- Ears
  - Position, rotation (e.g., low set, posteriorly rotated)
  - Pre- or retroauricular tags, pits, creases
- Neck
  - Length, shape (e.g., pterygium)
  - Hairline (e.g., low, inverse)
- Trunk
  - Shape of ribcage (e.g., pectus excavatum, pectus carinatum)
  - Nipples (number, shape [e.g., inverted], distance)
  - Fat accumulation and distribution
  - Sacral dimples
- Arms, legs
  - Length, flexure, symmetry
  - Proximal/distal proportionality
  - Joints (e.g., hypermobility, contractures)
- Hands, feet
  - Size, length
  - Shape (e.g., position, sandal gap)
  - Palmar creases (e.g., single transverse palmar crease)
  - Fingers and toes (e.g., syndactyly, polydactyly, clinodactyly, contractures)
  - Nails (e.g., hypoplastic, brittle, abnormal pigmentation)
- Genitals
  - Anatomy (e.g., ambiguous, hypospadias)
  - Size and proportionality (e.g., hypoplastic, clitoral hypertrophy)
  - Testes (e.g., size, location, whether they are descended)

12.4 Behavioral Abnormalities

Several genetic disorders manifest with specific behavioral phenotypes. For example, individuals with Smith-Magenis syndrome have sleep disturbances with multiple and often prolonged nocturnal awakenings and excessive daytime sleepiness associated with an aberrant circadian rhythm of melatonin secretion. Individuals with Williams syndrome tend to be very loquacious, a personality feature that leads the examiner to overestimate their cognitive abilities, while those with Angelman syndrome are typically nonverbal. A rather unspecific characteristic is autistic behavior or autistic behavior traits, which are present with several genetic diseases including fragile X syndrome. Some behavioral abnormalities are so typical that they count among the diagnostic criteria, and their absence renders a diagnosis questionable. An example is the self-mutilating behavior in Lesch-Nyhan syndrome. An overview of genetic diseases with specific behavior pathologies is provided in ◘ Table 12.1.

12.5 Additional Examinations

The medical history and the physical examination can be sufficient for the physician to suspect causes of genetic disorders and to order specific laboratory tests (e.g., fluorescence in situ hybridization [FISH] for a specific region of the genome, targeted DNA analysis, or enzyme

▢ Table 12.1. Genetic Diseases with Specific Behavior Abnormalities

Disease	Behavior Abnormalities
Fragile X syndrome	Autism (60%), hyperactivity, lack of eye contact (90%), fearful-aggressive behavior, abnormal hand movements (flapping)
Rett syndrome	Stereotypical hand movements (washing and kneading), respiratory problems (e.g., hyperventilation, apnea, Valsalva, etc.), autistic behavior, bruxism, sleep disturbances
Smith-Magenis syndrome	Temper tantrums even in older children and young adults (i.e., out of proportion to cognitive level), self-hugging behavior when pleased, self-injurious behavior (e.g., head banging, hand biting, nail ripping and extraction), severe sleep disturbances
Lesch-Nyhan syndrome	Distinct and severe self-mutilating behavior (e.g., biting, scratching) with seemingly normal pain tolerance
Angelman syndrome	Ataxic gait, happy demeanor and frequently unprovoked laughter, hyperactivity, excitability, short attention span, lack of speech in severely affected individuals
Prader-Willi syndrome	Hyperphagia, constant feeling of hunger, lethargy, sleep disturbances, obsessive-compulsive behavior, temper tantrums, stubbornness, unusual skill with jigsaw puzzles. Patients can be extremely resourceful in their search for food.
Williams syndrome	Hyperactivity, highly verbal ("cocktail party personality"), sociable, lack respect of personal space boundaries, excessive empathy, hoarse voice, sensitivity to noise, keen musical ability
Velocardiofacial syndrome	Hypernasal voice, schizophrenia, bipolar disorder, and anxiety disorder in adults

analysis for certain metabolic diseases). Should a syndrome be suspected yet an etiology not determined, the following studies may aid in the determination of an underlying diagnosis:

- Testing the structure and function of the viscera (e.g., abdominal ultrasound, echocardiogram)
- Brain MRI for children with microcephaly or neurological abnormalities
- Radiographic examination (e.g., complete skeletal survey with hands and feet, bone age)
- Some metabolic disorders have dysmorphisms as major symptoms (e.g., lysosomal storage diseases, peroxisomal disorders, disruptions of sterol synthesis, and congenital disorders of glycosylation). The indication for metabolic analyses therefore depends on the clinical presentation. Blood lactate should be analyzed on more than one occasion if a primary disorder of energy metabolism is suspected.
- Array comparative genomic hybridization for all children with ill-defined dysmorphisms
- Routine G-banded chromosome analysis, which is still useful in the evaluation for infertility and multiple spontaneous abortions, as it represents the best test to detect balanced translocations

Databases

Databases offer valuable help for the diagnosis and management of syndromic conditions. The following resources are routinely used by clinical geneticists and basic scientists interested in human disease:

- OMIM (*Online Mendelian Inheritance in Man*, www.ncbi.nlm.nih.gov/omim)

- GeneClinics (www.geneclinics.org)
- The London Dysmorphology Database (commercial database)
- POSSUM (*Pictures of Standard Syndromes and Undiagnosed Malformations*, commercial database)

Important

The following advice is given to all future "syndromologists":

- It is extremely important to always use the correct terminology. The individual symptoms may be very similar, yet the underlying developmental biological mechanisms may be totally different. For example, an **omphalocele** remains if, during the 10th week of gestation, the intestinal loops are not retracted from the umbilical cord into the abdominal cavity. The result is a membrane-covered sac with intestinal content, from whose center the umbilical cord arises. **Gastroschisis** is also a prolapse of the viscera of the abdominal cavity through a defect of the anterior abdominal wall. The defect, however, is located lateral to the umbilicus, and the prolapsed intestine is not covered by a membrane. Pathogenetically this is probably caused by a unilateral migration defect of abdominal wall cells. In contrast to omphalocele, gastroschisis is not associated with chromosomal anomalies or other serious malformations.
- Should a child have multiple anomalies, those that are rarely observed are especially meaningful. In most cases they have a much higher specificity, which is especially important when searching a database for the correct diagnosis. Hypertelorism is part of numerous syndromes and therefore not very specific. Ambiguous genitalia, however, is a rare condition and would be useful to enter as the main criterion of the search.
- Rather than making a false diagnosis, it is better not to make any diagnosis at all. We frequently meet patients who manifest multiple anomalies that we fail to add up to a "meaningful whole" (i.e., a diagnosis). A wrong diagnosis can have negative consequences for the patient and the family—wrong risk calculation in genetic counseling, wrong projections for life expectancy, and, in the worst-case scenario, the wrong therapy.

13 Malformations and Other Morphological Disturbances

LEARNING OBJECTIVES

1 Distinguish between the four categories of morphological defects (malformation, deformation, disruption, and dysplasia), and give an example of each.

2 Define the terms *sequence*, *association*, and *syndrome* as they relate to the etiology of genetic disease, and give an example of each.

3 List the four major groups of teratogens. Give an example of each teratogen group, and state at least two common features of each.

Abnormal anatomic development is the result of one or more pathogenically distinct processes, each resulting from a different mechanism and categorized by the genetic and embryologic bases of the disturbance. Important distinctions include:

— Whether a morphological disturbance is caused endogenously (genetically) or exogenously

— Whether it is an isolated occurrence or an occurrence in combination with other changes

— Whether it is a one-time disturbance or a chronic cell function disorder

When evaluating morphological differences in newborns, these distinctions should be taken into consideration, and an attempt should be made to determine when in early development the disturbance occurred.

13.1 Embryology

Human prenatal development has three phases:

— The **preimplantation and implantation phase**, which occurs from ovulation and fertilization until the end of the second week postconception (p.c.)

— The **embryonic period**, which occurs from the third to the eighth week p.c.

— The **fetal period**, which occurs from the ninth week p.c. until birth

> **Important**
>
> By convention, a pregnancy or gestation begins on the first day of the mother's last menstrual period. The first week postconception (p.c.) is referred to as the third gestational week, or the third week of pregnancy (postmenstruation [p.m.]).

Preimplantation and Implantation Phase

The fertilization of an egg cell occurs in the ampulla of the fallopian tube within 6 to 12 hours after ovulation. Fertilization results in the completion of meiosis II in the egg cell and the re-establishment of a diploid chromosomal complement. The conceptus (now called a **zygote**) undergoes a number of cell divisions within the fallopian tube and reaches the uterine cavity as a solid ball of cells called a **morula**. The differentiation of a morula into a **blastocyst** involves the loss of the zona pellucida and the development of a blastocyst cavity. The blastocyst differentiates further into an inner cell mass from which the embryo develops (**embryoblast**), and an outer cell mass from which the trophoblast originates. Between the fifth and sixth days, the blastocyst makes contact with the uterine mucosa and continues to penetrate into the endometrial wall during the second week of pregnancy. At the end of the second week, a simple uteroplacental cycle develops.

> **Important**
>
> The preimplantation and implantation phase are ruled by the **all-or-nothing principle**. Disturbances and defects that occur during this early phase of embryogenesis are inevitably fatal.

Embryonic Period

The embryonic phase spans the third to the eighth week p.c. At this time, all organ primordia are formed (organogenesis), and the external appearance of the embryo changes considerably. At the end of the second month p.c., much of the final body shape is recognizable. Most major malformations can be traced back to this developmentally important time period (◻ Fig. 13.1).

The formation of the germ layers, a process termed **gastrulation**, marks the beginning of the embryonic period. Three germ layers are formed: the ectoderm (exterior germ layer), the mesoderm (middle germ layer), and the endoderm (interior germ layer).

The **ectoderm** gives rise to the central and peripheral nervous systems; the sensory epithelium of the ear, nose, and eye; the epidermis and all its appendages; the pituitary gland; the mammary glands; and the dental enamel.

The **mesoderm** develops as an ectodermal fold from the region of the primitive streak and positions itself between the ectoderm and endoderm. The segmental structuring of the body originates from somites in the mesoderm. Myotomes differentiate into horizontally striated muscle fibers, sclerotomes differentiate into vertebrae and ribs, and dermatomes differentiate into skin segments, dermis, and subcutaneous tissue. The mesoderm also develops the loose, embryonic

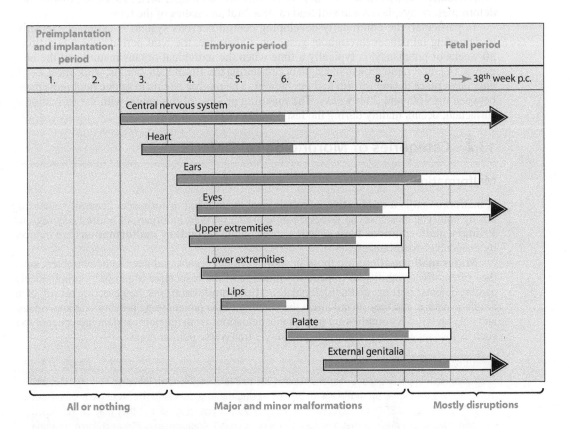

Blue bars indicate high sensitivity toward teratogens.

◻ **Figure 13.1. Milestones of Embryonic Development and Sensitivity to Teratogens.** The colored bands indicate particular sensitivities. (Modified from Clayton-Smith and Donnai 2002.)

connective tissue (mesenchyme), all of the remaining bones and cartilage, the pleura and peritoneum, the entire vascular and urogenital system, the adrenal glands, and the spleen.

The **endoderm** develops into the epithelial lining of the gastrointestinal tract, respiratory tract, bladder, tympanic cavity, and eustachian tube. Also of endodermal origin is the parenchyma of the tonsils, thyroid and parathyroid glands, thymus, liver, and pancreas.

During the third week p.c., the mesodermal notochord induces **neurulation** with the formation of the neural tube, which later differentiates into the brain and the spinal cord. The cranial end of the neural tube, called the anterior neuropore, closes on the 25th day p.c., and the caudal end (i.e., the posterior neuropore) 2 days later, on day 27. The large spectrum of neural tube defects, from anencephaly to spina bifida occulta (see Chapter 31, Fig. 31.4), originates from disturbances during neurulation.

The **neural crest** forms in the transition zones between the closing neural tube and the ectoderm. Cells of the neural crest travel laterally into the mesoderm, where they form segments that are induced by dermomyotomes. They form the spinal ganglia and the medulla of the adrenal glands, differentiate into melanocytes and Schwann cells, and play a role in the formation of the endocardial expansions in the conus and truncus regions of the heart. They travel ventrally into the pharyngeal arches and rostrally into the forebrain, eye sockets, and facial regions, where they form bones and connective tissues of the middle face and the pharyngeal arches. Migration disturbances of the neural crest cells are found in a multitude of dysmorphism syndromes.

Fetal Period

By the beginning of the fetal period, all organs of the human body have been formed and largely differentiated. At this time, primary dysmorphisms no longer arise. However, disruptions, deformities, or dysplasias can still lead to structural anomalies of the fetus.

In particular, the continually developing central nervous system is extremely sensitive to damaging influences throughout gestation. Otherwise, the fetal period, which constitutes 30 weeks of pregnancy, is typically a time when the individual organs mature and the body grows. The most rapid growth in length occurs during the 4th and 5th months, while most weight gain takes place during the 8th and 9th months. The mother begins to notice fetal movements between the 16th and 20th weeks. The maturing process of the lungs, with the formation of surfactant, occurs mainly during the last 8 weeks of pregnancy.

13.2   Categories of Morphological Defects

Malformation

A malformation is a **qualitative** morphological, primordial disturbance, generally occurring during embryogenesis. It can affect a single organ, parts of an organ, or entire body regions. **Primary malformations** have genetic causes, while **secondary malformations** are induced by exogenous disturbances.

Major malformations are those involving critical organs and need to be corrected, since they often affect viability or impede the function of the respective organ (e.g., omphalocele, cardiac defects, cleft lip, and/or cleft palate). **Minor malformations**, however, are mostly of an aesthetic nature, and they do not affect the viability of the patient (e.g., preauricular appendages and polydactyly). **Anomalies** are measurable deviations from the norm and include phenotypes such as low-set ears, hypertelorism, and single transverse palmar crease.

> **Important**
>
> Functionally important malformations occur in 2% to 3% of all newborns (baseline risk). Another 2% to 3% are diagnosed up to the age of 5 years, raising the total to 4% to 6%. A single anomaly can be found in up to 30% of newborns. Alone, they are not pathological, but they may be associated with other malformations that may be obvious or "occult." Approximately 3% of children with one anomaly also have a major malformation. The risk for having a major malformation increases to 10% when a child has two anomalies and to 20% when a child has three or more anomalies.

Deformation

Deformations are caused by extrinsic factors, including mechanical constraint, that impinge physically on normally developing organs, organ parts, or body regions. This generally occurs during the fetal period after completion of organogenesis. Some examples of relatively common deformations include clubfeet, plagiocephaly (asymmetric craniostenosis), and hip joint dysplasia. Frequent causes of these deformations are structural anomalies of the uterus, abnormal position of the fetus, or oligohydramnios. Oligohydramnios serves to demonstrate that deformations can have intrinsic (e.g., fetal anuria) as well as extrinsic (e.g., amnion rupture) causes. If an intrinsic factor is suspected, further evaluation is warranted, as there may be occult malformations present. Deformations occur in 2% of all newborns. After birth, when the child no longer has to endure the mechanical constraint, mild deformations either resolve spontaneously or can be corrected through physical therapy or the use of prosthetic devices such as orthotics or helmets (as in cases of clubfoot and plagiocephaly, respectively).

Disruption

Disruption impedes the normal development of organs through infection, ischemia, bleeding, or adhesion of injured tissues. Disruptions frequently occur in different tissues within a well-defined anatomical region (□ Fig. 13.2). For example, a breach of the integrity of the amniotic sac can cause strands of amniotic tissue, called *amniotic bands*, which can cause diagonal mouth–face creases that do not coincide with any ontogenetic raphe and simultaneously constrict several tissues (e.g., bones, muscles, and skin), leading to amputation or restriction.

> **Important**
>
> Deformations and disruptions affect structures that originally formed normally. Therefore, they are secondary morphological disturbances. Generally they are not associated with any increased risk of reoccurrence unless they are due to intrinsic causes or structural anomalies of the uterus.

Dysplasia

In contrast to malformations that are temporally and spatially defined, dysplasias are caused by an ongoing disturbance of the development or maturation of a particular tissue due to

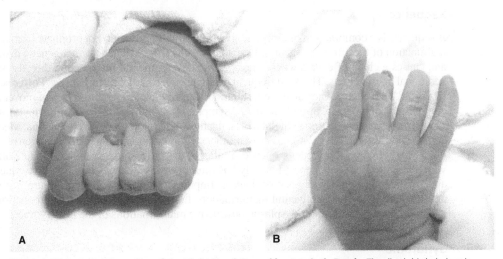

A   B

□ **Figure 13.2. A, B. Disruption of the Right Hand Caused by Amniotic Bands.** The distal third phalanx is constricted, yet not completely amputated by an amniotic band. The distal pharynx of the fourth digit is completely disrupted; no nail is present on this digit. Amniotic bands were noted on the fetal surface of the placenta. (Courtesy of Lorraine Potocki, Department of Molecular and Human Genetics, Baylor College of Medicine and Texas Children's Hospital, Houston.)

persistent cellular malfunction. This manifests itself in the cells' faulty organization, proliferation, differentiation, function, or degeneration, and it results in morphological or histological pathology. A dysplasia does not affect a distinct body region; rather, it affects a particular tissue or cell type. Thus, many dysplasias cause morphological changes throughout the body. Most dysplasias originate from genetic defects. During gene production, these can be enzymes (e.g., lysosomal storage diseases) or structural proteins (e.g., osteogenesis imperfecta). In some cases, the existing germline mutation has to have a second hit to inactivate the other gene copy before dysplasia actually occurs (e.g., neurofibromatosis). This explains why some tissues develop normally, others are dysplastic, and still others become abnormal later in life (e.g., an increasing number of neurofibromas with neurofibromatosis type 1). Additional mutations may continue to change the dynamics of some dysplasias (e.g., malignant degeneration in polyposis coli or neurofibromatosis). Some primary dysplastic disorders, such as Fanconi anemia, are associated with variable malformations caused by a disturbance of embryonal development.

Important

An important characteristic of dysplasia is its continual progression. This clearly differentiates dysplasias from other morphological disturbances, such as malformations, disruptions, and deformations, which are all pathogenetically temporal. They can have a long-term effect on the patient's health, but their progression is neither progressive nor continual. A dysplasia, however, can be lasting and/or progressive, as long as the affected tissue continues to exist and/or to grow.

13.3   Etiology of Multiple Morphological Defects

The occurrence of a distinct combination or pattern of seemingly independent, structural changes in multiple organs can have various causes. Depending on the pathogenesis, these are grouped as sequences, syndromes, or associations. If multiple malformations are present, possible **teratogen exposure** during pregnancy should be considered. A chromosome analysis, or ideally, a **DNA array analysis**, should be performed to exclude structural or numerical chromosomal abnormalities. Moreover, diagnostic imaging should be performed to identify possible **occult malformations**.

Sequence

A sequence is a combination of morphological abnormalities that do not originate from a cellular malfunction of the affected organ(s). Instead, it results from a genetic or nongenetic disturbance and causes a chain of events where one specific, developmental malfunction directly results in additional malfunctions. The most frequent example of this sort of disturbance is **Potter sequence** (◘ Fig. 13.3). It occurs when an extreme amniotic fluid deficiency results in lack of movement and compression of the fetus. Important clinical symptoms are clubfoot and other joint malformations, as well as facial deformation with flat facies, flat nose, and micrognathia/retrognathia. Mechanical compression also inhibits the expansion of the thorax, thus compromising fetal respiration of amniotic fluid. Many children with Potter sequence die after birth from respiratory failure. Oligohydramnios, which leads to Potter sequence, not only has multiple consequences in the Potter sequence but also can be the result of various disturbances. Important causes are amnion rupture, with loss of amniotic fluid or severe urogenital malformations that result in reduced urine production (renal agenesis, renal hypoplasia or dysplasia, obstructive malformations of the urinary tract).

Syndrome

A syndrome, in clinical genetics, is a combination of developmental abnormalities or malformations that share a common etiology. Historically, the term **syndrome** signified that the common origin was unknown (e.g., Down syndrome was named after John Langdon Down many years before the chromosomal etiology was elucidated); however, the term *syndrome* continues to be used

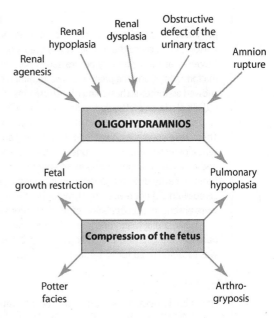

☐ **Figure 13.3. Potter Sequence.** (Modified from Jones 2006.)

in many conditions even after the etiology is discovered. Furthermore, as molecular diagnostic techniques become increasingly robust, many syndromes are now discovered by virtue of their common molecular etiology. The common origin need not be a single-gene defect, but it must include a shared, tightly linked pathogenic pathway (monogenic, chromosomal, epigenetic).

Association

In contrast to a syndrome, which is defined as having a common cause (even when the cause itself is not yet defined), an **association** is defined as a combination of independent malformations in which there is insufficient evidence to support a common pathogenetic basis. Any particular association is characterized by the occurrence of three or more individual malformations at a much greater frequency than would be statistically expected. The particular **pattern of malformations** varies from one association to the next, and patients with the same association often have varied clinical severity. While a pattern of inheritance is not usually discernable, the recurrence risk is typically low (1% to 2%). Establishing a diagnosis of a specific association allows the clinician to proceed with additional studies to search for other, possibly occult, abnormalities common to affected individuals.

■■■ **CHARGE Syndrome**

In many cases, the term **association** is used until the etiology of a disease is clearly established. A good example of this is CHARGE syndrome, a combination of **c**oloboma, cardiac (**h**eart) defects, choanal **a**tresia, mental **r**etardation, **g**enital malformations, and **e**ar anomalies. CHARGE was considered an association until 2004, when mutations in the *CHD7* gene, which encodes for a chromosomal domain helicase, were found in CHARGE patients.

VACTERL Association (VATERR Association)

The name VACTERL is an acronym formed by the first letters of the possible individual symptoms.

Case History

Mr. and Mrs. Forester visit the prenatal genetics clinic, because they terminated a previous pregnancy because of multiple malformations in the fetus. At this time, they want to know their risk of having a similarly affected pregnancy. The previous pregnancy progressed well in the first and second trimesters. An amniocentesis was performed, because the mother was 37 years old. The result was a normal, male chromosome complement. However, as the pregnancy progressed, a polyhydramnios developed. A high-level ultrasound showed many malformations, and the pregnancy was terminated (without genetic counseling). The postmortem examination showed asymmetric shortening of the forearms and anomalous hand shape. Radiographs identified right-sided radial aplasia and left-sided radial shortening, with hypoplasia of the first metacarpal bilaterally. The spinal column had agenesis of the 12th pair of ribs, as well as a synostosis of the 3rd and 4th lumbar vertebrae. There were anomalies in the lungs (asymmetry and hypoplasia of the lobes), in the heart (atrial and ventricular septal defects), and of the urogenital tract (an absence of the kidney, urethra, and renal artery on the left, and an oversized right kidney in an abnormal position). There was herniation of abdominal organs into the thoracic cavity due to a diaphragmatic hernia. A neuropathological examination of the cerebrum and the cerebellum did not reveal any pathological findings. Although tracheal, esophageal, and anal malformations were absent, the constellation of malformations allowed a diagnosis of VACTERL association.

While a diaphragmatic hernia is not a cardinal sign of VACTERL, it is found in 3.5% of the cases. The parents were counseled regarding a 1% to 2% recurrence risk in future pregnancies. A detailed sonography was recommended for all future pregnancies.

Epidemiology

VACTERL occurs as a sporadic combination of several abnormalities, with a frequency of 1 out of 6,000 newborns. Boys are affected twice as often as girls, with a male-to-female ratio of 2.2:1.

Clinical Symptoms

The clinical symptoms are displayed as the beginning letters of the acronym (□ Table 13.1).

Occasionally, the acronyms VATER or VATERR are used. VATER does not include a cardiac defect, while VATERR includes radial dysplasia instead of limb defects. Other more rarely associated malformations are genital anomalies (25%), ear anomalies (20%), single umbilical artery (30%), and cleft lip, jaw, or palate (5%).

There is one distinct familial disease, VACTERL-H syndrome (VACTERL plus hydrocephalus), which is heritable in either an X-linked or autosomal recessive manner. The hydrocephalus is caused by an aqueductal stenosis. The prognosis is poor.

Diagnosis

VACTERL is a **diagnosis by exclusion**, because there is no specific test to confirm the diagnosis. Since some, or all, of the features may be seen in a chromosomal syndrome such as trisomy 13, a chromosome analysis and an array analysis should be performed in patients with findings of VACTERL. Very few affected persons have all seven anomalies as listed in Table 13.1; on average, only three to four of these symptoms occur. **Minimal criteria** include one anomaly

□ **Table 13.1.** Chief Clinical Symptoms of VACTERL Association

		Frequency of Malformation
V	**V**ertebral defects	70%
A	**A**nal atresia (Fig. 13.4)	80%
C	**C**ardiac defects (congenital cardiac defects, mostly ventricular septal defects)	55%
TE	**T**rach**e**oesophageal fistula (esophageal atresia with tracheoesophageal fistulae)	70%
R	**R**enal anomaly (renal malformations)	55%
L	**L**imb defects (malformations of the limbs, such as radial dysplasia, polydactyly, and syndactyly; 25% defects of the lower limb)	65%

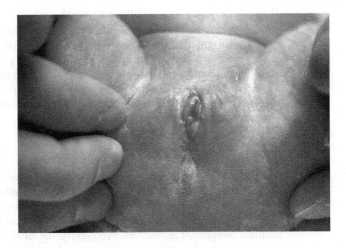

Figure 13.4. Anal Atresia and Hypoplasia of the Labia in a Newborn. (With permission of Universitäts-Kinderklinik Heidelberg.)

in each of the three possible body regions (thorax, limbs, and pelvis/lower abdomen) or at least two anomalies in two of these regions.

Therapy

The management of VACTERL association is complex. Each of the seven pathological malformations could require surgical intervention. Esophageal atresia and anal atresia need to be surgically corrected immediately after birth or within the first 2 days after birth.

Prognosis

The prognosis depends mostly on the severity of the various malformations. Between 5% and 25% of infants born with VACTERL association die within their first year. The prognosis is excellent if all existing malformations can be successfully corrected. These children generally have normal cognitive development.

13.4 Teratogenic Factors

Until the early 1940s, there was no scientific proof that exogenous factors could result in embryonic malformations. Teratology had its beginnings when the Australian ophthalmologist Norman McAlister Gregg found a causal link between rubella in early pregnancy and a typical pattern of abnormalities in the child, including inner ear deafness, cataracts, and cardiac defect. In 1961, the German pediatrician and human geneticist Widukind Lenz observed that thalidomide ingestion caused frequent defective development of the extremities, including phocomelia and amelia. This proved that medications could cross the placenta and cause malformations. To date, numerous additional substances have been identified as teratogens.

Teratogens can be divided into **four major groups:**
- Intrauterine infections
- Medications and drugs
- Physical causes
- Maternal metabolic diseases

Research and clinical studies have provided several general principles for the mechanism of action of teratogens:
- **Dosage:** The greater the dose of a teratogen and the longer the duration of its action, the greater the effect.
- **Sensitive phase:** The sensitivity to a teratogen depends on the developmental phase. Most organs go through developmental phases, during which they are especially vulnerable to

exogenous disturbances (Fig. 13.1). The most sensitive is the phase of organogenesis (i.e., the embryonic stage between the third and eighth weeks of gestation).

— **Genetic constitution:** Sensitivity to a teratogen depends on the genetic constitution of the organism. It was shown that mothers who had given birth to one child with fetal alcohol syndrome had a much higher risk of recurrence than mothers—with equal or comparable alcohol ingestion during pregnancy—who had previously given birth to a healthy child.

— **Specificity:** Each teratogen affects the cell in a specific way, resulting in a specific anomaly depending on the organ's predisposition.

Intrauterine Infections

Most teratogenic infectious diseases do not cause substantial signs or symptoms in an immunocompetent adult or child, yet often have devastating effects in the fetus when the mother is first exposed during her pregnancy. Although intrauterine infections are not genetic, they cause congenital anomalies in the fetus, so they are an important differential in a newborn with multiple congenital anomalies. Frequently, the mothers contract the infection from their own older children who attend playgroups or school. An exception is toxoplasmosis, which is typically contracted when a previously unexposed mother cleans the litter box of the family cat. When evaluating for congenital exposure to a pathological organism, the following questions should be considered:

— Are there antibodies that indicate an acute infection?
— During which week of pregnancy did the exposure occur?
— How likely is it that the infection will affect fetal development?

The most important infections are detected by **TORCH analysis** (an acronym for **to**xoplasmosis, **r**ubella, **c**ytomegalovirus infections, and **h**erpes simplex). If an intrauterine infection is suspected, TORCH titer analysis should be done as soon possible after birth to confirm an infection and causal link with the virus (an assay performed after the neonatal period cannot distinguish with certainty between pre- and postnatal infections).

Congenital Rubella Syndrome. The rubella virus is transmitted through the placenta during the viremia of first infections of pregnant women. The risk of congenital anomalies is up to 85% if the mother has her first infection (with manifest exanthema) within the first 12 weeks of pregnancy (p.m.). There is a 50% risk between the 13th and 16th weeks of pregnancy (p.m.) and a 25% risk toward the end of the second trimester. Congenital rubella syndrome frequently results in spontaneous miscarriage or stillbirth. If the embryo is infected before the completion of organogenesis, this typically results in a combination of sensorineural hearing loss, cardiac defects (typically pulmonary stenosis), eye abnormalities (cataracts, microphthalmia, and "salt and pepper retinopathy"), microcephaly, and growth retardation.

The MMR (measles, mumps, rubella) vaccine is a standard vaccine for all children in the United States and Europe. Completion of vaccination schedules before childbearing protects fetuses from congenital infections. Successful immunization is confirmed by a protective titer (greater than 1:32) and ideally should be confirmed prior to conception. Active immunization during pregnancy is contraindicated.

Cytomegalovirus Infection. Congenital cytomegalovirus (CMV) is usually caused by a primary infection of the pregnant woman. In 40% of cases, this results in a fetal infection during viremia. Approximately 15% of these children will manifest clinical pathologies. The risk of a fetal infection is higher during the first half of pregnancy. Characteristic symptoms of congenital CMV are microcephaly, intracerebral calcifications, blindness and retinochoroiditis, hepatosplenomegaly, and, sometimes, typical dental enamel defects.

Toxoplasmosis. Only if the first infection occurs in the mother during pregnancy will parasitemia be harmful to the fetus. The mother can be infected by ingestion of insufficiently cooked meat, contact with family pets (especially cats), or contact with dirt that is contaminated with feces. The risk of fetal infection is higher in later pregnancy. In the first trimester the risk is 15%, in the second trimester 45%, and in the third trimester 70%. However, the fetal symptoms are milder when the infection occurs later in pregnancy. Classic symptoms are the triad of encephalitis (with intracerebral calcifications and hydrocephalus), retinochoroiditis, and hepatitis. A suspected toxoplasma infection of a pregnant woman should be treated immediately with appropriate antibiotics.

Varicella. A primary varicella-zoster virus infection of the mother poses a risk of approximately 2% of fetal viremia with teratogenic effects. The highest risk is between week 13 and 20 of gestation (p.m.). Among the typical abnormalities are microcephaly, muscular atrophy, microphthalmia, malformations of the extremities (various types of hypoplasia), and skin anomalies, including scars, blisters, and epidermal hypoplasias.

Parvovirus B19. Infections with parvovirus B19, causing erythema infectiosum in children, are frequently asymptomatic in adults. If a pregnant woman and her fetus become infected, the fetus may have serious consequences such as anemia, hydrops fetalis, and possibly intrauterine fetal death. Between 25% and 50% of maternal primary infections that occur during pregnancy also result in fetal viremia. Hydrops fetalis develops in a small percentage of cases. Additional symptoms may be myocarditis, myositis, and arthrogryposis.

Medications and Drugs

Thalidomide. Between 1959 and 1962, thalidomide was available in many countries as an over-the-counter sedative. Since it was especially effective in combating morning sickness, it was often used during the first months of pregnancy. It took several years to notice that there was a dramatic increase in developmental defects of the extremities (e.g., phocomelia and amelia) in children whose mothers had taken thalidomide during early pregnancy (◘ Fig. 13.5). More than 10,000 children worldwide were affected. The risk of deformities from exposure was approximately 20%. Fetuses were particularly vulnerable when their mothers ingested thalidomide between days 35 and 50 p.m. The type of deformity closely correlated with the day the medication was taken. For example, typical peromelia occurred with ingestion between days 38 and 40 p.m., duodenal atresia correlated with ingestion between days 41 and 43 p.m., and cardiac developmental defects occurred with ingestion between days 43 and 47 p.m. The clinical picture of fetal thalidomide syndrome can be a phenocopy of the autosomal dominant condition known as **Holt-Oram syndrome** (e.g., phocomelia limited to the upper extremities, radial aplasia, cardiac defects, and normal intelligence; ◘ Fig. 13.6). It can also be a phenocopy of the autosomal recessive Roberts syndrome (e.g., phocomelia of all extremities, but also small stature; cleft lip or palate; and psychomotor developmental disturbances).

Peromelia: Congenital malformation of a limb (general term).

Amelia: Absence of a limb.

Phocomelia: Extreme shortening of the long bones of a limb, with a hand or foot close to the shoulder or hip.

Sirenomelia: The fusion of the legs, creating the appearance of a mermaid's tail

Phenocopy: A particular phenotype that is caused by exogenous factors (such as teratogens) and resembles the phenotype caused by genetic factors (such as a monogenic disorder).

Coumarins. Coumarins (e.g., warfarin and Marcumar®) are vitamin K antagonists that are used in the prevention of thromboembolic events. Coumarins, if taken during pregnancy, can lead to fetal defects, including disproportionately short stature, limb reduction defects, a hypoplastic nose, eye defects (e.g., cataracts and microphthalmia), and epiphyseal stippling. Coumarin embryopathy is a phenocopy of Conradi-Hünermann syndrome (e.g., chondrodysplasia punctata, X-chromosome dominant variant) (see Section 26.2).

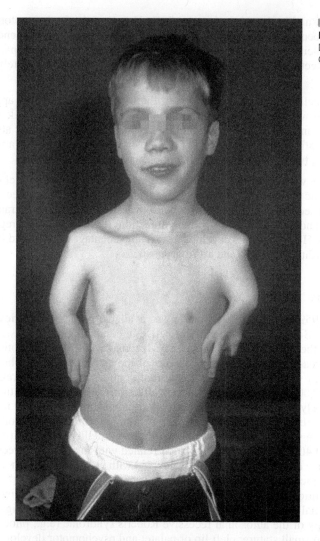

Figure 13.5. Thalidomide Embryopathy. (Courtesy of Hj Müller, Department of Medical Genetics, University Children's Hospital, Basel, Switzerland.)

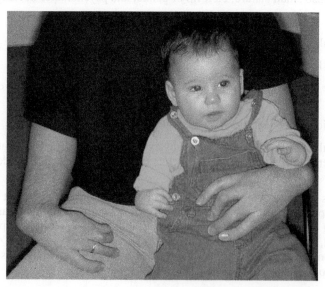

Figure 13.6. Holt-Oram Syndrome in Father and Son. The autosomal dominant malformation syndrome is an important differential diagnosis for radial developmental defects. Intelligence is normal.

> **Important**
>
> Phenocopies of medication-induced embryopathies:
> - Thalidomide embryopathy: Holt-Oram syndrome, Roberts syndrome
> - Coumarin embryopathy: Conradi-Hünermann syndrome

Antiepileptics. Children of mothers who suffer from epilepsy that requires treatment have a two- to threefold higher risk for malformations as compared to the general population. This risk is higher in women treated with antiepileptics but also exists when the mother is not taking medications during the pregnancy. The possible causes of the embryopathy are toxic epoxide metabolites and deficiencies of vitamin B_{12} and folic acid. If the mother is treated with phenobarbital, phenytoin, or carbamazepine during the entire pregnancy, the child has a 5% to 10% risk of developing pre- and postnatal short stature, microcephaly, intellectual disability, midfacial hypoplasia, and other anomalies. Less frequent developments are cardiac defects and cleft lip and/or cleft palate. Treatment with valproic acid results in a clearly heightened risk of neural tube defects and/or dysmorphism with trigonocephaly, small mouth, and dysplastic ears. Although there are teratogenic effects associated with antiepileptics, the risks are less than the risks associated with uncontrolled seizures in the mother. Early prenatal, and even preconception, care (including preconception folic acid supplementation to reduce the risk of neural tube defects) and close monitoring during pregnancy are essential.

Retinoids. Retinoids (vitamin A derivatives) are highly effective medications that are used in dermatology as a systemic treatment of severe psoriasis and acne. If a pregnant woman is treated beyond the 15th day p.c. with retinoids (especially isotretinoin), there is approximately a 35% risk for the development of craniofacial dysmorphisms with flat face, facial palsy, cleft palate, micrognathia, dysplastic ears, and deformities of the auricle of the ear. There are frequent internal malformations, including conotruncal cardiac defects, thymic hypoplasia, hydrocephalus, hypoplastic kidneys, and other urogenital anomalies. The affected children generally manifest developmental delay and intellectual disability.

Cytostatins. Chemotherapy with cytostatins intrinsically carries a teratogenic risk. Folic acid antagonists, such as methotrexate and aminopterin, and alkylating substances have been frequently reported as causing embryopathies. There is a 20% risk of severe malformation for monotherapy with a cytostatin during the first trimester.

Illicit and Nonillicit Substances

Cigarette smoking and alcohol and drug use cause substantial health risks to the mother and her fetus. While no amount of these substances is considered safe in pregnancy and effects vary from one person to the next, most health care professionals agree that there is a greater risk associated with higher amounts and prolonged exposure. Fetal alcohol syndrome is covered in detail in the next section. Nicotine exposure during pregnancy, either from cigarette smoking or excessive second-hand smoke, results in a low birth weight and is also associated with an increased risk of premature birth and perinatal mortality. Nicotine is not known to cause malformations. Cocaine use has substantial teratogenic effects and can result in embryopathy with growth defects of the extremities, various central nervous system (CNS) malformations (including porencephaly), severe intrauterine growth retardation, and urogenital and gastrointestinal malformations.

Fetal Alcohol Syndrome (Alcohol Embryopathy)

Alcohol consumption and smoking are the most widespread drug addictions in the Western world; however, it was not until the end of the 1960s that a scientific study elucidated the damaging effect of alcohol on embryonic development. In the 1970s, numerous subsequent studies convinced the scientific community and the general public of the teratogenic potential of alcohol use. Fetal alcohol syndrome is the most common teratogenic cause of intellectual disability worldwide, yet its true incidence is difficult to estimate due to variability of clinical features and the necessity of acquiring history of alcohol exposure.

Case History

A 2½-year-old girl is seen by a clinical geneticist because of developmental delay. She was born at term and was small for gestational age (SGA). Her weight and height eventually reached the low-normal range. Her milestones were not achieved in an age-appropriate manner, and her behavior was marked by increased hyperactivity and inattentiveness. Physical examination revealed mild microcephaly and distinct facial dysmorphisms, including bilateral epicanthic folds; small mouth with thin upper lip; a long, smooth philtrum; a short nose; and anteverted nares. There were no malformations of the inner organs. When asked specifically about her alcohol use during the pregnancy, the child's mother admitted to having four to five binge-drinking episodes during pregnancy, each resulting in loss of consciousness and hospitalization. She did not consume alcohol between these episodes. She had a history of alcohol abuse that had persisted for several years. The clinical diagnosis for the child is fetal alcohol syndrome. The recurrence risk is zero if the mother abstains from alcohol during subsequent pregnancies. Professional counseling, long-term therapy, and support groups are recommended for full recovery.

Epidemiology

Together with Down syndrome, fetal alcohol syndrome is one of the most frequent causes of intellectual disability worldwide. The actual prevalence is difficult to estimate; medical literature speaks of 1 in 1,000 to 1 in 3,000 neonates.

Clinical Symptoms and Progression

Fetal alcohol syndrome has three main characteristics (▢ Fig. 13.7):
- Pre- and postnatal growth deficiency, including microcephaly
- Developmental delay and intellectual disability, often with behavioral concerns
- Craniofacial dysmorphisms

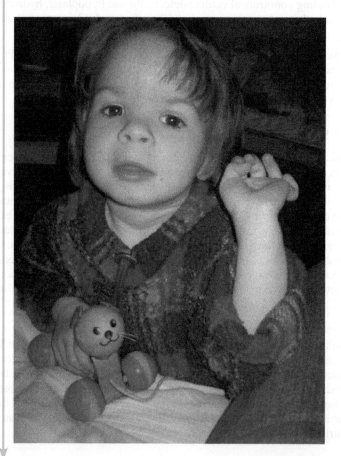

▢ **Figure 13.7. Fetal Alcohol Syndrome.**

The diagnosis of fetal alcohol syndrome or of fetal alcohol effect is often elusive due to sometimes subtle clinical features and lack of corroborating history from the mother. Affected children are typically SGA and often remain small throughout childhood. **Microcephaly** may be present at birth or develop during infancy and childhood.

The characteristic **craniofacial dysmorphisms** are not always obvious to the unexperienced examiner, nor are they specific for fetal alcohol exposure. Affected children typically have short, laterally down-slanting palpebral fissures. The nasal bridge is short and flat. Highly characteristic are the **smooth philtrum** (95% of the cases) and the **thin upper lip** (65%). Maxillary hypoplasia gives the middle face a flattened appearance. The ears, in many cases, are low set and can be slightly dysplastic.

Approximately 30% of the patients have a **congenital heart defect** (mostly ventricular septal or atrial septal defects). Another 30% have **genital anomalies** such as hypospadias, clitoral hypertrophy, and hypoplastic labia. Attention should also be paid to skeletal, genitourinary, and renal malformations (e.g., renal agenesis and duplication of the ureters).

The degree of **psychomotor retardation** depends, in part, on the amount of alcohol consumption during pregnancy. Speech and language development is especially deficient (speech delays in more than 90% of patients), as are logical and abstract thinking. During nursery school and kindergarten, many affected children are hyperactive, impulsive, boundless, eager to engage in risky behavior, and prone to mood swings. Fine motor skills are impaired, while gross motor function remains intact.

Etiopathogenesis

The complete picture of fetal alcohol syndrome exists only in children of chronic alcoholics. As stated earlier, no amount of alcohol is considered "safe" during pregnancy; however, fetal alcohol syndrome is unlikely to be diagnosed in a child whose mother consumed only one to two servings of alcohol during the pregnancy (many women admit to having had alcohol prior to the recognition of pregnancy). A "threshold dosage" is not known and depends on maternal metabolism of alcohol and its metabolites. **Fetal alcohol effects** (fetal alcohol spectrum disorder) can be seen in children of women who consume minimal or moderate amounts of alcohol during pregnancy, yet there are no established criteria for the diagnosis of the mild manifestations of fetal alcohol exposure. Maternal alcohol use can affect the fetus throughout gestation. As there is no placental barrier for ethanol, the embryo or fetus has the same blood alcohol levels as the mother. It is unclear, however, whether it is the ethanol itself or one of its metabolites (especially acetaldehyde) that has the teratogenic effect.

About 10% to 40% of the children of women with chronic alcoholism have typical fetal alcohol syndrome; between 50% and 70% manifest alcohol effects.

Diagnosis

Diagnosis is based on clinical examination and history of alcohol use in the pregnancy. If fetal alcohol syndrome is suspected, one should search for occult malformations (e.g., cardiac, renal, and urinary tract).

Therapy

Therapy is symptomatic. During the first weeks and months of infancy it is often necessary to hospitalize the infant in order to correct major malformations.

Important

In addition to the lifelong effects on the affected child and his or her family, fetal alcohol syndrome poses a substantial economic and social burden. The only way to effectively eradicate this condition is by **prevention** with therapy and counseling of women at risk and provision of support networks for women and their families.

II

Prognosis

The prognosis depends on the number and severity of organ malformations and the degree of intellectual disability. Most children with fetal alcohol syndrome require developmental and educational intervention. The psychosocial climate also influences the ultimate prognosis situation—many children with fetal alcohol syndrome are placed in foster care or with adoptive families, as their biological parents are unable to provide a nurturing environment.

Physical Causes

Ionizing Radiation. The teratogenic effects of ionizing radiation became evident after the explosions of atomic bombs at Hiroshima and Nagasaki toward the end of World War II. Women who were pregnant at the time of the explosion and survived had an abortion rate of 28%. Approximately 25% gave birth to children who died within their first year, while 25% of the surviving children had severe malformations, especially of the central nervous system. Ionizing radiation is teratogenic only at very high doses. Such high doses usually are not attained during radiological diagnostic evaluations or extensive examination during pregnancy (an exception is scintigraphic imaging where radionuclides are also transmitted to the fetal organs). The situation is different for therapeutic radiation, and guidelines have been established to limit toxic exposure, especially during the embryonic period. However, there are no threshold values for the carcinogenic effects of ionizing radiation, neither for organogenesis nor for cellular DNA damage in the embryo or the fetus. Therefore, treating pregnant women with ionizing radiation should always be limited to what is absolutely essential. There is no proof that air travel has teratogenic risks.

Maternal Metabolic Diseases

Maternal Diabetes Mellitus. Children of diabetic mothers have a 6% to 9% probability of developing congenital malformations, which is two to three times higher than in the general population. This is especially true for mothers with type 1 diabetes. In cases where the diabetes is untreated or severe, there is a 10% risk of **diabetic embryopathy**. The most frequent deformities are cardiac defects (especially conotruncal malformations), CNS malformations, and neural tube defects. Another typical malformation that usually occurs sporadically or as the result of maternal diabetes mellitus is caudal regression, which results in the absence or hypoplasia of the sacrum, coccyx, pelvis, and lower extremities and is accompanied with anal atresia and urogenital malformations. Sirenomelia (from the siren in Greek mythology) is the most severe form of caudal regression and is usually fatal due to renal agenesis among other problems (■ Fig. 13.8). Up to 50% of children with manifest diabetic embryopathy die secondary to their defects. It is crucial that blood sugar levels are regulated optimally before conception and during pregnancy, since this considerably reduces the risk of malformations.

■■■ Diabetic Fetopathy

Children of mothers with **gestational diabetes**, as a rule, have no increased risk of malformation, since most cases develop after the completion of the first trimester (i.e., completion of embryogenesis). Children of mothers with severe gestational diabetes are at risk for developing **diabetic fetopathy** (■ Fig. 13.9), which is characterized by infantile macrosomia, hyperinsulinemia, and hypoglycemia. Histological examination of the pancreas reveals hyperplasia of the islets of Langerhans.

Maternal Phenylketonuria. Elevated maternal phenylalanine levels, caused by maternal phenylketonuria (PKU) or hyperphenylalaninemia, are highly teratogenic. There is a direct correlation between the phenylalanine level in the mother's blood and the risk for congenital malformations in the developing fetus. Spontaneous abortions are seen in approximately 25% of women with poorly controlled phenylketonuria. Typical abnormalities in the newborn include microcephaly, growth deficiency, and cardiac defects; also, there is a high likelihood for behavioral problems and intellectual disability. Women with PKU need to be on a low-phenylalanine

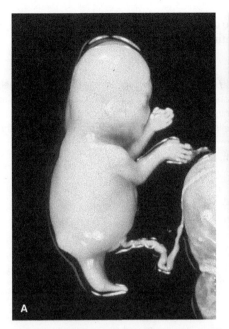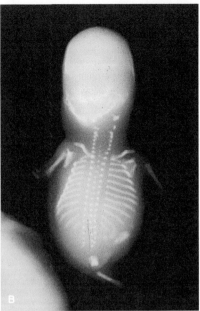

Figure 13.8. A, B. Sirenomelia in a Fetus. Sirenomelia represents the most severe end of the caudal regression spectrum and is associated with the teratogenic effects of maternal diabetes. (Photo courtesy of Halit Pinar of the Department of Pathology at Brown University and Women and Infants Hospital, Providence, Rhode Island, and Lorraine Potocki of the Department of Molecular and Human Genetics, Baylor College of Medicine and Texas Children's Hospital, Houston. © 2009 Core Curriculum Publishers, LLC. Used by permission.)

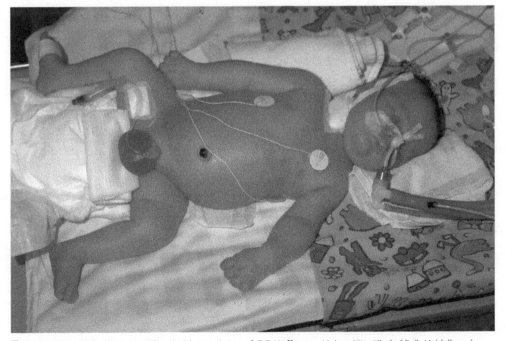

Figure 13.9. Diabetic Fetopathy. (With permission of G.F. Hoffmann, Universitäts-Kinderklinik Heidelberg.)

diet and achieve good control prior to conception. They need to have their phenylalanine levels monitored closely throughout the entire pregnancy.

Important

PKU and hyperphenylalaninemia are detected on the newborn screen; thus, most women with these disorders are followed by a metabolic specialist from infancy. While untreated PKU would be obvious, the clinical features of hyperphenylalaninemia can be subtle. If features of maternal PKU are present in an infant or child, a phenylalanine level measurement should be performed on the mother, especially (though not exclusively) if she was born at home or in a country where newborn screening (NBS) was not established at the time of her birth.

14 Risk Estimation and Calculation

Consider the following three classic counseling situations that can occur in clinical human genetics:

— A person seeking clinical advice is aware of a congenital disorder in the family and wishes to know the likelihood that he or she will be affected.

— A person seeking advice knows that he or she is a carrier for a certain disease-associated mutation and wishes to know the likelihood of his or her being affected by the disease.

— A couple seeking advice has a child with a heritable disorder and wishes to know the recurrence risk for future pregnancies.

These are three questions about the likelihood that an event will occur, three questions with a major impact on individual, as well as shared, life choices.

14.1 Probable or Improbable?

Calculation and Communication of Risk. One of the most important considerations of genetic counseling is calculating risk. Mathematics is only the first step; equally important is communicating the probability that the event will occur. It is crucial that the person seeking advice understands the calculated risk. In clinical counseling situations, we realize, on a daily basis, that different persons see risk numbers in different ways. This is due to various factors.

A Question of Wording. There are a number of ways to say that an event will not occur with absolute certainty: perhaps, probably, unlikely, possibly, not with certainty, likely, not to be excluded, etc. Studies have shown that these terms are understood and evaluated differently by different individuals. Another factor that varies between patients is that events are evaluated according to whether the result will be considered positive or negative and by which consequences they will have. For example, the probability that, beginning at age 45, mothers have a 5% risk of giving birth to a child with a chromosomal disorder is generally considered a high risk. In cancer, on the other hand, a survival chance of 5% is considered low.

Terms such as *risk*, *chance*, *possibility*, or *probability* also imply value judgments (e.g., risk = bad, chance = good), which may be perceived differently by different individuals. Therefore, the physician should use terms that are as neutral as possible or offer several terms for the same condition. Terms such as *luck* or *bad luck*, which each denote unequivocally strong value judgments, should not be used in genetic counseling situations.

It also is important to note whether the evaluation of a risk is expressed as a probability (e.g., 0.005), as a percentage (0.5%), or as an absolute (natural) number (1 in 200). Mathematically, there is no difference, since all three express the same value. Yet the difference in how these values are perceived can be considerable. In most cases absolute numbers (1 in 200) are easier to understand than percentages (0.5%), while small numbers of probability are hardest to comprehend. If in doubt, one should attempt to express a risk several ways, in order to be as clear as possible.

II

■■■ **Comprehensible Information**

Not every person seeking advice is adept in mathematics, and not everyone has equal intellectual abilities. If a person seeking advice lacks basic understanding of probability, the genetics professional needs to be especially careful to make sure he or she communicates risk in a manner that can be understood. Healthy parents with a first child diagnosed with phenylketonuria (PKU) are heterozygous carriers, and according to probability calculations, one of four of their children will be affected with PKU. For some patients, however, it is hard to understand that after one affected child, the next three children are not necessarily healthy. A possible way to explain this is to use the example of a bag full of equal numbers of blue and red marbles. If one grabs two marbles out of the bag and both are blue, the child will be affected; two red marbles would indicate an unaffected child who is not a carrier; and one red and one blue marble would indicate a carrier. If the bag is full of thousands of marbles, pulling out two blue marbles on the first try does not influence which marbles you pick on subsequent selections.

14.2 Rules of Risk Calculation

In order to provide appropriate risk calculations in the typical genetic counseling session, it is sufficient to be familiar with three basic mathematical principles: the addition rule of probability, the multiplication rule of probability, and Bayes theorem.

Addition Rule of Probability

If two events, A and B, are mutually exclusive, meaning they cannot occur simultaneously, these two events are called disjunctive. If the probability for event A occurring is P(A), and the probability for event B occurring is P(B), it can be deduced that the probability of either event A or event B occurring [i.e., $P(A \cup B)$] is P(A) + P(B):

$$P(A \cup B) = P(A) + P(B)$$

Example: Twins can be either monozygotic or dizygotic. The probability that twins are monozygotic is P(MZ) = 1/3 (Chapter 6). The probability that twins are dizygotic is P(DZ) = 2/3. According to the addition rule, the probability that twins are either monozygotic or dizygotic is $P(MZ \cup DZ)$ = 1/3 + 2/3 = 1. To put it briefly, the sum of all probabilities is one.

Multiplication Rule of Probability

The multiplication rule of probability applies if two events, A and B, are independent of one another. If event A occurs with probability P(A) and event B with probability P(B), the probability that both A and B occur is:

$$P(A \cap B) = P(A) \times P(B)$$

Example: The risk of a miscarriage in the absence of special risk factors is approximately one-sixth; this also applies to second pregnancies of couples who had a miscarriage in the first pregnancy. Therefore, the "random" chance that both the first and the second pregnancy end in a miscarriage is $P(A \cap B)$ = 1/6 × 1/6 = 1/36, which is equal to approximately 3%. This number is not particularly small; it also explains why the majority of couples with unexplained miscarriages have no risk factors, and subsequent pregnancies can be carried to term.

Another example for medical practice is the concurrence of two different disease pictures in the same patient. The lifetime probability for female breast cancer is approximately 8% (i.e., 0.08). Approximately 5% of breast cancer cases are associated with a familial cancer predisposition. The lifetime probability for ovarian cancer in the general population is approximately 1%; however, for women with familial predisposition, the risk is approximately 50%. The estimated prevalence of mutations in one of the two breast cancer genes, *BRCA1* and *BRCA2*, in women is about 0.5% (i.e., 1 in 200 or 0.005). If both breast cancer and ovarian cancer occur in the same woman, the probability that there is no cancer disposition (i.e., that both diseases occur independently) is $0.08 \times 0.01 = 0.0008$, which is equivalent to 1 in 1,250. The probability that the concurrence of the two types of cancer is due to a familial cancer disposition, however, is calculated as the product of the following: (prevalence of *BRCA1/BRCA2* mutation) $\times$ (lifetime risk for breast cancer if carrying such a mutation) $\times$ (lifetime risk for ovarian cancer). In other words, the risk equals $0.005 \times 0.8 \times 0.5 = 0.002$ or 1 in 500. The probability of an underlying cancer disposition, therefore, is more than twice as high as the random concurrence of the two types of cancer, but both are possible.

Bayes Theorem/Bayesian Analysis

In 1763, Thomas Bayes published this theorem, which today, almost 250 years later, is still the most important method used by clinical geneticists and general practitioners to calculate the risk of acquiring a disease. It is particularly important because it allows for readily available, additional information to be calculated into the risk. All people intuitively act according to the Bayes theorem in their daily lives, while practically no one, human geneticists included, remembers the exact mathematical formula. If we assume, for example, that the probability of rain during an average day in September is approximately 20%, we can be more precise in our prediction when we look at the sky in the morning. If there is a thick cloud cover, we will be more inclined to take along an umbrella than we would be in clear, sunny weather. The prior probability of 20% is changed by this additional information; as a result, the posterior probability of rainy weather is much higher.

> **Important**
>
> The Bayesian analysis contains three important steps:
> - Initially, an event has a certain prior probability that is based on various possible circumstances.
> - Additional information excludes some of the possible circumstances.
> - Considering the remaining possibilities, we can calculate an exact posterior probability.

The simplest example is the probability that a child from two parents who are carriers for an autosomal recessive disorder is also a carrier for this disorder. The prior probability is two-fourth or 50%. If the disorder is not present in the child, one-fourth of the possible situations (in this case, homozygosity for the mutation) can be excluded. The remaining three-fourths is then redefined as a new reference total (virtually a new 100%), and two of the three remaining possible situations would mean carrier status. Thus, the posterior probability of carrier status is two-thirds.

Complex problems require more elaborate calculations. The application of the Bayes theorem is based on two scenarios that are mutually exclusive (e.g., "affected" and "not affected"). These scenarios, and their probabilities, are compared. The prior probability of a scenario is established by its average prevalence, without consideration of additional information (although simple pedigree information is taken into account).

Prior probability: The probability of an event **before** taking additional information into account.

Conditional probability: The chance of something occurring, assuming that each event is true (e.g., the chance of a mother having four unaffected sons, assuming that she is a carrier for X-linked hemophilia A, is equal to $1/2 \times 1/2 \times 1/2 \times 1/2 = 1/16$).

Joint probability: The prior probability multiplied by the conditional probability.

Posterior probability: The probability of the event after taking into account additional information. It is calculated as the quotient of the joint probability divided by the sum of all of the joint probabilities.

Table 14.1. Risk Calculation Using Bayesian Analysis

	Event/Probability A	Event/Probability B
Prior probability (a + b = 1)	a (or 1-b)	b (or 1-a)
Conditional probability	c	d
Joint probability	ac	bd
Posterior probability	ac/(ac + bd)	bd/(ac + bd)

Example 1. The daughter of a confirmed maternal carrier for Duchenne muscular dystrophy has a 50% (0.5) prior probability of being a carrier herself. However, additional information (e.g., determination of the creatine kinase [CK] titers in the blood) can modify these early probabilities. These are used to calculate **conditional probabilities**, allowing a certain finding for both scenarios (e.g., predicting the probability of elevated CK values for carriers or noncarriers [normal persons]). In our example, we assume that 70% of carriers have elevated CK titers, but only 5% of noncarriers do. Calculating joint probabilities from prior probabilities and conditional probabilities is done according to the multiplication rule, which is easy to follow in the case of our example, because Mendel's laws and a blood test are independent of one another. With this information, a four-field table can be constructed; each field represents one of four possibilities (◘ Table 14.1). If the woman being tested has an abnormal CK, two fields that are not relevant would no longer be considered possible, thus leaving the two remaining fields to be added and used as a new reference (in the example of ◘ Fig. 14.1, this would be

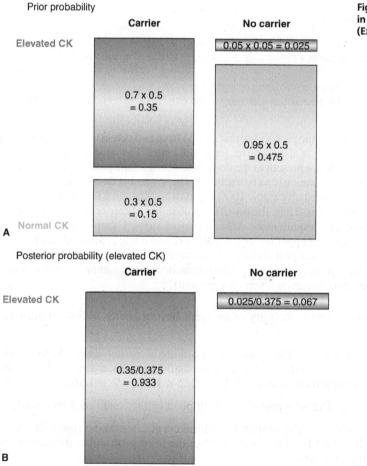

Prior probability

Carrier — No carrier

Elevated CK

0.05 x 0.05 = 0.025

0.7 x 0.5 = 0.35

0.95 x 0.5 = 0.475

0.3 x 0.5 = 0.15

A Normal CK

Posterior probability (elevated CK)

Carrier — No carrier

Elevated CK

0.025/0.375 = 0.067

0.35/0.375 = 0.933

B

Figure 14.1. Four-Field Table in a Probability Calculation (Example 1).

◘ Table 14.2. Calculating the Probability That Person B Is a Carrier for Duchenne Muscular Dystrophy (Example 2)

	B Is a Carrier	B Is Not a Carrier
Prior probability	½	½
Conditional probability (four healthy sons)	$(½)^4 = 1/16$	1
Joint probability	$½ × 1/16 = 1/32$	$½ × 1 = ½ = 16/32$
Posterior probability	$(1/32)/(17/32) = 1/17$	$(16/32)/(17/32) = 16/17$

0.375 in the case of elevated CK titers). The **posterior probability** (i.e., the probability that combines the original scenario with the additional information into one risk figure) results from the share of the combined probability in this reference figure (in this case, 0.35/0.375 = 0.933 for carrier status and 0.025/0.375 = 0.067 for a normal person, meaning that there is a 93% probability that a woman with elevated CK values is a carrier).

Example 2. A person seeking advice (referred to as person B) wishes to know whether she is a carrier for Duchenne muscular dystrophy. She is the daughter of an obligate carrier, since both her maternal uncle and her brother have Duchenne muscular dystrophy. This preliminary information allows us to calculate the prior probability for situation A (carrier) and situation B (no carrier). The probability for each of these situations is 1/2. The two events are mutually exclusive; therefore, their sum is 1/2 + 1/2 = 1.

The person seeking advice has four sons, all of them healthy. The conditional probability that four sons of a carrier are healthy is $(1/2)^4 = 1/16$ (with a probability of 15/16 that at least one of the sons would have been affected). Since the various pregnancies represent mutually independent events, the multiplication rule is applied. In the case that person B is not a carrier for muscular dystrophy, she would only have healthy sons. The conditional probability in this case is 1.

All this information is taken into account in the calculation according to the Bayes theorem as shown in ◘ Table 14.2. This results in an posterior probability of approximately 1/17 for situation A that she is a carrier, and in an posterior probability of 16/17 that she is not a carrier. This example demonstrates the considerable change in risk figures once all relevant information is taken into account.

14.3 Hardy-Weinberg Law

The Hardy-Weinberg law is used in population genetics and dates back to 1908 and 1909, when it was discovered independently by the English mathematician Geoffrey Hardy and the German physician Wilhelm Weinberg, respectively. The Hardy-Weinberg law makes it possible to determine the frequency of different genotypes in a diploid chromosomal complement (i.e., where two separate copies of a certain gene exist). In clinical genetics, it is mainly used for determining the frequency of heterozygosity in autosomal recessive heritable disorders when only the disease frequency is known.

The Hardy-Weinberg law rests on the assumption that there are two different alleles at a certain locus; these alleles are named "p" and "q" (i.e., a normal allele [traditionally p] and a variant allele [traditionally q]). Since there are only these two alleles, p + q = 1. If in humans the respective gene occurs in two copies on only one autosome, the frequency of the three possible genotypes is calculated from the binominal distribution $(p + q)^2 = pp + pq + qp + qq = p^2 + 2pq + q^2 = 1$. This can easily be represented as a square, where each side represents one chromosome (with the specific probabilities of the alleles p and q; ◘ Fig. 14.2).

In rare recessive disorders, the disease-causing allele occurs much less frequently than the normal allele, with q being close to zero and p close to 1. Therefore, q^2 is much smaller than p^2. In such cases, the frequency of heterozygosity (i.e., 2pq) depends mostly on the value of q, while p can be assumed to be 1. The frequency of heterozygosity in a population can be determined by

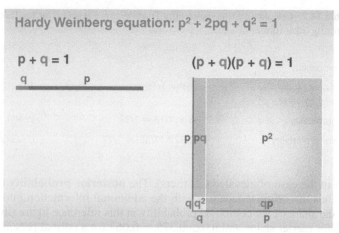

Figure 14.2. Graphic Representation of the Hardy-Weinberg Law. The different alleles p and q are represented as lines, the various genotypes as squares.

extracting the root of the frequency of a recessive disorder and multiplying it by 2. For example, if a disorder has an incidence of $q^2 = 1{:}40{,}000$, the theoretical carrier frequency is $2 \times (1{:}200) = (1{:}100) = 1\%$.

■■■ The Hardy-Weinberg Law

If two alleles, p and q, exist at one gene locus, the allele frequencies are:

$$p + q = 1$$

The frequency of the three possible genotypes AA, Aa, and aa results from the binomial distribution

$$(p + q)^2 = p^2 + 2pq + q^2 + 1$$

For autosomal recessive disorders

the incidence of the disorder is q^2.

For cases in which the disease-causing allele q is much rarer than the normal allele p,

frequency of heterozygosity is approximately 2q,

i.e., the square root of the disease frequency multiplied by 2.

In clinical practice, it occasionally makes sense to apply both Bayes theorem and the Hardy-Weinberg law, as is demonstrated in the following example (■ Fig. 14.3).

Example 3. Mr. and Mrs. Potter (I_1 and I_2) have two healthy children. Recently, they found out that the niece of Mrs. Potter has cystic fibrosis (CF). Now they are inquiring about the risk of cystic fibrosis in their third child.

— Step 1: What is the probability that Mrs. Potter is a carrier for cystic fibrosis? Since one of her parents is an obligate carrier, she herself has a probability of 50% (1/2) of being a carrier for a cystic fibrosis mutation.

Figure 14.3. Pedigree for Example 3.

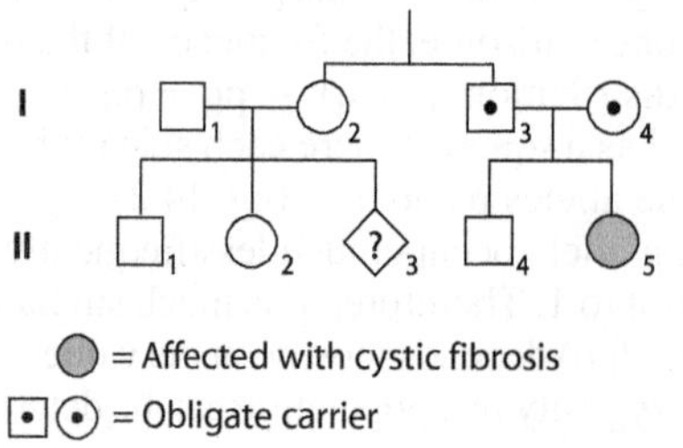

○ = Affected with cystic fibrosis

▣ ⊙ = Obligate carrier

Table 14.3. Bayesian Analysis for Example 3 (Cystic Fibrosis)

	I_1 and I_2 Are Both Carriers	I_1 and I_2 Are Not Both Carriers
Prior probability	½ × 1/25 = 1/50	1 – 1/50 = 49/50
Conditional probability (two healthy children)	$(3/4)^2$ = 9/16	1
Joint probability	9/800	49/50 = 784/800
Posterior probability	9/800 : 793/800 = 9/793 ≈ 1/88	784/800 : 793/800 = 784/793 ≈ 87/88

— Step 2: What is the probability that Mr. Potter is a carrier for cystic fibrosis? Mr. Potter has no relatives with the disorder (i.e., his risk is the same as that of the general population and can be calculated with the Hardy-Weinberg law). The incidence of cystic fibrosis in the general population (q^2) is 1 in 2,500. Based on this, the allele frequency q is calculated as $1/(\sqrt{2,500})$ = 1/50, and the frequency of heterozygosity (2q) is approximately 1/25 or 4%.

— Step 3: How large is the probability that they have an affected child, not taking into consideration the healthy children (the prior probability)? With a probability of 1/50 (1/2 × 1/25) or 2% that both partners are carriers and a probability of 1/4 that an affected child would be born to two recessive carriers, the prior probability is 1/50 × 1/4 × 1/200 (0.5%).

— Step 4: How large is the probability that they have an affected child if the healthy children are taken into consideration (i.e., what is their posterior probability of having a child with CF)? As can be seen from the calculations in ◻ Table 14.3, the probability that both parents are carriers is reduced to 1/88, and the disease risk for a future child to approximately 1/350 (0.3%).

A clearly more efficient way to modify the risk would be to do a molecular genetic test on Mrs. Potter. Mutation screening for CF identifies approximately 90% of CF carriers. A negative test result in Mrs. Potter would lower her carrier risk to approximately 1/20, and the disease risk for a future child would be 1/3,500, lower than the one for the general population. At that point it would no longer be necessary to test Mr. Potter.

■■■ **Factors That Affect the Hardy-Weinberg Equilibrium**
The Hardy-Weinberg law only applies to an "ideal population" that meets the following criteria:
— Mating within the population occurs randomly, with equal probability and equal success for the various genotypes.
— The population is large enough to prevent random events (gene drift) from affecting the allele frequency.
— There is no selection advantage or disadvantage for carriers of certain genotypes.
— There are no new mutations.
— There are no migration events that might alter the allele frequency.

The one factor that has practical implications among this group of criteria is random mating, since the Hardy-Weinberg law cannot be applied if there is frequent intermarriage. In such cases, rare recessive disorders occur with much greater frequency than would be expected from the frequency of heterozygosity. The other criteria are more relevant to whether or not the allele or genotype frequencies remain constant or whether the incidence of a disorder changes.

Factors That Affect Genotype Frequency but Not Allele Frequency

In humans, the consequences of **random mating** are only partially fulfilled or not filled at all. This does not primarily affect the allele frequencies (p and q) of the subsequent generations, but rather affects the frequency of the various genotypes (p^2, 2pq, and q^2). "Mating" does not occur

II

totally at random but according to certain characteristics. **Assortative mating** describes the tendency to select partners with phenotypically similar characteristics. This becomes clinically relevant when partners are selected who have similar medical problems (e.g., deafness, blindness, or short stature). If these medical problems are genetic, subsequent generations will have larger numbers of homozygous carriers in the population or, in the case of recessive heritable disorders, larger numbers of clinically affected persons. It should be noted that in some cases the same phenotypical characteristic can have etiologically different genetic causes; an example would be the various types of autosomal recessive heritable deafness (Section 30.1).

In many cultures, **consanguinity** is acceptable (typically between first-degree cousins, but also between uncle and niece). Sometimes this fulfills important social functions. This type of nonrandom mating between genetically related individuals also increases the share of homozygous genotypes in the population for the subsequent generation. The share of heterozygous genotypes, however, will be lower. When compared to the general population, the offspring of consanguineous partners have an increased risk of having recessive heritable disorders. The extent of the risk depends not only on the degree of relatedness of the consanguineous parents but also on the frequency of the disease-causing allele in the general population. If the homozygous disorder causes decreased reproductive fitness (i.e., there is less of a probability that an affected individual has children of his or her own), consanguinity, in the long term, also increases the **selection** of the normal allele (i.e., the disease-associated allele is eliminated faster from the population). Therefore, the probability of being a carrier for a rare recessive disorder is theoretically lower in cultures with a higher number of consanguineous marriages than in cultures where consanguinity is taboo. Hence, the risk of having a child with a recessive disorder is higher with the same degree of kinship if the partners come from a traditional nonconsanguineous culture than if they come from a traditionally consanguineous culture.

■■■ **Disease Risk for Offspring of Consanguineous Relationships**
In a marriage between first-degree cousins, the baseline risk typically only increases by 2% to 3%. The risk is higher if there is an autosomal recessive disorder in the family. Therefore, in order to clarify the disease risk for children with consanguinity, it is necessary to construct an exact pedigree.

Factors That Influence Allele Frequencies

Evolutionary factors such as genetic drift, mutation, selection, and migration alter the allele frequencies of a population.

Genetic Drift. The allele frequencies in the generation of parents are not completely identical to the allele frequencies in the generation of children; instead, they are subject to fluctuations. This probability effect, called genetic drift, is more significant in smaller populations. The reasons are statistical and can be demonstrated in the example of throwing a coin. Theoretically, heads and tails should show with equal frequency. Indeed, a 50:50 ratio is approached as the number of throws increases. With only very few throws, however, it is unlikely that heads and tails appear with the same frequency. So it is with small populations; they have larger fluctuations in allele frequencies caused by genetic drift than populations with many individuals.

Founder Effect. If a small group of individuals splits off from a population to establish a new population, random factors play an important role as to which alleles occur in the new group and which are absent. The smaller the number of founders, the more they fluctuate from the original population. These differences remain over numerous subsequent generations if the founder population grows in isolation from the original population or other populations. This is known as a **bottleneck effect**. The founder effect denotes a clearly limited number of genotypes as well as phenotypes in the founder generation as compared to the original population, because the founders only represent part of the gene pool of the original population. The founder effect further signifies that some disorders in the "new" population occur with great frequency, while other disorders are extremely rare. The frequent disorders in these populations are mostly caused by a few typical mutations.

A founder effect occurs if a population:
- is based on a small group of "founder fathers" and "founder mothers"
- grows in isolation from other populations

The founder effect results in the fact that:
- some heritable disorders occur with great frequency
- some heritable disorders, which occur frequently elsewhere, are extremely rare

■■■ Examples of Founder Effects in Human History

There are numerous examples of founder effects in mankind. Frequently cited are the descendents of Ana-baptists in the United States, today's Hutterites, Mennonites, or Amish. The Anabaptist movement started as a radical reform group in the 16th century in Zurich and soon spread in small sections into middle and Eastern Europe. Since they were frequently persecuted, some groups migrated in the 17th century to North America, founding new communities that grew in self-imposed isolation; some have maintained their culture over time. Among the best known are the **Amish** in Pennsylvania, who have preserved their traditional lifestyle (and German dialect) to this day. Strong social ties are the reason why marriages chiefly occur within their own population. They usually have many children, a fact that contributes to the strong growth of the religious group. Due to a very distinct founder effect, the Amish have a very high incidence of rare autosomal recessive diseases, such as glutaric aciduria type I and Ellis-van-Creveld syndrome. Interestingly, the disease-causing mutations of the Amish are still found in those central European regions where the founders originated, but with a much lower allele frequency.

Another example of founder effect is the **Ashkenazi Jewish** population of central and Eastern Europe (differing from Sephardic Jews of the Iberian Peninsula), where some otherwise rare autosomal recessive diseases such as Canavan disease or Tay-Sachs disease are especially frequent; they (and also cystic fibrosis) are caused by specific mutations. Finland also has numerous diseases that occur with great frequency (only) in that country. Other diseases that are frequent elsewhere, such as phenylketonuria, are very rare in Finland, which is the result of a negative founder effect (i.e., the absence of the respective disease-causing mutations in the founder population).

Mutation. Mutations change the alleles of a population by adding new (mutated) alleles to the gene pool. Mutations are random and can have positive or negative effects (or no effect at all) on the procreation of their carriers. They are responsible for the genetic diversity of a population.

Selection. The term **natural selection** goes back to Charles Darwin and signifies the natural selection of phenotypes in the sense of **survival of the fittest**. The *fitness* of an individual is defined as the ability to procreate and to have as many descendents as possible. Fitness therefore does not necessarily mean survival of the stronger. It can also include coopera-tion and altruism. What is important is transmitting the genes to the following generation. The term **sexual selection** signifies the fact that procreating partners favor the selection of certain phenotypes of their own type. Important for sexual selection is transmitting alleles that result in phenotypes that, in the subsequent generation, will again be preferred by pro-creating partners. An important positive selection factor in autosomal recessive disorders is a **heterozygous advantage** that, for example, has been identified for various hemoglobin-opathies (Section 21.5) and that is suspected in other disorders (Section 22.1, Why Is Cystic Fibrosis so Frequent?).

Migration (Gene Flow). The term *migration* signifies migration of partial populations to another environment (i.e., to a new biotope). Immigrants introduce new alleles into a popula-tion, increasing (as any mutation will do) the heterozygosity rate of the affected population. Identifying the same alleles in different ethnic groups demonstrates the effects of gene flow on the corresponding gene pools of the various populations.

■■■ Population Genetics

Population genetics or the identification of polymorphisms, haplotypes, or disease-triggering mutations in different countries allows the study of kinship between different populations. Large numbers of studies were done with genetic markers of mitochondrial DNA, which are exclusively transmitted maternally, and of the Y chromosome, which is exclusively transmitted paternally. This helped explain, for example, the expansion of mankind from Africa (out-of-Africa hypothesis) and their settlement in the various continents. Migration events, however, can also be shown in autosomal recessive disorders. Of special interest is the example of **phenylketonuria.** This is one of the most frequent genetic disorders in Europe (to be explained by a yet unidentified heterozygosity advantage); yet, in different countries it is caused by mutations of different frequencies. By far the most frequent mutation in Denmark, IVS12+1G>A, is also the most frequent mutation in England, pointing to the fact that the establishment of the Anglo-Saxon state in Britain between the 4th and 6th centuries CE was accompanied by a considerable gene flow from what is now Denmark and northern Germany (the home of the Angles and the Saxons). In Ireland, this mutation is relatively rare, which points to the fact that the anglicization of the local Celtic population was achieved by political force and not by immigration. On the other hand, PKU mutations from the Norwegian Atlantic coast are not infrequent in Ireland, pointing to the considerable migration of Vikings between the 7th and 9th centuries, which resulted in the founding of the most important Irish cities. The Mediterranean and also Germany have a very broad range of mutations, as can be expected in areas with significant migration over the centuries.

15 Methods for Laboratory Diagnostics in Genetics

LEARNING OBJECTIVES

1 Compare and contrast the techniques of G-banded chromosome analysis and array DNA analysis, including the advantages and disadvantages of each method.

2 Describe the types of mutations that can be detected by direct DNA sequencing.

3 Explain why polymerase chain reaction (PCR) testing is essential when performing preimplantation genetic diagnosis.

15.1 Cytogenetics

The term *cytogenetics* refers to the study of chromosomes, their structure, and their inheritance mechanisms. In 1956, Tijo and Levan discovered that a human somatic cell had 46 chromosomes (◘ Fig. 15.1), and since then cytogenetics has been the reference point for subsequent genomic discoveries and the premiere diagnostic test for patients with various genetic conditions.

Chromosome Analysis

Although for many indications routine chromosome analysis is now largely replaced in the diagnostic laboratory by DNA array analysis, it still continues to be a useful diagnostic tool. In addition, all genomic loci are referenced by their cytogenetic location; therefore, understanding the basic principles of cytogenetics is an asset for medical practice. Chromosome analysis involves examination of chromosomes of a dividing cell by **light microscopy** following induced cell cycle arrest during metaphase or prometaphase during mitosis (Fig. 15.1).

Testing Material. Usually **lymphocytes** are obtained from venous whole blood (3 to 10 mL blood mixed with sodium heparin). Chromosome analysis can be performed in any cell that has a nucleus (e.g., skin, placenta, amniocyte, and bone marrow). The tissue selected depends on the clinical or analytical question.

Culture. In vivo, neither the blood nor human skin contains sufficient mitotic cells for analysis; therefore, cells are first placed in tissue culture medium, and division is stimulated with phytohemagglutinin, a polysaccharide of plant origin.

Colcemid Treatment. Lymphocytes reach their peak rate of mitosis after approximately 72 hours. The dividing cells are arrested in metaphase with chemicals that inhibit the mitotic spindle (e.g., colcemid, a derivative of colchicine, which is the toxin contained in *Colchicum autumnale*, commonly known as autumn crocus).

Preparation. Approximately 10 to 60 minutes after colcemid treatment, the cells are sedimented by centrifugation and treated with a hypotonic (0.075 M) potassium chloride solution to release the chromosomes from the nuclei. Chromosomes are then fixed (methyl acetic acid removes parts of the histone proteins), spread onto slides, and stained by one of several techniques.

Banding/Staining. Cytogenetic banding techniques have been used since the 1970s. With the aid of banding patterns, each of the 46 chromosomes can be positively identified, and the 23 pairs of homologous chromosomes are easily sorted. Numeric chromosomal

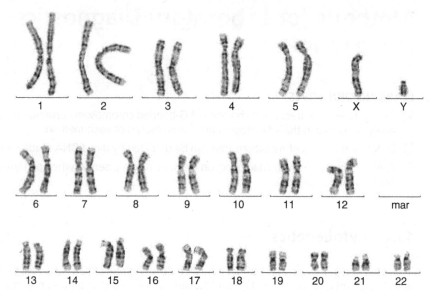

Figure 15.1. Normal Male Karyotype 46,XY. Resolution approximately 400 bands. (Courtesy of H.-D. Hager, Institut für Humangenetik Heidelberg.)

abnormalities are recognized when the number of chromosomes in a cell is anything other than 46 (e.g., 47,XX,+13). Structural chromosomal abnormalities can be recognized through a change in the banding pattern. The most common method is **G-banding**. In this process, the chromosomes initially are treated with a proteolytic enzyme (e.g., trypsin) that removes some of the chromosomal proteins. Next the chromosomes are stained with a Giemsa dye, resulting in visible alternating light and dark bands along the length of each chromosome. Each chromosome has a specific banding pattern—any divergence represents a structural anomaly in the individual. A chromosome band has an average size of 7.5 million nucleotides (7.5 Mb). A higher resolution (i.e., *high-resolution banding*) is possible with prometaphase chromosomes, yielding *fewer* nucleotides per band. At that point, the chromosomes are not as condensed, and many segments, which show as a single band in the metaphase, are found to be two or three distinct bands. Under optimal conditions, between 550 and 850 bands can be differentiated. For the purpose of investigating developmental disturbances in childhood, a resolution of 500 bands or more should be achieved (Fig. 15.2). Besides G-banding, there are other banding techniques available; however, their clinical application is rapidly becoming historical due to the application of DNA array analysis.

Cytogenetic Nomenclature

The term *karyotype* refers to the number and appearance of the chromosomes in an individual's cell as determined by comprehensive chromosome analysis. The components of a karyotype are the total number of chromosomes and the specific sex chromosomes, followed by any specific numerical abnormality and/or structural abnormality that is present. A normal karyotype in a female is 46,XX, and in a male, 46,XY. A male with Down syndrome is depicted as 47,XY,+21.

According to international convention, the short arm of a chromosome, which is located above the centromere, is the "p" arm (for petite), and the long arm, which is located below the centromere, is "q" (the next letter in the alphabet). The bands of a chromosome are labeled much like the streets of a town—the town center being the centromere. Band p10 or p11 is the closest to the centromere on the short arm (analogous to North 1st Street) and q10 or q11 is its counterpart (analogous to South 1st Street). The numbering of bands and subbands is sequential from the centromere to the telomere of each chromosome (Fig. 15.2).

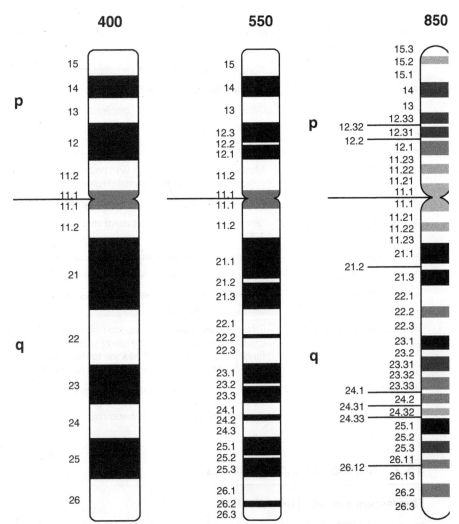

Figure 15.2. Different Band Resolutions and Corresponding Ideograms of Chromosome 10. Resolution of approximately 400, 550, and 850 bands. Notice that at a resolution of 550 and 850 bands, band 10q21 is further defined to 10q21.1, 10q21.2, and 10q21.3. (G-banded chromosomes courtesy of H.-D. Hager, Institut für Humangenetik Heidelberg. Ideograms of chromosome 10 adapted from ISCN [International System for Human Cytogenetic Nomenclature].)

Important

Karyotype Nomenclature

The cytogenetic finding (Table 15.1) is notated as follows:

— Number of chromosomes
— Constellation of sex chromosomes
— Numeric variations
— Structural variations

Important acronyms for variations are t = translocation, rob = robertsonian translocation, del = deletion, dup = duplication, ins = insertion, der = derivative chromosome, mos = mosaic, up = uniparental disomy, mat = maternal, and pat = paternal. For structural variations, the chromosome is indicated in parenthesis, followed by the region(s) or band(s), which are also in parenthesis. For translocations, the two chromosomes involved are separated by a semicolon in the first parenthesis, while the corresponding regions/bands are separated by a semicolon in the second parenthesis. The centromere determines with which chromosome the structurally altered chromosome will be grouped.

Table 15.1. Examples of Cytogenetic Findings

Karyotype	Finding
46,XX	Normal female chromosome complement
46,XY	Normal male chromosome complement
69,XXY	Triploidy (triple chromosome complement)
47,XXY	Klinefelter syndrome
45,X	Monosomy of the X chromosome, results in Turner syndrome
mos 45,X [17]/46,XX [3]	Mosaic monosomy X, 17 cells with pathological chromosome complement, 3 cells with normal chromosome complement
47,XY,+21	Male with trisomy 21 (results in Down syndrome)
46,XX,del(5)(p13)	Terminal deletion of the short are of chromosome 5 beginning at band 1.3.
46,XX,inv(3)(p25q21)	Pericentric inversion with breakpoints in 3p25 and 3q21
46,XX,inv(3)(p21p25)	Paracentric inversion with breakpoints in 3p21 and 3p25
46,XY,t(4;12)(p14;q13)	Reciprocal translocation between chromosomes 4 and 12 with breakpoints in 4p14 and 12q13
45,XX,rob(14;21)(q10;q10)	Balanced Robertsonian translocation involving the long arms of chromosomes 14 and 21. The loss of each of the short arms is functionally not relevant. In addition to the derivative chromosome, there is a normal chromosome 14 and a normal chromosome 21.
46,XX,rob(14;21)(q10;q10),+21	Trisomy 21 with unbalanced robertsonian translocation of chromosomes 14 and 21. Besides the derivative chromosome, there are one normal chromosome 14 and two chromosomes 21.

15.2   Molecular Cytogenetics

Fluorescence In Situ Hybridization

By the mid-1990s, further development of cytogenetic diagnostics resulted in the introduction of fluorescence in situ hybridization (FISH) into the clinical laboratory. The FISH technique combines cytogenetic and molecular genetic approaches and offers the possibility of showing chromosome segments in color under the fluorescence microscope (□ Fig. 15.3). Locus-specific DNA probes allow reliable detection of small microdeletions that are not visible in traditional G-banded chromosome analysis.

When compared to conventional banding techniques, FISH analysis can produce a far superior resolution but is limited to a specific area of interrogation (e.g., normal hybridization for a FISH probe of the 22q11.2 region excludes only the diagnosis of velocardiofacial syndrome or DiGeorge syndrome). Stained with fluorescent dyes, DNA probes are hybridized at complementary chromosome segments. FISH technique, as all other hybridization techniques, relies on the complementarity of the DNA molecule. Hybridization occurs in situ, directly on the chromosome or the nuclear cell preparation of the patient. Both FISH analysis and conventional chromosome analysis utilize the same chromosome preparation. Metaphase FISH is performed on metaphase chromosomes and provides information about the location of the genomic region in question. Interphase FISH interrogates cells in which the DNA is dispersed within the nucleus. It is possible to perform interphase FISH on nonmitotic cells from a swab of the oral mucosa or from an uncultured specimen from amniocentesis. The latter provides a much more timely analysis of an amniocentesis specimen. It is necessary to culture amniocytes for a routine chromosome analysis of the sample, which often yields a result in 10 to 14 days. However, partial (yet extremely important) information can be obtained from direct analysis

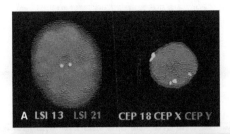

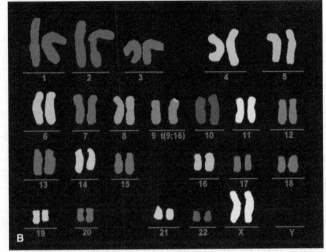

☐ **Figure 15.3. Fluorescence In Situ Hybridization (FISH) Diagnostics. A.** In prenatal diagnostics, a rapid FISH test of interphase nuclei reveals three copies of the chromosome 18 centromere, indicating either trisomy 18 or partial trisomy 18 in a male fetus. **B.** Multiplex-FISH (M-FISH) analysis with combination stained "painting" probes for all human chromosomes shows an unbalanced translocation of (9)t(9;16). The short arm of the derived chromosome 9 (in blue) shows additional material of chromosome 16 (green). (Courtesy of Dr. Jauch Institut für Humangenetik Heidelberg.)

of interphase cells obtained at amniocentesis, providing results in less than 24 hours! Most often, chromosomes 13, 18, 21, X, and Y are analyzed in this manner, thereby excluding the most frequent numeric chromosomal anomalies (trisomy 21, trisomy 18, trisomy 13, numeric alterations of sex chromosomes).

■■■ **Staining of DNA Probes**

Staining of the DNA probes occurs through a process called *nick-translation reaction*. The enzyme DNAse I places single-strand breaks (so-called *nicks*) in the DNA probe. The enzyme DNA polymerase I and the requisite nucleotides are then added, replacing deoxythymidine triphosphate (dTTP) with a chemically modified nucleotide (e.g., Cy3-depoxyurdine triphosphate [dUTP] or biotin-dUTP). Due to its exonuclease activity, DNA polymerase begins to digest nucleotides beginning at the 5′ end. In the subsequent repair synthesis polymerase simultaneously incorporates the chemically modified nucleotide in place of dTTP. The DNA probe is now stained with fluorescent dye or with a reporter molecule.

15.3 DNA Array Analysis—The Bridge between Cytogenetics and Molecular Analyses

Over time, cytogenetic techniques have increasingly pushed the limits of resolution—from nonbanded chromosome analyses, to G-banding, to FISH. However, this resolution, as well as the number of loci that can be interrogated in a single assay, pales in comparison to that of DNA microarray analysis, which, in most diagnostic laboratories, can cover the entire genome at an

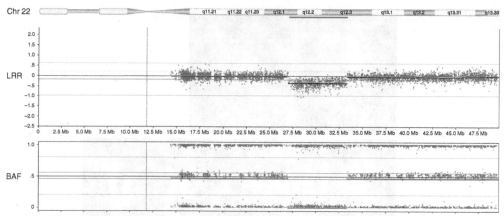

Figure 15.4. SNP array analysis in an 18-year-old patient with intellectual disability and dysmorphic features reveals a 6.2 Mb interstitial deletion of the long arm of chromosome 22. SNP arrays provide two types of information: copy number information and genotype information. Copy number information is given as log R ratio (LRR), the logged ratio of observed probe intensity to expected intensity (Norm = 0). Genotype information is given as B allele frequency (BAF), with homozygosity for the arbitrary "B" allele indicated by BAF = 1, homozygosity for the arbitrary "A" allele indicated by BAF = 0, and heterozygosity A/B indicated by BAF = 0.5. In the present example, the upper diagram shows a clear loss of signal intensity in the deleted region (red bar), while the lower diagram shows loss of heterozygosity in the same region (absence of the BAF = 0.5 dots). This deletion was not visible by routine G-banded chromosome analysis. (Courtesy of Christine Fauth, Human Genetics Innsbruck.)

average resolution of 30 kb with increased coverage at disease loci and the telomeres. With a single test, the DNA array can detect any numerical abnormality and any unbalanced structural abnormality that is represented by the DNA probes on the array. These probes include all of the loci for the well-known microdeletion and microduplication syndromes, the centromeric and subtelomeric regions of all chromosomes, hundreds of specific disease genes, and the mitochondrial genome in some laboratories (■ Fig. 15.4). The frequently used **oligonucleotide array** assay uses genomic DNA from a patient and compares the sample to a control. Patient and control DNA is differentially labeled, combined into a single sample, and hybridized to the complementary region-specific oligonucleotides. Results are analyzed by using quantitative imaging and analytical software. Differences in copy number between the patient and control samples (as detected by the array) are then usually confirmed by FISH analysis or quantitative polymerase chain reaction (PCR) of the respective chromosomal region. Other systems (e.g., **SNP arrays**) directly type single nucleotide polymorphisms (SNPs), thereby providing additional sequence information and detecting abnormalities such as uniparental disomy and large expansions of absence of heterozygosity (AOH) as observed in children of consanguineous parents. The limitations of DNA arrays are that they do not detect low-level mosaicism or balanced rearrangements such as inversions or balanced translocations. They also do not detect small deletions or duplications, point mutations, or triplet repeat expansions; consequently, the DNA arrays are not suitable for the diagnosis of most monogenic disorders.

> **Important**
>
> **General Indications for Requesting a DNA Array Analysis**
> — Multiple malformations or unknown dysmorphism syndrome
> — Unexplained fetal demise, especially if history of more than one fetal demise or stillbirth
> — Psychomotor developmental delays, especially in the context of short stature, dysmorphism, and/ or multiple malformations
> — Growth disturbances in girls; quite often, these are caused by Turner syndrome/monosomy X
> — Increased risk for a fetal chromosomal disturbance during pregnancy (e.g., advanced maternal age, as well as prior child or fetus with chromosomal abnormality)
> — Positive family history for chromosomal abnormality; a copy of the abnormal chromosomal report should be reviewed

> **Important**
>
> **Indications for Requesting a G-Banded Chromosome Analysis**
> - Recurring unexplained miscarriages or stillbirths. If two or more unexplained miscarriages occur, the parents should undergo a G-banded chromosome analysis, which will detect balanced rearrangements.
> - Infertility, especially when planning invasive fertilization techniques such as intracytoplasmic sperm injection (ICSI), to exclude a balanced translocation or sex chromosome abnormality
> - First-line testing when Down syndrome, Turner syndrome, Klinefelter syndrome, or autosomal trisomy is suspected. A G-banded analysis will detect robertsonian translocations, whereas a DNA array analysis would only detect increased dosage. G-banded analysis will also detect low-level mosaicism.
> - Characterization of malignant tumors. Almost all neoplasias manifest chromosomal aberrations. A chromosomal analysis of tumor tissue can be of diagnostic, prognostic, and/or therapeutic value.

15.4   Molecular Genetics

Molecular genetics refers to all diagnostic methods that examine changes of genetic information in extracted DNA or RNA. This diagnostic area of human genetics has grown rapidly in the past 25 years, largely due to the invention of PCR in 1983, which permits a focused replication of small DNA fragments (see special section Polymerase Chain Reaction). Following PCR, the amplification products can be further examined with respect to sequence, size, and quantity.

Obtaining the Test Material. While cytogenetic analysis typically requires cells that are mitotically active or ones in which mitosis can be induced in cell culture, molecular genetic testing only requires DNA. The DNA can be obtained from any cell and, except for cases of mosaicism, is expected to have the same sequence in all cells from a single individual. A sample of whole blood, obtained via venipuncture, and placed in a tube with ethylenediaminetetraacetic acid (EDTA) is usually sufficient. The genomic DNA is extracted from nucleated cells of the blood (lymphocytes). Various techniques and commercial kits are available for this purpose. Other common test materials are skin cells (fibroblasts), cells of the oral mucosa (from saliva or buccal swab), and amniotic fluid cells or fetal cells from chorionic villi biopsies in prenatal diagnostics. The high sensitivity of polymerase chain reaction makes it possible to obtain valid results from a minimal amount of test material. This is the case in preimplantation diagnostics, wherein a single cell is removed from the dividing zygote and serves as the test material for molecular genetic diagnostics.

In contrast to DNA analysis, RNA testing requires cells in which the respective gene is expressed. An organ biopsy may be necessary (e.g., liver biopsy), and the cells need to be processed rapidly, since RNA is unstable. Numerous techniques and commercial kits are also available for RNA extraction. RNA is translated in the laboratory into complementary DNA (cDNA) and analyzed in the same way as genomic DNA (e.g., sequenced). RNA testing has several advantages over genomic DNA testing. For example, introns are not present in RNA, and mutations that disrupt the splicing of pre–messenger RNA are easily identified. This process, however, is subject to flaws, and additional problems can occur if, for example, mutant RNA is completely absent due to nonsense-mediated decay (see Section 2.4). Consequently, in most cases molecular genetic diagnostics is performed on genomic DNA.

Selecting the Best Methods. Selecting the appropriate molecular genetic method for detecting mutations largely depends on the type and frequency of the suspected mutation. Point mutations and very small deletions are easily accessible for PCR-based methods such as direct sequencing, but larger deletions, duplications, or triplet repeat expansions require special methods for genomic quantification or Southern blot analysis. On the other hand, imprinting mutations in which the genomic imprinting is defective need to be identified with special methylation tests.

Occasionally, the quality and quantity of the test material is of importance. PCR-based tests require only a tiny amount of possibly dried or degraded test material (as is the case in forensic medicine and criminology). DNA can also be extracted from decade-old paraffin-fixed histological materials and has even been successfully extracted from the tissues of Egyptian mummies or bone fragments from the Stone Age. A Southern blot analysis, however, requires larger amounts of intact highly molecular DNA in relatively pure condition.

Important Methods for Detecting Mutations

Mutation Screening Methods. These test a limited number of specific mutations in a gene (□ Fig. 15.5A). They are indicated in diseases for which few yet frequent mutations are known (e.g., cystic fibrosis). There are some low-cost commercial kits available. However, one should consider the limited sensitivity of the test. In addition, the ethnic background of the patient must be considered, since allele frequencies can vary considerably among different populations. In some cases, results can only be adequately evaluated when taking into account the patient's ethnic origin(s). The physician requesting such an analysis is responsible for passing this information on to the laboratory.

Mutation Scanning Methods. These tests examine a gene for all possible mutations and can therefore detect both known and unknown mutations. They are based on the analysis of physical or chemical characteristics of single or double strands after PCR amplification (e.g., the melting temperature at which a double strand separates into its individual strands). These methods make it possible to predict, for example, the presence of a point mutation, although they cannot exactly localize the base exchange. Abnormalities need to be confirmed by sequencing. These methods were very useful in the past, when DNA sequencing was relatively expensive. Now, however, they are less relevant despite still being used to analyze very large genes.

Examples of mutation scanning methods are **SSCP** (single-strand conformation polymorphism), **DGGE** (denaturing gradient gel electrophoresis; Fig. 15.5B), and **dHPLC** (denaturing high-capacity liquid chromatography).

Direct Sequencing. This method continues to be the "gold standard" for mutation detection (Fig. 15.5C). Sequencing allows reliable authentication of mutations and prediction of their effects on the amino acid sequence and the secondary structure of the coded protein. The technique is limited (as with most PCR-based methods) in detecting larger deletions and genomic rearrangements. Disease-relevant mutations outside of the tested segments (e.g., in large introns) are not detected.

Southern Blotting. This method makes it possible to determine the length of a specific DNA fragment (Fig. 15.5D). It is a classic molecular genetic method that was first described in 1975. At this time, Southern blotting is used especially to detect large repeat extensions in triplet repeat disorders (see Fig. 3.8).

Genomic Quantification. Determination of the number of copies of a specific DNA locus allows the molecular genetic detection of larger deletions or duplications in a gene or chromosome segment. *Multiplex ligation-dependent probe amplification* (**MLPA**) allows simultaneous analysis of at least 40 different loci (e.g., 40 exons in Duchenne muscular dystrophy or all subtelomeric regions) with definitive detection of deletions as well as duplications. MLPA has largely replaced multilocus FISH analysis, because it is easier and duplications are hard to detect with FISH. **DNA microarrays** (i.e., DNA chips) are increasingly used in large-scale genomic quantifications and can test many (10,000 to 100,000) DNA sequences simultaneously. In many centers, DNA microarrays have replaced classic chromosome analysis for most, but not all, indications.

■■■ Polymerase Chain Reaction

Polymerase chain reaction has revolutionized molecular genetics since its invention by Kary Mullis in 1983. Exceptionally potent, it allows the in vitro exponential amplification of specific DNA fragments. For testing material, one needs only the smallest amounts of amplifiable DNA, as **primer** two single-stranded oligonucleotides (approximately 20 base pairs [bp]) that are complementary to the forward or backward strand of the DNA and that respectively contain the amplifiable region in the 3' direction of the primer, as well as a DNA polymerase. Beginning in 1998, the use of a heat-stable **Taq DNA polymerase** from the bacterium *Thermus aquaticus* allowed repeated PCR reactions without replacing the enzyme after each denaturation step. The primer can be extended at temperatures between 66°C and 75°C in the presence of free nucleotides (deoxyadenosine triphosphate [dATP], deoxycytidine triphosphate [dCTP], deoxyguanosine triphosphate [dGTP], dTTP) and is not denatured by heating to 95°C. The amplifiable segment generally is between 150 and 500 bp in size, while sometimes reaching more than 20,000 bp.

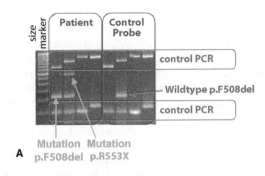

A. Mutation p.F508del   Mutation p.R553X

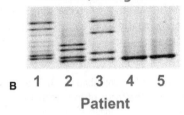

Exon 7, *PAH* gene

B. 1 2 3 4 5

Patient

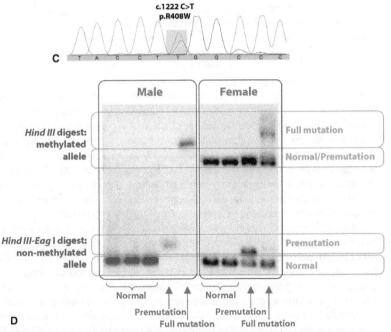

C. c.1222 C>T p.R408W

D. Normal / Premutation / Full mutation

◘ Figure 15.5. Important Techniques for Mutation Detection. A. Screening a patient for 29 frequent cystic fibrosis mutations shows compound heterozygosity for p.F508del and p.R553X. (Courtesy of B. Janssen, Institut für Humangenetik Heidelberg.) **B.** Screening of exon 7 of the *PAH* gene with denaturing gradient electrophoresis. Patients 4 and 5 are homozygous for the wild-type allele, patients 2 and 3 each are heterozygous, and patient 1 is compound heterozygous for variants in this exon. **C.** Detection of the most frequent phenylketonuria mutation p.R408W (c.1222C>T) heterozygous by sequencing. **D.** Molecular analysis for fragile X syndrome involves methylation-dependent digest of genomic DNA and visualization by Southern blot. In males, there is only one allele that is nonmethylated in normal individuals or individuals with a premutation, but this allele is methylated in patients with a full mutation. Females show two alleles (active and inactive X chromosome) and thus have two bands representing both methylated and nonmethylated copies of the gene; a full mutation is always methylated.

PCR is a repetitive three-step process. It consists of denaturation of the double strands (94°C), hybridization of the primer (annealing, 50°C to 65°C), and extension of the primer (extension, 72°C), whereby each step of the standard PCR takes 30 to 60 seconds. At the end of the third step, the DNA region that is to be synthesized has doubled in concentration. By repeating this process, an exponential amplification of DNA between the oligonucleotides can be achieved, since the newly synthesized strands are also amplified. After the usual 30 to 35 cycles, the segment covered by the two primers has been copied billions of times (theoretically amplified 2^{30} times). Utilizing a thermostable DNA polymerase has the advantage that all components (DNA, primer, deoxynucleotide triphosphates [dNTPs], enzyme, buffer) are combined in one single reaction, and numerous reaction cycles can be fully automated.

Extremely high sensitivity and exponential amplification are the major advantages of PCR. However, this advantage also makes the process vulnerable to contamination, especially through amplification of waste products from previous PCR tests. The slightest contamination, such as those carried over in pipetting aerosols, can lead to a false-positive result. Therefore, a negative control, a positive control, and good protection from contamination are important components of every PCR experiment.

■■■ Southern Blotting

This molecular genetic method was first described in 1975 by the geneticist Ed Southern as a technique for the detection of genetic variants. The focus of this technique is fractionating genomic DNA with specific **restriction endonucleases** (restriction enzymes). These enzymes occur naturally in bacteria, where they form a prokaryotic defense mechanism to digest foreign DNA. They recognize and cut specific sequences of DNA (restriction sites, mostly palindromic sequences of 4 to 8 bp in length), which is why they are being used as "enzymatic scissors." For example, the restriction enzyme EcoRI (from *Escherichia coli*) specifically cleaves the sequence 5'-GAATTC-3', and HindIII (from *Haemophilus influenzae*) the sequence 5'-AAGCTT-3'.

The first step in a Southern blot analysis is enzymatic cleavage of genomic DNA by a restriction endonuclease. The respective DNA fragments are fractionated electrophoretically on an agarose gel. The larger a fragment, the greater is its molecular weight and the slower is its movement in the gel. This results in fractionation of the fragments in the gel. In the second step, the actual "blotting," the DNA is transferred from the gel to a nitrocellulose (or alternatively nylon) membrane and subsequently immobilized by ultraviolet (UV) irradiation. Next, short, single-stranded, radiolabeled DNA probes (e.g., the cloned cDNA of a gene) can be hybridized onto the DNA that is bound to the membrane. The probes specifically bind to only complementary DNA sequences on the membrane; all nonspecifically bound probes are removed by stringent washing. Then the position of the bound probes is documented by exposure of an X-ray film to the labeled membrane. The film shows a specific band pattern, where each band corresponds to a genomic fragment that represents precisely the applied probe. Since the DNA is immobilized onto the membrane the way it was fractionated in the gel, the height of the band indicates the size of the DNA fragments.

If a specific restriction site in a gene is altered by a polymorphism (or a disease-causing mutation), this will alter the banding pattern in the Southern blot analysis of a suitable probe. This is known as **restriction fragment length polymorphism** (RFLP). Many years before PCR was invented, Southern blot analysis allowed for reliable detection of point mutations. Today, this complex method is no longer used for detecting simple genetic variants (PCR does that much more efficiently). It is, however, still the method of choice for detecting large changes in DNA length, such as large repeat expansions in trinucleotide repeat diseases (Section 3.6).

With respect to Southern blot analysis of DNA by electrophoretic fractionation and its specific representation after transfer to a nitrocellulose membrane, the corresponding examination of RNA is called **Northern blot** and that of proteins is called **Western blot**. To continue the play on words, the term *Eastern blot* and variations on this term are used to denote methods for the detection of various other biological materials (e.g., lipids and glycoconjugates).

■■■ DNA Sequencing

The most important method for sequencing specific DNA segments is the enzymatic dideoxy **Sanger method**. The Sanger method is based on the concept that, by utilizing the four different dNTPs, the DNA polymerase enzyme is capable of copying a single-stranded DNA beginning at a double-stranded point of departure (e.g., a primer bound to a DNA strand) and ending at a complementary, antiparallel double strand. In this process, the formation of phosphodiesters between the 5' phosphate and the 3' OH groups of dNTPs is catalyzed.

Also important is that DNA polymerase has the capability of utilizing **dideoxynucleotide triphosphates** (ddNTPs, also called terminators, which are not naturally occurring) as a substrate. These are deoxygenated at the 2' and 3' position of the ribose sugar. Therefore, they can be inserted at their 5'-phosphate residue into an emerging DNA chain and bring the extension of the chain to a halt because they lack the 3'-OH group necessary to link to the phosphate of the next nucleotide. The sequencing reaction requires both dNTPs as well as (in much smaller concentration) ddNTPs. The occasional random insertion of a ddNTP into the cloning chain generates shortened fragments whose length is determined by the sequence of the template DNA strand. These fragments are electrophoretically separated and visualized.

In order to obtain analyzable sequencing, it is necessary to first amplify the relevant DNA segment through PCR. The actual **sequencing reaction** for each amplifiable fragment was initially carried out in four different reaction tubes, each of which contain all four dNTPs but only one specific ddNTP (either ddATP, ddGTP, ddCTP, or ddTTP). In each tube, this always results in breaks in the chain that are specific to one particular nucleotide. The reaction products are applied in four parallel tracks onto a polyacrylamide gel and visualized by isotope labeling on an X-ray film. Radioactive sequencing has now been replaced by sequencing with **fluorescently labeled ddNTP terminators**, which are inserted into the synthesized fragment. The product can be visualized with the help of a laser and a system of light-sensitive detecting diodes imaged in an automated sequencing apparatus. Each of the four nucleotides is represented by a different color, and the sequencing reaction can be performed in a single tube.

While Sanger sequencing is considered the "gold standard" of single-gene diagnostic sequencing, high-throughput sequencing technologies (**next-generation sequencing**) have been developed that parallel the sequencing process, producing millions of sequences at once. SOLiD sequencing, 454 pyrosequencing, and Solexa sequencing are some of the widely used next-generation sequencing techniques that make it technically, analytically, and economically feasible to sequence whole human genomes (or *exomes*, focusing on the coding regions of the human genome). Currently, the false-positive and false-negative rates of next-generation sequencing are still higher than that of standard Sanger sequencing. Data analysis represents one of the biggest challenges of next-generation sequencing, as 5 to 10 gb of mappable sequence is generated per individual in whole exome sequencing. Still, whole exome sequencing is currently being introduced as a clinically available test.

Indirect Diagnostics and Linkage Analysis

Frequent polymorphisms, such as single nucleotide polymorphisms (Section 3.1) or microsatellites (Section 2.3), can be useful in establishing an exact definition of various alleles at a given gene (or chromosomal locus). **Linkage analysis** is based on the fact that disease-causing mutations are inherited jointly (linked) with the genetic markers located in their immediate vicinity on the same chromosomal strand. Human genetics can benefit from this in two different ways:

— **Identification of disease-related genes:** In the many genetic diseases, the respective genes are identified by way of linkage analysis. Such an analysis is possible when a disease occurs in several persons within one family. It is necessary to do a genomic analysis of polymorphic DNA markers in all family members. In the case of an autosomal dominant heritable disorder with an assumed penetrance of 100%, for example, one examines which alleles are present in all family members with clinical symptoms of the disease and which alleles never occur when the family member is healthy. In other words, one searches for the alleles that, in this family, are always transmitted together with the disorder (segregate with the disorder). Thus, one tries to identify the genomic (chromosomal) locus to which the disorder is linked. Since a linkage between gene and marker can be lost through recombination and since linkage can be a spurious chance effect (especially in small families), such an analysis can only result in probabilities. Such probabilities are represented by way of a logarithm or the *logarithm of the odds* score (**LOD score**). The higher the LOD score, the larger is the probability that a disease-causing gene is present in this region.

— **Indirect diagnostics of a family:** If it is known which gene or which chromosomal locus is linked to a given disorder, yet there is no available method to test the gene itself, familial segregation analysis can predict whether a person is a carrier for the disorder. In order to do this analysis, DNA must be available from a sufficiently large number of affected and unaffected family members, and the markers used must be closely linked to the gene to minimize the potential for recombination. Due to the rapid progress that has taken place in the development of the previously mentioned techniques for mutation detection, this approach has decreased in importance.

Clinical Evaluation of Molecular Genetic Findings

In the past few years, molecular genetic tests have become a central element of diagnostics in all medical disciplines. Diagnostic analyses for dozens (if not hundreds) of single-gene disorders are now available in clinical genetic laboratories. Many individuals with intellectual disabilities, autism, and/or syndromic disorders can now benefit from high-resolution DNA-based testing for submicroscopic chromosomal aberrations, and the analyses of the genetic alterations in malignancies have improved substantially. However, despite the completion of the Human Genome Project and the development of advanced technologies in molecular diagnostics, there is a relative paucity of diagnostic tests for common disorders that affect a large proportion of the population. Even for those disorders that are now testable in the diagnostic laboratory, consideration must be given to utility of these studies in improving health and well-being.

Gain of Information. Mutation analyses are only a part of a very large diagnostic repertoire and should be used selectively. The question of which technique to use is not as relevant as the question of how much information can be gained and when this information will be available. Before requesting molecular genetic testing, one should always ask what information this test will (or could) provide and what effect this will have on the patient. Of special concern should be the potential predictive nature of genetic diagnostics. For example, there is no difference (except in cost) between diagnosing sickle cell anemia with a blood smear and electrophoresis or with mutation analysis; however, only mutation analysis would provide a diagnosis in utero. There is a substantial difference, however, between diagnosing Huntington disease *clinically* in a 50-year-old or *predictively* in a 20-year-old.

Cost and Benefit. Selecting a molecular genetic technique depends on the type of mutation and the consideration of costs and benefits. For example, a clinically unequivocal diagnosis of neurofibromatosis type 1 need not be confirmed by molecular genetic testing to provide optimal clinical care of the patient. Molecular diagnosis would be necessary to perform prenatal testing or to clarify the diagnosis in clinically ambiguous cases. Sometimes specific mutations are associated with special clinical manifestations. In addition, there is a role for molecular analysis in the research setting to gain understanding of genotype–phenotype correlations.

Interpretation of Test Data. In order to adequately judge the findings of a molecular genetic test, the geneticist must be familiar with the mutation spectrum of the tested gene and the clinical background (and also genotype–phenotype correlations). Evaluating "new" genetic variants can be especially difficult, since frequently we cannot say with certainty whether these are disease relevant or not (*unclassified variants*). This needs to be discussed in the laboratory report.

Limited Sensitivity. As with every diagnostic test, molecular genetic testing should be of high specificity and sensitivity. There are several factors that determine the sensitivity of molecular genetic techniques, including the specific technique being used, the specific gene being tested, and the ethnicity of the patient undergoing the analysis. Even with very extensive testing, most disorders will not reveal all disease-associated mutations. Sensitivity is especially relevant in mutation screening techniques that test for few yet frequent mutations in the respective gene. In case of a negative test result, the test report should always include a statement about the technique's sensitivity.

Compound Heterozygosity. A special situation occurs if, in a recessive disorder, two different heterozygous mutations (of the same gene) are detected. One speaks of compound heterozygosity if these two mutations occur in *trans* (i.e., on the two separate chromosome strands). This is to be expected in a recessive disorder; however, there are occasions whereby the two identified mutations stem from the same parent and are located in *cis* (i.e., on the same chromosome strand). In such a circumstance, one parent will harbor both mutations but not be affected with the disorder. If the patient is truly affected with the disorder in question, another mutation (even if not detectable in the laboratory) must be present.

No Laboratory Is Perfect. All clinical diagnostic laboratories in the United States undergo periodic inspection and performance testing and are subjected to the regulations of the Clinical Laboratory Improvement Act (CLIA). Despite this oversight, errors in reporting and technique are possible. Therefore, if a molecular genetic finding is unexpected or does not corroborate with clinical assessment, the clinician should contact the laboratory and discuss options for repeat analysis.

16 Metabolic Diagnostics and Newborn Screening

LEARNING OBJECTIVES

1 Discuss the rationale for newborn screening, and give at least two examples of disorders that are asymptomatic in the neonate but cause severe neurological impairment in the untreated child.

2 Describe the three clinical laboratory tiers as they relate to the diagnosis of metabolic disorders.

3 Describe the Guthrie test, and contrast this method to current methods in the newborn screening laboratory.

Inborn errors of metabolism constitute a broad group of disorders that are characterized by the inability of the body to convert or break down one substance (substrate) to another (product). These disorders are typically due to the absence or insufficiency of crucial enzymes or cofactors and are usually inherited in an autosomal recessive or X-linked manner. As many of these disorders are easily diagnosed in the laboratory and can be treated effectively, they are represented on newborn screening panels in the United States and Europe. This chapter discusses the basic principles of metabolic diagnosis as well as newborn screening. See Chapter 24 for a detailed discussion of clinical, diagnostic, and therapeutic aspects of inborn errors of metabolism.

16.1 Metabolic Diagnostics

The laboratory diagnosis of metabolic disorders can be divided into three tiers of testing. The first tier includes the basic analyses that are available at all hospitals on an emergency basis. The results of first-tier testing are useful in the acute management of the patient, but alone they would not provide a definitive diagnosis. The second tier of tests consists of those analyses that are typically available only at reference laboratories. In a routine setting, the results of the second-tier analyses may not be available for several days; however, they may be able to identify the specific pathway that is affected. The third tier of testing consists of specific enzyme analyses and DNA testing, which implicate the deficient enzyme and/or the mutated gene that is causing the patient's illness.

Tier One: Basic Diagnostics. Several laboratory studies are essential in the evaluation of a critically ill patient who presents with cardiorespiratory compromise, sepsis, acute gastrointestinal illness, change in mental status, or even failure to thrive. These first-tier tests should be obtained on an emergency basis within minutes of presentation and include **electrolytes**, **blood glucose**, **pH** (venous or arterial), **lactate**, **ammonia**, and **urinary ketones**. The results will direct acute management and may point to a particular category of metabolic disorders.

Tier Two: Selective Screening. These studies are often obtained simultaneously with tier one testing when there is a medium to high index of suspicion of an underlying inborn error of metabolism. Obtaining the samples at presentation (i.e., before stabilization of the patient) is necessary, as some metabolic disorders can only be detected when the patient is in an acute crisis. At most hospitals, the results will not be available for at least 3 to 5 days, as most institutions send these tests to reference laboratories. However, when the results of tier one testing clearly indicate an inborn error of metabolism, the physician should make arrangements to promptly deliver these specimens as emergency samples to a laboratory that can process and interpret the sample in a more timely manner (possibly even as rapidly as a few hours from receipt). Among the most important selective screening techniques are:

- **Organic acids in urine:** provides evidence for organic acidemias, fatty acid oxidation defects, aminoacidopathies, mitochondrial disorders, etc.
- **Amino acids in plasma:** especially useful for diagnosing aminoacidopathies and urea cycle disorders, as well as other metabolic disorders
- **Acylcarnitine profile in plasma or dried blood on a filter paper card:** useful for diagnosing fatty acid oxidation defects and organic acidemias

Tier Three: Enzyme and DNA-Based Analysis. Many genetic enzyme defects can be diagnosed with certainty by specific identification of enzyme activity in appropriate cells. Often a blood sample (lymphocytes) or a skin biopsy (fibroblasts) is sufficient; occasionally, it is necessary to perform organ biopsies (e.g., liver biopsy). Enzyme analysis (from blood or skin cells) can be preferable to molecular genetic methods in some cases; however, DNA-based tests have become available for most inborn errors of metabolism. Molecular analyses will secure a specific diagnosis and provide information that can be used in carrier testing and prenatal diagnosis.

Function Tests. Some metabolic disorders are best detected by a daily metabolic profile (i.e., by measuring relevant metabolites, including glucose, lactate, and amino acids, during the course of the day). A daily profile can also contribute to the significance of external factors and optimize treatment. While not as frequently used because of advances in molecular diagnoses, it may be necessary to perform stress tests to establish controlled metabolic situations that are of critical importance for the diagnosis. For example, delivering an increased protein load would unmask a late-onset urea cycle disorder such as partial ornithine transcarbamylase (OTC) deficiency, and a prolonged fast would be expected to induce hypoglycemia in a person with a fatty acid oxidation disorder. These tests may be life-threatening and should only be done in specialized metabolic clinics or inpatient units.

16.2   Basics of Newborn Screening

Universal newborn screening was introduced in the 1960s with the **Guthrie test** for early detection of phenylketonuria and was soon expanded to include other treatable disorders, including congenital hypothyroidism and galactosemia. Over the last few years, the introduction of a new laboratory technique, tandem mass spectrometry, has considerably improved diagnostic possibilities. **Expanded newborn screening** helps diagnose many other treatable metabolic diseases, such as medium-chain acyl-coenzyme A dehydrogenase (MCAD) deficiency (Section 24.3), before the onset of symptoms or acute metabolic crises. This expanded screening also detects metabolic "abnormalities" that may not be clinically relevant. Newborn screening for cystic fibrosis, which uses immunoreactive trypsinogen (IRT) from dried blood spots, has been implemented in most of the United States and many other countries. On the horizon is the development of newborn screening for other nonmetabolic disorders such as fragile X (Chapter 31) and deletion 22q11.2 syndrome (Chapter 21). To be sure, newborn screening programs require the collaborative efforts of physicians who are expert in metabolic disorders, public health departments, hospitals, and government agencies. While advanced technologies promote more efficient and comprehensive testing, they also invoke challenges with regard to interpretation of the samples and, most importantly, to the delivery of health care for the children who are subjected to screening. Also, the early diagnosis of conditions with limited or no treatment options, or the identification of variants of uncertain clinical relevance, poses challenges.

■■■ Historic Perspective: The Guthrie Test
The Guthrie test is named after the pediatrician and microbiologist Robert Guthrie who had a niece with untreated phenylketonuria (PKU) and an intellectually disabled son (not caused by PKU). Searching for a cost-effective and feasible technique that would detect PKU before the onset of symptoms, he developed a **bacterial inhibition assay** that, for the first time, made it possible to universally test newborns. The test is based on the growth-inhibiting effect of the antimetabolite β-2-thienylalanine, which competitively inhibits enzymes

for which phenylalanine (Phe) is the substrate. A drop of blood is placed onto a filter paper card ("Guthrie card"). In the laboratory a small disk is punched out of the dried blood spot and placed on a nutrient plate containing β-2-thienylalanine and incubated with *Bacillus subtilis*. The Phe diffusing from the blood creates a growth spot whose size depends on the Phe concentration in the blood. Similar bacterial inhibition tests were developed for other disorders; since the 1980s, these have been replaced by other analytic techniques. The concept of universal testing of all newborns for diagnosing a relatively rare genetic disorder was initially controversial, but by the end of the 1960s it had become accepted in most Western countries and permitted normal development for thousands of children with PKU and other diseases.

16.3   Methods of Newborn Screening

For the actual screening, a few drops of capillary blood are obtained by pricking the inner or outer rim of the heel with a safety lancet. Blood from the umbilical cord should not be used. The blood is dropped onto standardized filter paper specimen cards. Instead of using capillary blood, one can also use untreated venous blood; ethylenediaminetetraacetic acid (EDTA) blood, however, is not suitable.

The American Academy of Pediatrics recommends that the first sample not be collected until the newborn is at least 24 hours old, **optimally on day 3** (i.e., 49 to 72 hours after birth), and no later than the fifth day. A specimen taken prior to 24 hours is useful as a screening test for some conditions (e.g., galactosemia, biotinidase deficiency, sickle hemoglobin, and cystic fibrosis), but will not reliably detect disorders like PKU, wherein the deleterious effects are due to an accumulation of a toxic metabolite. Some states (e.g., Texas) require a second screening test for all infants, typically performed between the ages of 10 and 14 days. A second sample is also required if the infant is discharged prior to 24 hours of life or if the birth was premature (i.e., less than 32nd week of pregnancy). Formal guidelines are available for testing premature infants as well as newborns who require blood transfusion and/or total parenteral nutrition.

16.4   Major Disorders Detected by Newborn Screening

Hypothyroidism

With an incidence of 1 in 3,000 newborns, congenital hypothyroidism is the most frequent congenital endocrinopathy. Nonspecific symptoms in the newborn include hypotonia and pro-longed jaundice; however, clinical features may be mild or absent, and an abnormal newborn screen (NBS) may be the only indication of disease. If untreated in early infancy, congenital hypothyroidism causes psychomotor retardation, growth failure, and irreversible cognitive and intellectual impairment. Late manifestations of untreated hypothyroidism include ataxia and sensorineural hearing loss. Features that do improve, even with delayed therapy, include dry skin, macroglossia (large tongue), hoarse voice, bradycardia, and constipation.

The newborn screening test measures the thyroid-stimulating hormone (TSH) level from the blood spot, which is elevated in congenital hypothyroidism. In case of positive test results, blood is drawn for the quantitative identification of thyroid hormones; this is immediately fol-lowed by oral administration of L-thyroxine.

Congenital Adrenal Hyperplasia

Congenital adrenal hyperplasia (CAH; incidence 1 in 10,000; Section 25.2) is a group of autosomal recessive disorders that involve enzyme defects of steroid metabolism, leading to a deficiency of mineralocorticoids and glucocorticoids and an excess of male sexual hormones. More than 95% of the cases result from a deficiency of 21-hydroxylase. This "classic" type of CAH is detected in newborn screenings. At birth, affected females (46,XX) often have ambigu-ous or completely masculinized external genitalia. However, affected males (46,XY) may have only a subtle hyperpigmentation of the external genitalia or a large penis—escaping clinical diagnosis in the first days or weeks of life. Diagnosis is achieved by detection of elevated 17-OH progesterone in the blood sample. Within the first 24 hours, the titers for 17-OH progesterone can be physiologically elevated; therefore, confirmation is only possible after the first day of life. Rapid analysis is important, since a proportion of affected infants develop adrenal crisis with salt wasting and hypovolemic shock. Long-term treatment consists of mineralocorticoid and glucocorticoid administration over the life span.

Phenylketonuria

As there are no symptoms of untreated phenylketonuria (incidence 1 in 8,000; Section 24.1.3) in the first months of life, the NBS is essential for diagnosis and initiation of treatment, which prevents the devastating effects of infantile hyperphenylalaninemia. The screening method detects elevated titers of the amino acid phenylalanine (Phe) in the blood. A positive test result (Phe greater than 150 µmol/L) prompts the physician to begin a phenylalanine-restricted formula and requires a confirmatory quantitative Phe level. If confirmatory testing is abnormal, a diagnosis of PKU is established, and the patient is referred to a metabolic specialist for dietary management and genetic counseling.

Maple Syrup Urine Disease

With an incidence of 1 in 100,000, maple syrup urine disease (MSUD) is rare even among the inborn errors of metabolism. However, the distinct sweet odor, similar to that of maple syrup, distinguishes this condition as one of the more recognizable metabolic disorders. It is caused by deficient oxidative decarboxylation of α-keto acid metabolites of leucine, isoleucine, and valine. Affected infants can become symptomatic during the first days of life, with poor feeding, lethargy, seizures, and occasionally coma. Milder forms of MSUD may present later in life, with developmental delay and intellectual disability. Maple syrup urine disease is primarily treated by diet but also by avoiding circumstances that increase catabolism such as high fever and dehydration. If a metabolic crisis occurs, emergency treatment in a hospital is necessary to stabilize the patient.

Organic Acidemias

Extended newborn screening permits diagnosis of various organic acidemias (Section 24.1.3). Organic acidopathies can manifest under conditions that lead to increased catabolism (e.g., infectious disease, fever, or dehydration) and present with severe metabolic acidosis and circulatory collapse. These events then cause damage to the brain and other organs, with variable recovery. Untreated glutaric academia type I (GA I) can be misdiagnosed as non-accidental trauma because patients often present with large bilateral subdural hematomas. This encephalopathic crisis can also result in a severe and irreversible movement disorder with dystonia and dyskinesia if not recognized and treated early. Treatment involves administration of carnitine and riboflavin, and a low protein diet (lysine, tryptophan, and hydroxylysine restricted).

Biotinidase Deficiency

The enzyme biotinidase provides the coenzyme biotin, which is important for carboxylation reactions. Affected newborns are asymptomatic, but after a few months of life, they show progressive developmental delay, regression of milestones, neurological abnormalities, eczema, and hair loss. This disorder is also rare (incidence, 1 in 80,000), yet it is easily treatable by simple administration of biotin; thus, it is clearly indicated for newborn screening that tests the activity of the enzyme biotinidase.

Disorders of Fatty Acid Oxidation and the Carnitine Cycle

Deficiency of the enzyme **MCAD** (Section 24.1.2) is the most frequent (incidence, 1 in 10,000 to 1 in 15,000) fatty acid oxidation disorder. It typically causes severe, nonketotic hypoglycemia in fasting situations, and if undiagnosed the deficiency has a mortality rate of 25% during the first manifestation. Treatment is very simple: avoidance of prolonged fasting (4 to 12 hours depending on age), especially during illness. Compliance allows for completely normal development and a normal life span without other health concerns. MCAD deficiency is detected on the NBS by tandem mass spectroscopy–based acylcarnitine analysis in dried blood spots and may be confirmed by molecular analysis (common mutation in the *ACADM* gene). Other disorders detected on the NBS within the same metabolic pathway are disturbances in the mitochondrial import of long-chain fatty acids via the carnitine cycle and deficiencies of long-chain fatty acid oxidation enzymes. These metabolic disorders present with liver failure or cardiomyopathy, in addition to nonketotic hypoglycemia in the neonatal period or later; patients with attenuated enzyme deficiencies may show stress-related rhabdomyolysis in older age.

Galactosemia

Galactosemia is a disorder of galactose metabolism that has an incidence of approximately 1 in 40,000. Galactose is one of the components of lactose, a glucose-galactose disaccharide. Classic galactosemia results from a deficiency of galactose-1-phosphate uridyltransferase (GALT), which converts galactose-1-phosphate into uridine diphosphate (UDP)-galactose. The accumulating galactose-1-phosphate is especially toxic for the liver, kidneys, and central nervous system (CNS). If untreated, the disease is fatal because of complications of gram-negative sepsis and/or hepatic and renal failure. Absence of GALT activity can be detected any time after birth. It is essential to obtain results promptly, because children with classic galactosemia can have a life-threatening crisis within the first few days after birth. Infants with a positive result are placed on a lactose-free formula, and confirmatory testing is accomplished by measuring specific metabolite concentrations and enzyme activity in erythrocytes. Molecular diagnosis is also available on a clinical basis. A lifelong lactose-free, galactose-restricted diet ensures a favorable prognosis. Despite early diagnosis and compliance regarding dietary restrictions, individuals with galactosemia often show learning disabilities and abnormalities of motor function, including tremor, incoordination, and gait disturbances. Women with galactosemia are at increased risk for premature ovarian failure.

■■■ **Duarte Variant Galactosemia**

In classic galactosemia, GALT enzyme activity is less than 5% of control values; in Duarte variant galactosemia, GALT enzyme activity is between 5% and 20% of control values. The D1 variant (LA variant) of the *GALT* gene is due to a point mutation (N314D), and the D2 ("true Duarte") variant is due to the same point mutation (N314D) *plus* a deletion in the 5′ carbohydrate response element, which reduces *GALT* expression. Persons who are homozygous for the D2 allele (or compound heterozygous for the D2 allele and a classic galactosemia mutation) are often detected on NBS. Depending on metabolite profile, individuals with the Duarte variant do not usually require treatment but are typically followed up for at least the first year of life. Thus, identification of such individuals may be regarded as an incidental finding (adverse effect) of newborn screening.

17 Prenatal Genetic Evaluation

LEARNING OBJECTIVES

1 Differentiate between screening tests and diagnostic tests, and give at least two examples of each.

2 List five reasons why a woman would elect to undergo invasive prenatal testing.

3 Describe the advantage of chorionic villus sampling over amniocentesis.

Prenatal testing for genetic conditions began in 1966 when Mark W. Steele and W. Roy Bregg demonstrated that the chromosomal constitution of a fetus could be examined with cultured amniotic fluid cells. Prenatal diagnostics is now a major medical subspecialty that relies on the expertise of obstetricians, clinical geneticists, and genetic counselors to deliver prenatal (and in some cases preconception) counseling for women and couples. The methods of prenatal diagnostics have advanced considerably and involve all aspects of fetal diagnosis, including maternal serum screening, fetal imaging, amniocentesis, chorionic villus sampling, and pre-implantation diagnosis.

> **Important**
>
> **■■■ Baseline Risk of Congenital Abnormalities**
> Every pregnancy—regardless of family history, maternal health, or parental age—has a baseline risk of 3% for a congenital abnormality to be detected in the perinatal period. Various factors, including maternal medical illness, medication or drug use, twin gestations, advanced maternal and/or advanced paternal age, and family history of heritable disorders, will add to this risk. Although a normal prenatal history and diagnostic evaluation provides reassurance to the couple, a baseline risk remains.

Most couples do not consider the baseline risk when planning a pregnancy, and most will deliver a healthy infant. However, if an abnormality is detected prenatally or found upon birth of the infant, the resulting emotional stress is often substantial. Prenatal diagnosis offers earlier detection and affords the couple various options in the management of the pregnancy and delivery. The physician or genetic counselor will discuss the benefits, limitations, and risks of prenatal tests; however, the choice to undergo testing, and the decisions made upon the receipt of the results, rests with the couple. For example, some couples would choose to terminate a fetus diagnosed with trisomy 21; others would plan to deliver the infant in a tertiary care center for rapid intervention should gastrointestinal and/or cardiac malformations be detected; others would opt not to undergo any prenatal diagnostic procedures unless there was a clear benefit to the health of the fetus. All of these scenarios are valid and should be respected by the health care team.

Prenatal testing can be either noninvasive (e.g., fetal echocardiogram) or invasive (e.g., chorionic villus sampling). The results of prenatal testing may be **diagnostic** (e.g., chromosome analysis) or may provide information regarding **risk** (e.g., maternal serum screening). Diagnostic genetic analyses require fetal tissue to perform chromosome analysis or DNA-based assays, and the means to obtain these tissues involve **invasive** techniques. Certain **noninvasive** techniques can also provide diagnoses regarding structure (e.g., conotruncal malformation observed by fetal echocardiography); however, the underlying molecular etiology (e.g., deletion 22q11.2) would depend on analysis of a sample obtained by invasive means. Diagnostic prenatal genetic testing is recommended if an abnormality is detected by noninvasive methods, if the family history is positive for a genetic condition amenable to DNA testing or specific enzymatic analyses, or if the results of testing would provide a diagnosis or assist in the management of severe maternal complications (e.g., HELLP syndrome in the mother secondary to a fatty acid oxidation disorder in the fetus).

17.1   Noninvasive Methods

Maternal Serum Analysis

Throughout gestation, the concentration of various proteins in maternal blood is influenced by the fetal placental unit. The first biochemical marker used to predict possible abnormalities in the fetus was α-fetoprotein (AFP), which is normally produced in high concentration in the fetal liver. Investigators determined that average maternal serum AFP (msAFP) not only increases in a predictable manner with increasing gestational age and with multiple fetuses but also is disproportionately elevated when the fetus has an open neural tube defect, an abdominal wall defect, or any other malformation that compromises the integrity of the fetal integument. Interestingly, msAFP was found to be low more often when the fetus had trisomy 21, trisomy 18, or impending fetal demise. Presently, several different proteins can be measured during the pregnancy, including AFP, PAPP-A (pregnancy-associated plasma protein A), β-hCG (β subunit of human chorionic gonadotropin), unconjugated estriol, and inhibin A. Testing these proteins and comparing them to reference levels at specific time points in the first and second trimesters of pregnancy permits the calculation of a **probability** for the fetus to have a chromosomal abnormality. When combined with findings of a first-trimester ultrasound to evaluate for nuchal translucency and with second-trimester ultrasounds, these studies can provide added reassurance to a couple or indicate referral for further diagnostic analyses. Importantly, none of these studies provides a definitive diagnosis as they are **screening tests**; however, as such, they do not pose an increased risk to the fetus.

First-trimester combined screening (between weeks 11 and 13, postmenstruation [p.m.]) consists of the measurement of the fetal **nuchal translucency** (◻ Fig. 17.1) and analysis of **PAPP-A** and **hCG**, in conjunction with maternal age, to provide information regarding the risk for fetal trisomy 21 and trisomy 18. This screening test has a nearly 90% sensitivity for the detection of fetal trisomy 21 and 90% to 95% sensitivity for trisomy 18.

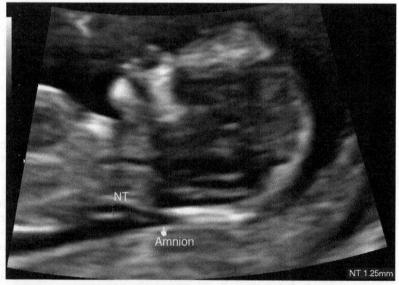

◻ **Figure 17.1. Measurement of Nuchal Translucency (NT).** The measurement is taken from a sagittal view of the fetal cervical and thoracic spine with angle of insonation perpendicular to the NT space. The fetus is away from the amnion and occupies over 50% of the image. The tip of the nose should be clear in fetal profile. The third and fourth ventricles of the fetal central nervous system (CNS) are frequently seen. The NT measurement is the distance in the echo-free space between the skin and soft tissue of the neck. The margins of the fetal skin edges and facial structures should be crisp and clean with the calipers place "edge to edge." The NT measurement in this 13-week chromosomally normal fetus is 1.25 mm. (Courtesy of Anthony Johnson, DO, Texas Children's Fetal Center, Baylor College of Medicine, Houston TX, USA.)

Second-trimester screening (between weeks 15 and 20, p.m.) involves the evaluation of either three (triple screen: AFP, hCG, and unconjugated estriol) or, more frequently, four (quadruple screen: AFP, hCG, unconjugated estriol, and inhibin A) "markers" in maternal serum. Ideally, this analysis is interpreted in conjunction with the results of the first-trimester screening; however, many women do not present for prenatal care until the second trimester. Although the triple screen and the quadruple screen have the same detection rate for trisomy 18 (70%, which means that 70% of fetuses with trisomy 18 will have an abnormal screen) and neural tube defects (85%), the quadruple screen has a higher detection rate for trisomy 21 (80%). An abnormal screening test is an indication for an ultrasound to determine if there are multiple fetuses and to help confirm dates. Even with accurate dating, the false-positive rate for these tests is approximately 5%, meaning that approximately 5% of fetuses with normal chromosomes will have an abnormal multiple marker screening test.

Ultrasonography

Prenatal ultrasonography is typically recommended for all pregnant women, since it poses no known risk to the fetus. During the **first trimester** ultrasonography provides proof of an intact intrauterine pregnancy, confirms gestational age (by measuring the length from head to coccyx and the biparietal diameter), and may detect embryonic developmental defects. Later in gestation, an ultrasound is more sensitive for the detection of fetal anomalies and growth disturbances. Importantly, the sensitivity is greatly dependent on the equipment itself as well as the expertise of the technician and physician who are performing and interpreting the study. High-resolution ultrasonography is recommended if any anomalies are detected; however, it should be clearly noted that while a normal ultrasound may provide reassurance, it cannot exclude the possibility of all anomalies.

When used alone, a nuchal translucency of 4 mm indicates an approximately 20-fold increased age-related risk for trisomy 21; a 5-mm nuchal translucency raises this risk to nearly 30-fold (▣ Fig. 17.2). For values between 3 and 5 mm, trisomy 21 is the most frequent underlying

▣ **Figure 17.2. Dorsal Nuchal Edema in a Fetus with Trisomy 21.**

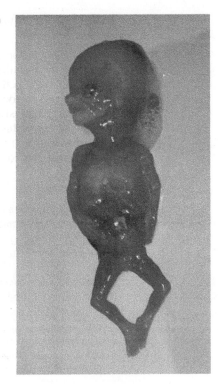

chromosomal disorder, while for higher values (6 mm and above), trisomy 18, trisomy 13, or Turner syndrome (45,X) can all be expected more frequently. Although the pathogenetic relationship between an increased nuchal translucency and a chromosomal disorder has not been completely resolved, it is likely that hemodynamic factors or the formation of the lymphatic vessel system plays a role in the development of the nuchal edema, since fetal heart defects are seen in more than 75% of cases wherein the nuchal edema is greater than 4 mm.

Ultrasonography in the **second and third trimesters** assesses fetal growth, organ development, the amount of amniotic fluid, and the position of the placenta. Fetal weight can be reliably estimated by ultrasound by the 24th week of pregnancy. High-resolution ultrasonography, color Doppler flow studies, fetal echocardiography, and fetal magnetic resonance imaging (MRI) will allow further delineation of fetal anatomy and may be indicated if abnormalities are detected on routine ultrasound. There are numerous sonographic findings such as cardiac defects, brain malformations, and/or gastrointestinal anomalies that, if present, modify the individual risk for a chromosomal disorder or other genetic disease. The presence of one or more or these findings and/or the determination that the fetus has intrauterine growth restriction are indications for further prenatal testing.

■■■ Other Sonographic Markers

The following findings often regress spontaneously over the course of the pregnancy, and *in isolation* may not require additional invasive testing:

— Elevated nuchal translucency (11 to 14 weeks p.m.)
— Hyperechogenic bowel (second trimester)
— Short femur (second trimester)
— Intracardiac echogenic foci (ICEF) (second trimester)
— Bilateral renal pelvis ectasia (second trimester)
— Single umbilical cord artery
— Umbilical cord cyst
— Choroid plexus cysts (second trimester)

17.2   Invasive Test Methods

Testing for specific genetic or chromosomal disorders requires fetal cells. While there is active research regarding the isolation of fetal cells from maternal circulation or from Pap smear samples, at this time fetal cells can only be obtained by invasive techniques. Complications of invasive techniques include infection, preterm labor, bleeding, and miscarriage; therefore, the decision to undergo invasive testing rests with the pregnant woman. The decision is often based on several factors, including the actual risk for a genetic abnormality (e.g., 50% risk if a parent has an autosomal dominant condition vs. a "screen positive" risk of 1% for trisomy 21), the risk of the specific procedure, and the moral attitudes and beliefs of the couple.

Important

■■■ Indications for Invasive Prenatal Diagnostics
— Evaluation for a fetal chromosomal disorder in the case of:
    — Advanced maternal age
    — Elevated risk after first- or second-trimester screening
    — Abnormal ultrasound, fetal echocardiogram, or MRI
    — Previous child with de novo chromosomal abnormality
    — Structural chromosomal rearrangement in a parent
    — Maternal choice to undergo testing
— Evaluation for mutation(s) for a suspected monogenic disorder
— Evaluation for specific biochemical analysis for a suspected genetic disorder
— Evaluation for an open neural tube defect
— Evaluation for fetal infection

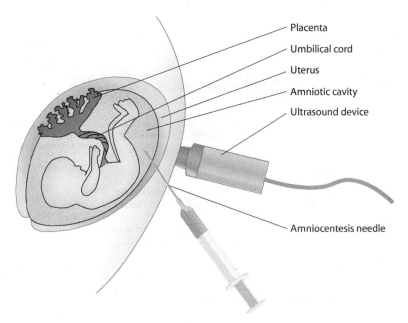

Placenta
Umbilical cord
Uterus
Amniotic cavity
Ultrasound device

Amniocentesis needle

Figure 17.3. Chorionic Villus Biopsy (Transabdominal Approach).

Chorionic Villus Sampling

Chorionic villus sampling (CVS) is usually performed between 10 and 12 weeks p.m., either transcervically or transabdominally, with or without local anesthesia (Fig. 17.3). At least 15 to 20 mg of villus tissue is obtained (more if multiple studies such as DNA array and/or mutation analysis will be conducted). The sample is examined under the microscope, and decidua and blood are removed. Further testing for maternal cell contamination is performed if tissue will be processed for anything other than G-banded chromosomes. In addition, laboratories that perform DNA array analysis require the simultaneous submission of blood samples from the biological parents to investigate the significance of copy number variation if present in the fetal sample. The major advantage of CVS is that it allows the results to be available at an earlier stage of pregnancy. However, chromosomal mosaicism in the fetal-placental unit may yield ambiguous results when CVS is performed, prompting recommendation for a follow-up amniocentesis in approximately 2% of cases. In addition, CVS does not provide information regarding open neural tube defects. The risk of miscarriage following CVS is approximately 1%.

Amniocentesis

Amniocentesis can be performed after the 14th week of pregnancy (p.m.), optimally at the end of the 15th week. At this time point, approximately 150 to 200 mL of amniotic fluid has accumulated. Under continuous ultrasound surveillance, 20 to 30 mL of amniotic fluid is removed by transabdominal puncture (Fig. 17.4). The amniotic fluid sample is centrifuged, and the cells (70% trophoblasts, 20% epithelial cells, and 10% fibroblasts) are cultured, allowing for DNA extraction for array analysis and molecular genetic analysis. Just as with chorionic villus sampling, blood samples from both biological parents are required for timely interpretation of prenatal DNA array analyses. The supernatant is used to measure AFP and acetylcholinesterase (AChE), both of which are elevated in open neural tube defects and abdominal wall defects (AFP only). The risk of miscarriage following amniocentesis is less than 1%. The advantages and disadvantages of chorionic villus sampling and amniocentesis are summarized in Table 17.1.

II

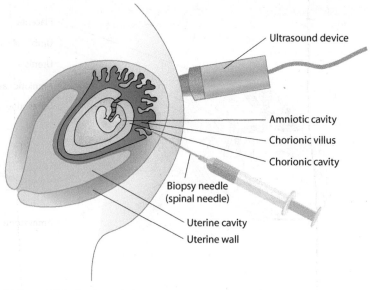

Ultrasound device

Amniotic cavity

Chorionic villus

Chorionic cavity

Biopsy needle
(spinal needle)

Uterine cavity

Uterine wall

Figure 17.4. Amniocentesis.

Umbilical Cord Blood Sampling (Cordocentesis)

Cordocentesis may be performed after the 18th week of gestation and is usually done to evaluate for fetal infection. Sampling fetal blood also allows for much more rapid genetic analysis—albeit starting from a later time period during the pregnancy. Other possible indications for umbilical cord puncture include ambiguous cytogenetic findings after chorionic villus biopsy or amniocentesis and/or clarification of a hydrops fetalis with simultaneous intrauterine blood transfusion. This procedure carries a higher risk of miscarriage (up to 2%) than either CVS or amniocentesis.

Table 17.1. Comparison of Amniocentesis and Chorionic Villus Biopsy

Criteria	Amniocentesis	Chorionic Villus Biopsy
Time when test is performed	From the 14th week of pregnancy (p.m.)	From the 11th to 13th weeks of pregnancy (p.m.)
Need for local anesthesia	Not usually	Occasionally for transabdominal approach
Success rate in obtaining adequate sample	>99%	~95% (depending on the position of the placenta)
Complication of miscarriage	Approximately 0.5%	Approximately 1%
Is chromosome analysis possible?	Yes	Yes
Are DNA-based tests possible?	Yes	Yes
Is rapid FISH possible?	Yes	Yes
Is measuring AFP and AChE of the amniotic fluid possible?	Yes	No

18 Ethical Concerns in Medical Genetics

LEARNING OBJECTIVES

1 List the four basic bioethical principles, and give examples of each.

2 Discuss "negative selection" as it relates to prenatal diagnosis.

3 Discuss situations where genetic information should be disclosed to a patient's family.

4 Discuss direct-to-consumer testing.

5 Define GINA, and discuss the protections this law provides.

Over the past century there have been tremendous discoveries in medical genetics and molecular biology. Since the double helical structure of DNA was elucidated in 1953 and the genetic code deciphered, these disciplines have grown exponentially. The resulting advancements have had very practical applications in the treatment of disease, the determination of disease risk, the response to pharmacologic agents, and the interpretation of clinical laboratory data. Associated with the advancement of genetic technologies is the emergence of ethical concerns regarding the application of these technologies to promote health and wellness. Volumes of literature have been written on biomedical ethics regarding genetic testing, genomic research, informed consent, disclosure of genetic information, and protection of genetic health information. This chapter will briefly discuss the major ethical concerns regarding genetics that affect the practicing physician. Predictive genetic diagnosis and genetic testing of children are discussed in Chapter 11.

18.1 Ethical Principles

Biomedical ethics is the study of moral controversies provoked by advances in biology and medicine. One of the first areas addressed by modern bioethicists was that of human experimentation. The National Commission for the Protection of Human Subjects of Biomedical and Behavioral Research was established in 1974, and the fundamental principles announced in the Belmont Report in 1979 have guided individuals and professional organizations in the decision-making processes that are subject to moral interpretation across a wide range of issues. Currently, four ethical principles are broadly accepted in the biomedical field. These ethical principles are highly relevant when applied to concerns regarding medical genetics.

> **Important**
>
> **Principles of Biomedical Ethics**
>
> *Autonomy*
> Autonomy relates to maintaining respect for the individual and his or her ability to make decisions regarding his or her health and medical care. This includes allowing the individual to take action (or not) based on his or her personal values and beliefs. The role of the health care professional is to provide information so the individual can make informed decisions (**informed consent**) and the duty of the health care provider is to maintain **confidentiality**. In a genetics context this applies to the decision to undergo genetic testing for adult-onset disorders such as Huntington disease.
>
> *Beneficence*
> The principle of beneficence refers to actions that promote the well-being of the patient and others. In the genetics context, this may be applied to the recommendation by the geneticist for the patient to disclose results of genetic testing results (e.g., *BRCA1* mutation) to at-risk family members.
>
> *Nonmaleficence*
> ***Primum non nocere***—"First, do no harm." The principle of nonmaleficence dictates that health care professionals do not intentionally cause harm or injury to the patient and implies a fundamental

commitment for the professional to protect the patient from harm. In the genetics context, this may be broadly applied to the avoidance of unnecessary genetic testing in an individual; however, one can see that "unnecessary genetic testing" may be interpreted differently by various individuals.

Justice

Justice can be defined as the fair distribution and equal availability of health care and genetic testing for all of society. Unfortunately, this principle is far from being realized in the United States. The disparity is even more apparent for the availability of anything but the most basic of genetic assays, as the results of most are still not considered crucial information for the medical management of many disorders.

18.2   Prenatal Diagnosis and Abortion

Following the US Supreme Court decision of *Roe v. Wade* in 1973, a woman, in consultation with her physician, can choose to legally terminate a pregnancy up to and including the 24th week (postmenstruation [p.m.]). Some states currently require parental consent for women younger than 18 years.

Prenatal genetic testing allows the identification of various medical and developmental diagnoses during pregnancy, and many couples choose to terminate a pregnancy when the fetus is found to be affected. The geneticist's role is to provide nondirective yet informative counseling regarding the diagnosis and prognosis and respect the autonomy of the woman and couple.

18.3   Preimplantation Genetic Diagnosis

While the goal of prenatal screening and diagnosis (see Chapter 17) is to detect medical or developmental abnormalities in the fetus, usually with the option of termination of pregnancy, the purpose of preimplantation genetic diagnosis (PGD) is to identify embryos with severe genetic disorders prior to the onset of a pregnancy and thereby avoid the need for termination. Those embryos found to be free of a detectable abnormality can then be transferred, usually 3 to 5 days postfertilization, with the timing depending in part on the techniques used for PGD. Additionally, unaffected embryos can be cryopreserved, while affected embryos are usually discarded.

Not unexpectedly, some couples pursue PGD with the intent to select *for* a given genetic condition (also known as negative selection), as, for example, hereditary deafness. Inherent in PGD is the preliminary step of in vitro fertilization (IVF), which itself raises ethical concerns regarding the moral status of the embryo. Furthermore, most PGD centers recommend prenatal diagnosis of the fetus after successful transfer and implantation of the embryo. Suffice it to say that PGD is an extremely controversial procedure despite the fact that the goal of PGD is most often to prevent the birth of a child affected by a lethal or otherwise devastating genetic disorder.

18.4   The Duty to Inform

The medical geneticist, as well as any subspecialist involved in the care of a patient with a heritable and treatable condition, has the obligation to discuss not only the *patient's* risk for disease but also the risk for other members in the patient's nuclear and extended family. In these situations, ethical as well as legal dilemmas exist as the duty to warn (beneficence and nonmaleficence) may outweigh the patient's right to confidentiality and autonomy. Most often, the practice is to encourage the patient to inform other family members and encourage them to contact clinical geneticists for more detailed discussion and testing. While this approach is adequate in many circumstances, there are barriers to its effectiveness, as many individuals report that informing family members can be mentally challenging and discomforting, leaving some relatives completely unaware of a serious genetic condition segregating in the family. Many geneticists will provide the patient with a letter to give or mail to at-risk relatives. This letter is devoid of information that identifies the patient, but it has specific information about the risk and genetic mutation (when known). However, under exceptional circumstances the physician may warn at-risk relatives. These circumstances are when (a) attempts to encourage disclosure on the part of the patient have failed; (b) the harm is highly likely to occur and is serious, imminent, and foreseeable; (c) the at-risk relative is identifiable; and (d) the disease is preventable or treatable, or medically accepted standards indicate that early monitoring will reduce the genetic risk. Clearly, disclosure for diseases that are neither treatable nor preventable would not be permissible. In every case, the harm from failing to disclose should outweigh the harm from disclosure.

18.5 Direct-to-Consumer Testing

Historically, genetic testing has been used selectively to diagnose monogenic or chromosomal disorders. Additionally, it has been used to evaluate the risk of developing or passing on single-gene disorders. Presently, genetic testing is increasingly being used to modify therapeutics, determine prognosis, and even provide probabilistic risk assessment for the development of common/complex disorders. Because of advances in technology and the availability of high-throughput sequencing, it is now possible to examine thousands of loci of an individual's genome at a relatively low cost and in a timely manner. The broad availability of this technology and the move toward consumer-driven health care has fostered the growing commercial industry of direct-to-consumer (DTC) genetic services. DCT genetic tests are advertised directly to consumers, are purchased through consumer-initiated requests, and provide results directly to the consumer without any involvement of the consumer's health care provider.

However, while the technologies used in genetic testing have advanced remarkably, the significance of the findings in assessing an individual's health is not always clear. When it comes to complex disorders, the results of analyzing the coding sequence of the individual's genome may only provide a subset of risk factors, while other factors related to noncoding DNA sequences, epigenetic modifications, and the environmental and behavioral components of health and disease will not be represented by the analysis. Besides the scientific concerns, the ethical concerns generated by DTC services are myriad and are being vetted by professional organizations and governmental agencies.

Concerns that have been identified include (a) the lack of federal (U.S. Food and Drug Administration) regulation of the laboratories and assays, (b) the lack of evidence of clinical validity and/or clinical utility for most DTC genetic tests, (c) privacy and research protection for consumers using DTC services, and (d) knowledge about genetics among consumers and/or inadequate training of health care providers who are being presented with DTC results by their patients.

A position statement regarding DTC has been published by the American College of Medical Genetics and calls for four minimum requirements for any genetic testing protocol:
1. A knowledgeable professional should be involved in the process of ordering and interpreting a genetic test.
2. The consumer should be fully informed regarding what the test can and cannot say about his or her health.
3. The scientific evidence on which a test is based should be clearly stated.
4. The clinical testing laboratory must be accredited by appropriate state and federal agencies.

The ultimate goal of professional organizations and governmental agencies is to protect the consumer.

18.6 The Genetic Information Nondiscrimination Act

The Genetic Information Nondiscrimination Act (GINA) was signed into law in 2008, was enacted in 2009, and protects residents of the United States from unfair treatment due to differences in DNA that may affect health. Under GINA, individuals may undergo genetic testing and participate in genetic research without fear of being discriminated against by their health insurance carriers or their employers; however, GINA's protection does not extend to life, disability, or long-term care insurance. While GINA represents a major step forward in US health care policy, critics argue that it falls short of regulating health insurers' and employers' access to all health-related information, such as fasting lipid profiles and electrocardiogram tracings, which can be equally as perilous. As stated previously, GINA also fails to protect the individual from discrimination when he or she is trying to obtain other insurance products such as life, disability, long-term care, and mortgage insurance. The effect of GINA on clinical practice, and its effect and benefits to the population at large, remains to be determined.

18.7   Professional Organizations

The ethical and legal concerns regarding genetic testing and counseling are vast, and the education and experience of the majority of health care providers are often inadequate to fully address the nuances of the applications of ethical principles toward societal issues. Fortunately, several professional organizations are actively involved in developing position statements, policies, and guidelines. Resources provided by these organizations, in addition to consultation with the hospital or medical center ethics committee and/or the center or department of ethics within most universities or colleges of medicine, are available to the academic and community physician and health care provider and should be consulted when there is a question relating to the basic ethical duties inherent to patient care.

Clinical Genetics

19 Multiple Congenital Anomalies

LEARNING OBJECTIVES

1 Describe at least three different etiological mechanisms that cause multiple congenital anomaly syndromes, and provide one specific example of each.

2 Prepare a 15-minute counseling session for parents of a newborn diagnosed with Down syndrome.

3 Describe physical features that would help you discriminate between trisomy 13 and trisomy 18 in a newborn patient. Outline your diagnostic evaluation, including molecular genetic tests and imaging studies that you would recommend.

4 Discuss the phenotypic effects of numerical aberrations of the sex chromosomes and hypothesize why 45,X might cause multiple congenital anomalies while 47,XXX and 47,XXY would not.

5 Define the term *contiguous genes syndrome,* and discuss it critically in regard to two microdeletion syndromes of your choice.

Newborns with multiple congenital anomalies (MCAs) or malformations represent a common cause for genetics consultation. Please refer to Sections 13.2 and 13.3 for important definitions, including malformation, deformation, and disruption.

Important

Multiple congenital anomalies are defined as either:
1. Two or more major malformations (e.g., neural tube defects, congenital heart defects, and anal atresia)
2. Three or more minor malformations (e.g., syndactyly, clubfoot, and preauricular tag)

The etiology of multiple congenital anomaly syndromes is diverse and includes chromosomal abnormalities (e.g., aneuploidy, microdeletions, and microduplications, as seen for trisomy 21, Williams syndrome, and Potocki-Lupski syndrome), single-gene defects (e.g., mutations of *CREBBP* that cause Rubinstein-Taybi syndrome), maternal infections, metabolic disorders, and substance abuse (e.g., fetal alcohol syndrome and maternal phenylketonuria [PKU] syndrome).

The evaluation of an infant with multiple congenital anomalies warrants a detailed pregnancy history, birth history, and family history and thorough physical examination. The latter should include the search for other associated physical features and minor malformations. Additional imaging studies that look for occult malformations should be considered (e.g., renal ultrasound, echocardiogram, head ultrasound, or brain magnetic resonance imaging [MRI]).

Occasionally, the combination of anomalies suggests a very specific diagnosis (e.g., atrioventricular [AV] canal and duodenal atresia would suggest Down syndrome; holoprosencephaly and cutaneous syndactyly of the second and third toes would suggest Smith-Lemli-Opitz syndrome). Whenever the combination of clinical features is not suggestive of a specific etiology, an **array analysis** should be done in order to identify cases of chromosomal aberrations, including microdeletions and microduplications. Once whole exome (or whole genome) sequencing becomes available on a clinical basis, another important genetic screening test for cases of multiple congenital anomalies will be available.

19.1 Numerical Chromosome Abnormalities

Abnormal Number of Autosomes

Only three **autosomal trisomies** are viable after birth: trisomies 13, 18, and 21. Exceptions are partial trisomies or mosaics of trisomic and normal cell lines. **Monosomies** of autosomal chromosomes result in a very early, spontaneous miscarriage, often before the pregnancy is identified.

Down Syndrome (Trisomy 21)

In 1866 the English physician John Langdon Haydon Down was the first to describe what has since become known as Down syndrome. He named the syndrome *Mongolian idiocy*. The term *mongolism* was widely adopted at the time, but is now long-abandoned and has been replaced by *Down syndrome* or *trisomy 21* (after Lejeune et al. discovered the true pathogenesis in 1959).

Case History

Marcus is a 4-year-old Caucasian boy. He was born at term to a 30-year-old G2P2 mother by vaginal delivery. Pregnancy was uneventful; an ultrasound scan did not reveal any thickening of the posterior nuchal folds. His weight at birth was 6.6 lb (10th to 25th percentile), his body length 20.5 inches (50th to 75th percentile), the Apgar score 10/10, and arterial cord blood pH 7.30 (all values within the normal range). The head circumference of 12.6 inches was below normal (less than third percentile). The nurse practitioner examining Marcus noted dysmorphic facial features, suggestive of Down syndrome, and blood was sent for chromosome analysis. The karyotype was reported as 47,XY,+21 in all cells examined. Marcus had a small atrial septal defect that did not require surgery and that corrected itself after a period of about 6 weeks. No other defects were found. The eye examination and hearing test were normal. Marcus was enrolled in ECI (Early Childhood Intervention) and has been receiving physical therapy for muscular hypotonia since age 4 months. Developmental milestones have been delayed; he walked at 28 months, and during his last visit, at age 3½, he spoke only a few words.

Epidemiology

Trisomy 21 is the most frequent chromosome abnormality diagnosed in newborns (approximately two-thirds of all cases). At the same time, it represents the most frequent cause of intellectual disability in the population. The **incidence** is estimated to be about **1 in 650**. The risk for giving birth to a child with trisomy 21 increases with the **mother's age**. While the likelihood of giving birth to a child with trisomy 21 is less than 1 in 1,000 up to age 30 years, it increases to 1 in 350 live-births at age 35 years, to 1 in 85 at age 40 years, and to 1 in 30 at age 46 years. Most children with trisomy 21, however, have mothers younger than age 35 years, since younger women tend to have more children and be less likely to undergo any invasive prenatal diagnostic testing. Of all zygotes with trisomy 21, 75% die prenatally, usually during the first trimester. For purposes of genetic counseling, it is important to note that if trisomy 21 was diagnosed through chorionic villus sampling (CVS, after the 11th week of pregnancy), there is still a 35% chance of spontaneous miscarriage. In case the diagnosis was made by way of amniocentesis (after the 14th week of pregnancy), the chance of miscarriage is still approximately 20%.

The average **life expectancy** for individuals with Down syndrome rose from 25 years in 1983 to 49 years in 2002. This increase is due to several factors, including early diagnosis and treatment of congenital cardiac defects and intestinal malformations, and more appropriate continued care, including anticipatory guidance from infancy to adulthood. Currently, approximately 15% of children with Down syndrome die within the first year. Mortality depends, in part, on external factors, such as the availability of tertiary medical care and the country in which the child is born. Major causes for death are severe cardiac defects and large gastrointestinal malformations.

Prenatal Diagnostic Testing

Historically, a maternal age of 35 years or older at the time of delivery has been used to identify women at highest risk of having a child with Down syndrome, and these women have been offered genetic counseling and amniocentesis or CVS. Aside from maternal age, abnormal findings on routine prenatal ultrasounds, including increased nuchal translucency (first-trimester scan), fetal hydrops, short femur, flat facial profile, duodenal stenosis, and cardiac defects (especially AV canal), may raise suspicion for trisomy 21.

In the 1980s, a biochemical serum screening for Down syndrome was introduced, as fetal trisomy alters the concentration of various **proteins in maternal blood**.

For first-trimester screening, decreased levels of pregnancy-associated plasma protein A (PAPP-A) and increased levels of free β-human chorionic gonadotropin (β-hCG) have been associated with an increased risk of Down syndrome. For second-trimester screening, decreased levels of maternal serum α-fetoprotein (AFP) and unconjugated estriol (uE3) and elevated levels of hCG and dimeric inhibin A (DIA) have been associated with an increased risk of Down syndrome.

It is important to realize that the test results of all noninvasive methods merely change the **probability** of trisomy 21, meaning they aim at identifying individuals in the general population that are at increased risk. The definitive diagnosis needs to be done by chromosome analysis of fetal cells (usually by amniocentesis or CVS).

Clinical Features

Down syndrome is most frequently suspected because of typical phenotypic features, postnatally. **No single phenotypic finding is pathognomonic for Down syndrome**, but in most cases the combination of dysmorphic features is easily recognizable.

Physical Abnormalities

- **Typical dysmorphic facial features** include a round face, **brachycephaly, flat facial profile** with a flat nasal bridge and midface hypoplasia, upslanting palpebral fissures (more pronounced when the baby cries), epicanthal folds, and small mouth (Fig. 19.1). The muscular hypotonia causes typical facial expressions with an open mouth and protruding tongue.
- Also typical are a short neck, hypoplasia of the middle phalanx of the fifth finger, clinodactyly of the fifth finger, a **single transverse palmar crease** (Fig. 19.1), and a wide gap between the first and second toes (sandal gap, Fig. 19.2).
- **Cardiac defects** occur in 45% of patients with Down syndrome. Of these defects, 40% are **AV canal** defects (i.e., atrioventricular septal defect [AVSD]), with faulty closure of the endocardial cushion as well as the atria and the ventricles and anomalies of the AV valves. Less frequent are isolated ventricular septal defects (VSDs), isolated atrial septal defects, and patent ductus arteriosus.
- **Gastrointestinal defects** occur in 12% of children with trisomy 21. These defects include **duodenal atresia** (occurs in 2% to 15% of all children with Down syndrome; conversely, 20% to 30% of all children with duodenal atresia have trisomy 21) and **Hirschsprung disease** (occurs in 2% of all children with trisomy 21; conversely, 10% to 15% of all patients with Hirschsprung disease have trisomy 21).

 Figure 19.1. Trisomy 21. Typical facial features include flat nasal bridge and epicanthal folds, distinct shortening of the fingers, and broad hands with a single transverse palmar crease of both hands.

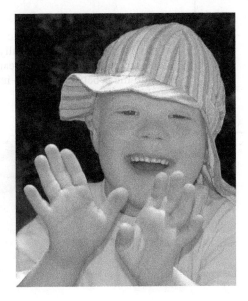

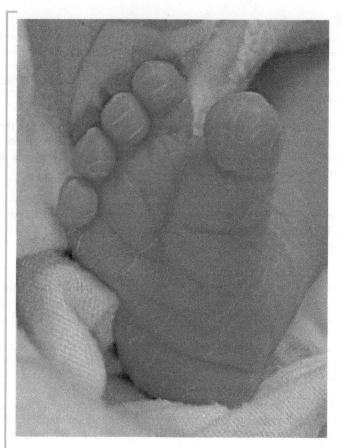

Figure 19.2. Sandal Gap Deformity in Trisomy 21.

— Anomalies in the **eyes** occur in 61% of children with trisomy 21; frequently occurring of these anomalies are myopia, nystagmus, strabismus, obstruction of the nasolacrimal duct, and Brushfield spots (white spots in the iris; Fig. 19.3).

Developmental Medical Problems:

— Birth weight, size, and head circumference are typically within the lower normal range. Following birth, there is usually mild **postnatal growth retardation**. Height at 1 year of age is often 3 SD below the mean; the expected final adult height for individuals with Down syndrome is between 4 feet 6 inches and 5 feet 3 inches.

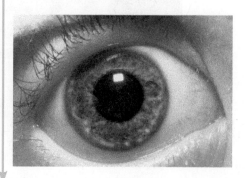

Figure 19.3. Brushfield Spots of Trisomy 21. In an adolescent with trisomy 21, the margin of the blue iris has a rosary of small white, stromal tufts, eponymically Brushfield spots. These are more evident in persons of European ancestry and rare among native Africans. In individuals without Down syndrome, the same anomalies, with no functional or visual significance, are called Wölfflin-Krückmann spots after the two German ophthalmologists who described them as incidental variants a century ago. (With permission by R. Lewis, Baylor College of Medicine, Houston.)

◻ Figure 19.4. Down Syndrome.
With the advent of enhanced
curricula and availability of special
education and vocational training,
changes in society's attitude toward
children with special needs, and
further refinements in medical
care, most individuals with Down
syndrome are now able to complete
high school. Typically, adults with
Down syndrome are able to find a
job and live in a semi-independent
setting. This young woman with
Down syndrome works full time
in the cafeteria of an academic
institution. (Photo courtesy of Rick
Guidotti, www.positiveexposure.org.)

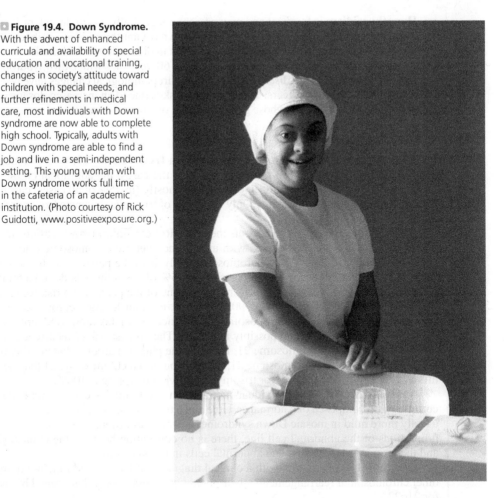

— **Motor and speech development are delayed**, but most children reach all developmental milestones. Intellectual disability is a constant feature, although there is great variability in the ultimate cognitive level in persons with Down syndrome (◻ Fig. 19.4). Behavior is sometimes said to be particularly friendly and open but may be regarded as just normal.
— **Epilepsy** develops in 10% of cases.
— Children with Down syndrome have altered immunological parameters, with an increased tendency toward infections. There is slightly less than a 1% risk of developing **leukemia** (a 20-fold increase compared to the general population). Although acute lymphoblastic leukemia (ALL) is more common than acute myeloid leukemia (AML) in children with Down syndrome, the risk of megakaryoblastic leukemia (M7) is increased 400-fold. An underlying diagnosis of Down syndrome or mosaic Down syndrome is often expected when an infant presents with M7 leukemia, even if physical features are not particularly suggestive of this diagnosis. Approximately 10% of newborns with Down syndrome have a transient myeloproliferative syndrome.
— Pubertal development is usually normal. Fertility in males with Down syndrome is decreased, owing to hypogonadism.

Complications in Adulthood

— Between 40% and 75% of patients develop **hearing loss** in one or both ears, primarily caused by recurring ear infections. Sensorineural hearing loss is also more common than in the general population.

- **Hypothyroidism** is frequent and may present congenitally, in childhood, or in adulthood. More than 30% of adults with Down syndrome have antithyroid autoantibodies.
- Early-onset **Alzheimer disease** is very common in older adults who have Down syndrome. Approximately 10% of 50-year-olds and 75% of 60-year-olds with Down syndrome develop clinical symptoms of the disease. The typical neuropathological changes have been found in patients as young as 40 years. This increased risk is due to an increased dosage of amyloid precursor protein (APP), whose gene is located on chromosome 21.

Genetics

In 95% of cases, Down syndrome is caused by a **free trisomy 21**, giving a karyotype of 47,XX,+21 or 47,XY,+21. In more than 90% of the cases, the additional chromosome 21 originates from oogenesis. Pathogenically, this is mostly (in 75% of all cases) caused by non-disjunction during the first meiosis. Only about 5% of trisomies originate from nondisjunction during spermatogenesis.

In approximately 4% of the patients there is a **Robertsonian translocation**, whereby the additional chromosome 21 is fused with another acrocentric chromosome (most frequently chromosome 14). In these cases, chromosome analysis of the parents is extremely important for precise calculation of the recurrence risk. In 75% of cases this is a de novo translocation. If, however, the translocation was transmitted by one of the parents, the risk for recurrence is high for subsequent pregnancies. In 90% of cases, the translocation chromosome originates from the mother; balanced chromosome disturbances in males more frequently result in a defect in spermatogenesis and possibly infertility. The highest risk of recurrence occurs with the presence of an **isochromosome 21**. If one of the parents harbors a balanced chromosome complement with an isochromosome 21, there is no normal chromosome 21 that can be transmitted to children, and the risk for trisomy 21 in living offspring is 100%.

Approximately 1% of individuals with Down syndrome have a **mosaic chromosomal complement**, composed of a normal cell line and a trisomic cell line. The clinical phenotype is usually more mild in mosaic Down syndrome; however, as different tissues may have varying proportions of the abnormal cell line, there is no correlation between the clinical phenotype and the proportion of normal and abnormal cells in blood or skin.

Less than 1% of children with a clinical diagnosis of Down syndrome are found to have other chromosomal rearrangements; their phenotype is essentially determined by the trisomy for 21q22.

Therapy

Therapy is symptomatic. Complications must be diagnosed early and corrected surgically if necessary. It is important for optimal psychomotor development that the children be enrolled in early intervention developmental and education programs. Most children with Down syndrome can be enrolled in inclusion programs or integrated classrooms with other children who do not have intellectual disabilities. Life skills education is employed in later years to allow the adult with Down syndrome to lead a semi-independent lifestyle.

Management and Anticipatory Guidance

The American Academy of Pediatrics (AAP) publishes management guidelines, which are designed to assist the pediatrician caring for children with the diagnosis of Down syndrome. Recommendations include:
- Complete blood count (CBC) at time of diagnosis
- Echocardiogram at time of diagnosis
- Thyroid function tests at diagnosis, at 6 months, at 12 months, then annually
- Annual ophthalmologic evaluation
- Annual audiologic evaluation
- Radiographs of the C-spine in flexion and extension once between ages 3 and 5 years (to evaluate for atlantoaxial instability)

Trisomy 18 (Edwards Syndrome)

Important

Remember: **E**ighteen-**E**dwards.

Case History

Jonas was diagnosed with trisomy 18 prenatally, after ultrasound scans in the 28th week of pregnancy (third trimester) had revealed excessive levels of amniotic fluid (polyhydramnios). The detailed ultrasound examination showed a heart defect (high ventricular septal defect with polyvalvular heart disease, meaning pulmonary and aortic valve defects), an enlarged ureter (suspected megaloureter), and a single umbilical cord artery. Fetal chromosome analysis following amniocentesis showed that all tested cells had a karyotype 47,XY,+18. Jonas was born spontaneously in the 40th week of pregnancy. Body length and weight were in the low-normal range, and the head circumference was approximately 0.8 inches below the third percentile. Dysmorphic features suggestive of trisomy 18 included microcephaly, low-set and posteriorly rotated ears with pointed helices, overlapping fingers, and rocker-bottom feet. The cardiac and genitourinary malformations were confirmed postnatally. Jonas's condition remained stable; at 4 weeks of age he was discharged home. Over the next few weeks, he experienced repeated apneic episodes and died at 7 weeks. The parents later reported that the discrepancy between the obviously poor prognosis and the lack of visibly life-threatening features of the condition was very stressful for them. Especially after the baby's discharge from the hospital, they found it difficult to cope with the conflicting emotions of hope, despair, and the uncertainty of how long their child would live. They would have liked to have been better prepared for being at home with a seemingly normal child and to have had more counseling and support from the physicians.

Epidemiology

With an incidence of approximately **1 in 6,000 live births**, trisomy 18 is the second most common aneuploidy in neonates. As with other autosomal trisomies, there is a close correlation with maternal age unless the trisomy is due to an unbalanced translocation. Trisomy 18, diagnosed by chromosome analysis or array analysis of amniotic fluid after suggestive findings on of prenatal ultrasound examinations (malformations or growth retardation), is the most frequent fetal chromosome aberration (with an incidence that is 50% higher than Down syndrome). It is estimated that only 5% of all conceptions with trisomy 18 survive to birth. After trisomy 18 is diagnosed through amniocentesis, the risk for spontaneous miscarriage is 70%. There is a gender mismatch among newborns with trisomy 18 (male:female ratio = 1:4). The causes for this observation are not clear. The average life expectancy for an infant with trisomy 18 is 15 days. Approximately 10% of patients survive until their first birthday, and 1% survive until age 10.

Clinical Features

Prenatally, there is usually **intrauterine growth retardation** accompanied by **morphological abnormalities**, including increased nuchal translucency, malformations of the brain (e.g., choroid plexus cysts), or cardiac defects (polyvalvular heart disease, meaning malformations of more than one valve, is found in more than 90% of patients with trisomy 18; other frequent cardiac defects include VSDs and outflow tract malformations). The average birth weight is approximately 5 lb. The placenta is frequently hypotrophic (small).

Craniofacially, the affected children have **microcephaly** with prominent occiput (dolichocephaly). The **ears** are especially conspicuous; they are low-set, rotated backwards, and typically dysplastic with a pointed helix. The mouth and chin are small (micrognathia, shown in ▢ Fig. 19.5). Specific **dysmorphisms of hands and feet aid the diagnosis**; the fingers have contractures and typically overlap (the index finger overlaps the middle finger, the fifth finger overlaps the fourth; ▢ Fig. 19.6). The big toes are short and dorsiflexed, and the feet have a prominent calcaneus and rounded plantar surfaces ("rocker-bottom feet"; ▢ Fig. 19.7). Frequent **malformations** include heart defects (especially polyvalvular heart disease), umbilical hernia or diastasis recti, a short sternum, and genitourinary abnormalities.

II

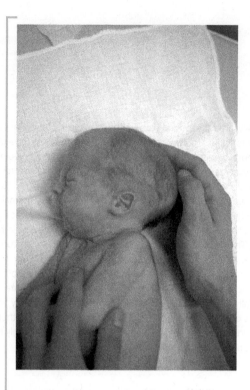

Figure 19.5. Trisomy 18 in a Newborn.
Dolichocephaly with prominent occiput, dysplastic ears, microretrognathia. (Courtesy of Universitäts-Kinderklinik Heidelberg.)

Cytogenetics

The **definitive diagnosis** for trisomy 18 is confirmed pre- and postnatally by chromosome analysis or array analysis of the amniotic cells, chorionic villi, or lymphocytes. Chromosome analysis of skin fibroblasts may be indicated if the chromosome analysis of blood is normal and a mosaic trisomy 18 is being considered.

In approximately **80 %** of cases, there is a **free trisomy 18**, and the extra chromosome 18 is usually transmitted by the mother (in greater than 90% of cases). In contrast to Down syndrome, however, the cause is more frequently a nondisjunction in the **second meiotic division**. Occasionally there is **mosaicism** of trisomic and normal (disomic) cell lines for chromosome 18. A low percentage of trisomic cell lines results in a milder clinical picture and longer survival.

A few cases of **translocation trisomies** of chromosome 18 have been described; in such cases a chromosome analysis of the parents is imperative to find balanced translocations. As with all other chromosomes, there are also **partial trisomies 18**. If the trisomy occurs on the short arm of chromosome 18, a mild and nonspecific phenotype presents, often without intellectual disability. A trisomy of the long arm of chromosome 18, however, may be clinically indistinguishable from a full trisomy 18.

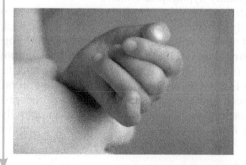

Figure 19.6. Trisomy 18. Typical finger position. (Courtesy of Universitäts-Kinderklinik Heidelberg.)

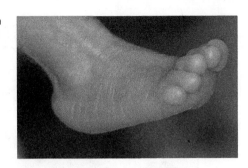

Figure 19.7. Trisomy 18. Typical "rocker-bottom" foot in a neonate. (Courtesy of Universitäts-Kinderklinik Heidelberg.)

Therapy and Prognosis

The overall prognosis for neonates with trisomy 18 is poor. After genetic counseling, most parents decide for supportive care rather than aggressive medical interventions. If the infant's condition stabilizes (mostly in neonatal intensive care), correction of severe malformations (including cardiac defects) can be considered. Clinical management focuses on feeding (often tube feeding), gastroesophageal and esophagotracheal reflux, immune deficiency with recurring infections, vision and hearing defects, epilepsy, and progressive severe scoliosis.

Following cytogenetic confirmation of the diagnosis, the counseling should emphasize that in rare instances children with trisomy 18 can live into adolescence, although most have severe impairments spanning motor, language, and intellectual function. Discharge from the hospital should be planned, and home nursing and hospice care should be arranged before discharge, as the transition to home care is often overwhelming to the parents. Even when parents comprehend the gravity of the diagnosis and poor prognosis for their child, most find it extremely difficult to cope with the uncertainty of knowing how long the child will live.

> **Important**
>
> As always in the medical field, one should be cautious about giving a prognosis for life expectancy; this also applies to infants with the most severe genetic diseases. It is impossible to accurately predict the **life expectancy** of a patient. Whoever ignores this principle (e.g., stating, "Your child will not live to his first birthday") not only loses the trust of the parents but also takes away their opportunity to prepare for a life with their child (which might be longer or shorter than expected).

Patients with trisomy 18 who survive the first year have profound psychomotor impairment. Most of them will never be able to walk independently or learn more than a few words. Communication, however, is possible through visual contact and gestures, and audio-visual communication devices should be considered.

Trisomy 13 (Pätau Syndrome)

Case History

Mr. and Mrs. Wagner visit the genetics clinic for a consultation concerning a recurrence risk for trisomy 13. Their first child, Verena, had been diagnosed with this chromosome disorder. Mrs. Wagner reports that, while the pregnancy was initially normal, fetal growth retardation was noted at around 7 months' gestation. At birth (during the 37th week of pregnancy), all body measurements were below the 3rd percentile. Verena had a severe cardiac defect (large ventricular septal defect) and a cleft lip. There were distinct dysmorphic features, including microcephaly, upward-slanting palpebral fissures, a flat nose with a broad root, micrognathia, and low-set ears. Verena was transferred to a tertiary care center for further evaluation and management. Once the clinically suspected diagnosis of trisomy 13 was cytogenetically confirmed, the parents decided against aggressive therapeutic measures. Verena was discharged into her parents' care with close supervision by the local pediatrician. She died at 5 weeks from respiratory arrest. During the counseling session, the Wagners are told that the chance of recurrence is approximately 1%, since Verena had had a free trisomy. The parents are informed about available prenatal diagnostic tests, including chromosome analysis and array analysis on CVS or amniotic fluid.

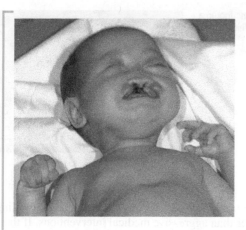

Figure 19.8. Trisomy 13. A newborn with microcephaly, a flat nasal bridge, a broad nasal root, bilateral cleft lip/cleft palate, and dysplastic ears. (Courtesy of Universitäts-Kinderklinik Heidelberg.)

Epidemiology

The incidence of trisomy 13 is between **1 in 10,000 and 1 in 20,000** live-born neonates. The risk for trisomy 13 increases with maternal age. Only 1 in 40 conceptions with trisomy 13 is carried to term. The average life expectancy of only 7 days is worse than for trisomy 18. More than 90% of the children die within the first year. The surviving children have profound psychomotor retardation, frequently have intractable epilepsy (often with hypsarrhythmia), and usually fail to thrive.

Clinical Features

It is not rare that an ultrasound examination, between the 20th and 22nd week of pregnancy, reveals the typical malformations, suggesting a possible chromosome disturbance, especially trisomy 13. **Holoprosencephaly** (Section 31.2.1) can be found in about two-thirds of patients. Mostly this is an alobar form without corpus callosum, septum pellucidum, and fornices, and is often accompanied by arrhinencephaly (missing olfactory bulbs as seen in 70% of individuals with trisomy 13). **Facial deformities** associated with holoprosencephaly can also be detected prenatally, especially synophthalmia, anophthalmia, or facial clefts (often bilateral or midline **cleft lip/cleft palate**) (◻ Fig. 19.8). Another frequent malformation is **postaxial polydactyly** (◻ Fig. 19.9). **Cardiac defects** (mostly VSD), as well as **renal abnormalities** (hydronephrosis, polycystic kidney, and renal hypoplasia), are seen. The birth weight of affected children is typically low for gestational age (mean 5.7 lb). Typical **cutaneous scalp defects** (◻ Fig. 19.10) can be helpful in narrowing the differential diagnosis. The clinically suspected diagnosis is confirmed by chromosome analysis.

Cytogenetics

In the majority of cases, individuals are found to have a **free trisomy 13**. The extra chromosome typically originates from oogenesis (85% of the cases). Roughly 25% of trisomy 13 cases are

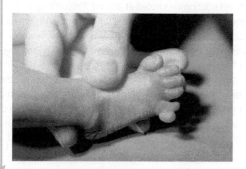

Figure 19.9. Trisomy 13. Postaxial polydactyly of the right foot of a newborn. (Courtesy of Universitäts-Kinderklinik Heidelberg.)

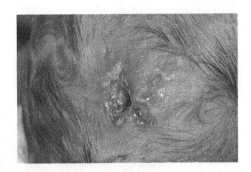

Figure 19.10. Trisomy 13. Typical cutaneous lesions on the scalp of a 3-year-old child. (Courtesy of Universitäts-Kinderklinik Heidelberg.)

caused by an unbalanced **Robertsonian translocation**, mostly rob(13q:14q). As a balanced translocation, it is found at a frequency of 1 in 1,500 in the general population. The clinical picture of mosaic cases (5%) is highly variable.

Therapy and Prognosis

More than 80% of children with trisomy 13 die within the first month, while 5% to 10% live to their first birthday. Survival depends primarily on the severity of the cardiac, renal, and cerebral malformations. As for all severe genetic disorders, decisions for surgical intervention should be made in close consultation with the parents. Surprisingly, the severity of holoprosencephaly has little influence on life expectancy. A few children with alobar holoprosencephaly (the most severe form) may live through adolescence and adulthood, though with profound intellectual disability. Children with trisomy 13 are frequently blind and deaf, and many have intractable epilepsy. Difficulty swallowing makes feeding often problematic and may require G-tube placement.

Abnormal Number of Sex Chromosomes

Numerical abnormalities of the human sex chromosomes cause relatively mild phenotypes, unlike numerical abnormalities of the autosomes. The human cell primarily utilizes the genetic information of one X chromosome and, therefore, can largely compensate for the loss of a Y chromosome or the second X chromosome, as well as additional X chromosomes (by way of X inactivation, Section 2.8). As a result, numerical sex chromosome abnormalities in newborns rarely lead to severe physical changes, and in most instances, do not cause substantial intellectual disability. **Monosomy X** is the only viable monosomy in humans.

Turner Syndrome (Ullrich-Turner Syndrome, 45,X Syndrome)

Case History

After an uncomplicated pregnancy, Sandra was born by spontaneous vaginal delivery in the 41st week of pregnancy. Although there were no medical concerns in the neonatal period, her parents noticed that she had puffy hands and feet. While the swelling slowly resolved over the first 4 to 6 months of life, a well-child check at 2 years of age revealed delayed growth and physical symptoms of Turner syndrome (including a low posterior hairline and widely spaced nipples). A chromosome analysis was initiated, which confirmed a mosaic Turner syndrome complement. Of the 50 tested metaphases, 28 had a normal female karyotype, while 22 had a monosomy X. This result prompted further evaluation. An echocardiogram revealed a small ventricular septal defect that did not need surgical intervention. Sandra was started on recombinant growth hormone. During the last physical examination, at age 6 years, the height of 42 inches was approximately 1 inch below the third percentile. Developmental milestones and socialization skills were normal.

Epidemiology

Turner syndrome has an **incidence of 1 in 2,500 to 1 in 3,000** newborn females. However, prenatally it occurs much more frequently; 20% of all miscarriages caused by chromosomal

III

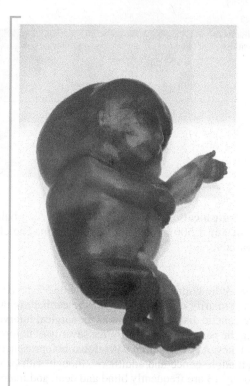

Figure 19.11. Turner Syndrome. Hydrops fetalis.

aberrations manifest a monosomy X. Thus, calculating backwards, a surprising **99%** of all zygotes with monosomy X end in a **miscarriage**, and only 1% of these pregnancies is carried to term.

Clinical Features

The classic **prenatal** manifestation of Turner syndrome is cervical lymphedema (cystic hygroma) or generalized edema (ascites or chylothorax, also hydrops fetalis) toward the end of the first trimester (■ Fig. 19.11). Subsequently, detailed ultrasound examinations may reveal cardiac and renal defects.

Newborns frequently display lymphedema of the backs of the hands and feet, which gradually disappears during infancy. A physical examination may reveal **pterygium colli** (webbed neck)

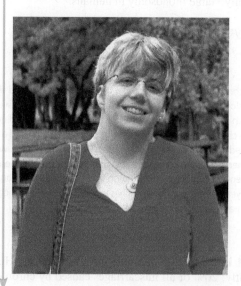

Figure 19.12. Turner Syndrome. This 4 foot 11 inch tall young woman had the pterygium colli surgically reduced at a young age, because it interfered with turning her head.

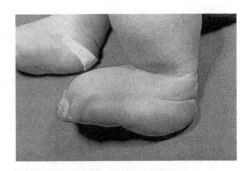

Figure 19.13. Turner Syndrome. Edematous swelling of the back of the foot in a newborn girl. (Courtesy of Hj Müller, Department of Medical Genetics, University Children's Hospital Basel, Switzerland.

or simply excessive nuchal skin as well as a **shield-shaped thorax** with increased internipple distance. The pterygium colli often persists into adulthood (Fig. 19.12).

> **Important**
>
> **Lymphedema** of the backs of the hands and feet (Fig. 19.13) in a newborn girl may be the only phenotypical sign of Turner syndrome; a chromosome analysis is indicated, as a diagnosis of Turner syndrome requires specific clinical management and intervention.

Some of the girls with Turner syndrome have **congenital heart defects**, almost always of the left side of the heart. Frequently seen are bicuspid aortic valve (30%), **coarctation of the aorta** (10%), valvular aortic stenosis, and mitral valve prolapse. Later there is an increased incidence of aortic dissection. The phenotype of Turner syndrome also includes a low, inverse nuchal hairline; a high-arched palate; a shortened fourth metacarpal (sometimes also the fourth metatarsal; Fig. 19.14); and numerous pigmented nevi. More than 50% of individuals with Turner syndrome have renal malformations (mostly horseshoe kidney) and hearing loss due to sensorineural deficits.

The clinically most relevant defect of Turner syndrome is **proportional short stature**. While the length of most neonates is still near the fifth percentile, height drops significantly

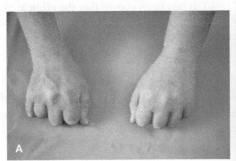

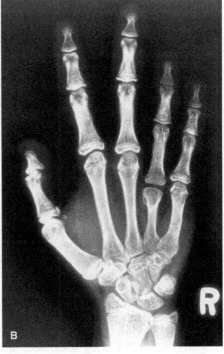

Figure 19.14. Turner Syndrome. Shortened fourth metacarpal. This is especially evident **(A)** with a clenched fist or **(B)** in a radiograph of the hand. (Courtesy of Hj Müller, Department of Medical Genetics, University Children's Hospital Basel, Switzerland.)

during the following months and years. By the time they reach third grade, the girls are often the smallest in the class. Some girls are not seen by a geneticist until the absence of puberty is noticed. The average **adult height** of women with Turner syndrome who have not received treatment is approximately 4 feet 11 inches (150 cm).

Gonadal dysgenesis is one of the most common features of Turner syndrome. The large majority of women with Turner syndrome have rudimentary ovaries with streaks of fibrous tissue ("streak gonads"). The degeneration of functional ovarian tissue, including oocytes, begins during the fetal period. This has been called "premenarchal menopause." Most women do not go through puberty (because of hypergonadotrophic hypogonadism) and have primary amenorrhea. Only 2% to 5% experience spontaneous menstruation. Dysfunctional ovaries and degeneration of the oocytes result in primary sterility.

Women with Turner syndrome usually are of normal intelligence, although IQ scores are typically 10 to 15 points lower than average. Often, there are partial deficiencies, for example, concerning spatial perception; the verbal IQ is usually higher than the operational IQ. Women with structural anomalies of the X chromosome more frequently manifest learning disabilities.

Cytogenetics

Approximately **40%** of women with Turner syndrome are found to have a karyotype 45,X in their blood lymphocytes. These women typically manifest with the "full clinical picture" of Turner syndrome, showing excessive nuchal skin and perinatal lymphedema. In most cases, the X chromosome in an individual with Turner syndrome is maternal in origin. Resulting from nondisjunction in spermatogenesis or as a postzygotic event, Turner syndrome is not associated with maternal or paternal age. It usually occurs sporadically; subsequent siblings have no significantly increased recurrence risk.

Roughly **30%** have **mosaic Turner syndrome** (mostly 45,X/46,XX). These women often have a milder phenotype and are more likely to experience spontaneous menarche. All reported cases of spontaneous pregnancy in women with Turner syndrome were identified to be mosaic.

The remaining women with Turner syndrome have **structural abnormalities** of the X chromosome, among them an isochromosome Xq (15% to 20% of all cases), a deletion Xp (2% to 5%), or a ring chromosome X (5%). It has been shown that the clinical phenotype of Turner syndrome correlates primarily with the loss of the short arm of the X chromosome. Short stature is caused by a haploinsufficiency of the *SHOX* gene in the pseudoautosomal region of Xp.

> **Important**
>
> About 6% of women with Turner syndrome have a **mosaic 45,X/46,XY**. In these cases there is a significant **risk of malignant transformation** of the streak gonads into a gonadoblastoma. Early surgical removal of these gonads is indicated.

Therapy and Management

In adolescence and adulthood, weight gain and obesity are frequent problems for women with Turner syndrome. Dietary counseling, in conjunction with an exercise program, is beneficial.

The standard therapy for short stature involves treatment with **growth hormone** replacement. Treatment can begin as early as 2 years of age. This treatment is applied, despite the fact that women with Turner syndrome do not actually lack growth hormone. Consequently, growth hormone is administered in superphysiological doses. Success is moderate, resulting in an average gain in height of 2 inches.

In order to initiate pubertal development of secondary sex characteristics, **sex hormone** (estrogen) is given beginning at age 14 years. An earlier start of sex hormone treatment is not advisable, because it decreases the effectiveness of growth hormone on height by inducing closure of the growth plates.

Approximately 5% to 10% of individuals with Turner syndrome have **hypothyroidism** in childhood. During adulthood, this increases to 30%. **Hearing loss** is commonly seen in individuals with Turner syndrome. This might be secondary to recurrent middle ear infections, but in addition, a progressive midfrequency sensorineural hearing loss often occurs.

Women with Turner syndrome manifest an increase in anomalies in the portions of the aorta close to the heart. These include congenital coarctation of the aorta, dilatations of the ascending aorta in adulthood, and a markedly increased risk for aortic dissection. **Echocardiograms**, at regular intervals of 3 to 5 years, are recommended. The administration of beta-blockers may be considered.

Turner syndrome is the only numerical sex chromosome aberration that would be considered a "multiple congenital anomaly syndrome." Additional X or Y chromosomes cause little to no physical anomalies.

47,XXX: Women with karyotype **47,XXX** have normal physical development, normal gonadal function, and normal puberty and fertility. They are frequently very tall (mostly above the 80th percentile) and display relative microcephaly (average head circumference between the 25th and 35th percentile). Delays in reaching milestones of motor development are frequently reported, as are coordination disturbances. Partial cognitive deficiencies are mainly evident in speech (e.g., expressive language and verbal learning). The birth of a child with karyotype 47,XXX is not associated with an increased probability of recurrence in future pregnancies, nor does the risk of aneuploidy increase for children of affected women (see Section 38.2 for a case report of a woman with 47,XXX).

Polysomy X: The occurrence of two or more additional sex chromosomes results in a lower IQ and an increase in morphological abnormalities. Women with karyotype 48,XXXX have an average IQ of 60 (range of 30 to 75). Morphological abnormalities are frequent, yet variable. They include midfacial hypoplasia, hypertelorism, epicanthal folds, upslanting palpebral fissures, and clinodactyly of the fifth finger; the facies sometimes resembles Down syndrome.

47,XXY: Klinefelter syndrome is the most common numerical sex chromosome aberration (incidence 1 in 500 to 1 in 1,000 newborn males). It is a frequent cause of male infertility and will be discussed in detail in Section 33.1.

47,XYY: Affected boys mostly have normal growth, normal body shape, normal gonadal function, and normal fertility. Occasionally there are behavioral problems, including moodiness, hyperactivity, and low frustration tolerance, especially during childhood and adolescence. The IQ is usually normal, but partial deficiencies in the verbal area may be seen (expressive language and speech reception). Slight deficiencies in motor function (e.g., defects in fine motor skills and slight intention tremor) have repeatedly been described.

19.2 Copy Number Variants and Structural Chromosome Abnormalities

Copy number variants (CNVs) are deletions and duplications of genomic sequence, ranging in length from a kilobase to multiple megabase pairs. They are known as major contributors to human genetic diversity. CNVs are known to influence both normal and disease variation. Structural chromosome abnormalities can occur via numerous mechanisms. The clinical severity largely depends on the size of the respective chromosome segments. Deletions usually have more serious consequences than duplications. There are a handful of larger deletion syndromes that have been described in detail for many years. These syndromes are typically structural chromosomal abnormalities that are large enough to be visualized under the microscope (limitation around 5 Mb). Cri-du-chat syndrome (deletion 5p) and Wolf-Hirschhorn syndrome (deletion 4p) are two such specific genetic syndromes that can be detected by standard chromosome analysis. The era of molecular cytogenetics, with newer molecular methods of genomic quantification (e.g., fluorescence in situ hybridization [FISH] and array analysis), led to the molecular characterization of additional genetic syndromes. If a genetic syndrome is caused by a deletion that is not visible by light microscopy, this is called a **microdeletion syndrome**. Occasionally, a microdeletion causes haploinsufficiency of several adjacent genes, of which two or more are associated to distinct genetic disorders, including *TSC2* (causing tuberous sclerosis; see Section 32.6) and *PKD1* (causing autosomal dominant polycystic kidney disease; see Section 27.2) on chromosome 16p13. The term **contiguous genes syndrome** has been coined for these situations.

1p36 Deletion Syndrome

With an estimated incidence of 1 in 5,000 to 1 in 10,000, 1p36 deletion syndrome represents one of the most common microdeletion syndromes. It is characterized by facial features, such as straight eyebrows, deep-set eyes, and midface hypoplasia. The majority of patients have microcephaly and delayed closure of the anterior fontanelle. Multiple congenital anomalies seen in this condition include structural brain malformations, congenital heart defects, ophthalmologic abnormalities (e.g., strabismus, refractive errors, cataract, and coloboma), genitourinary malformations, and skeletal anomalies (e.g., scoliosis, limb asymmetry, rib anomalies). All individuals affected with 1p36 deletion syndrome have intellectual disabilities (90% severe/profound, 10% mild/moderate). Muscular hypotonia is seen in 95% of all cases and may be associated with severe feeding difficulties during infancy and early childhood.

Several different mechanisms can lead to the deletion of the 1p36 chromosome region. The deletion can be terminal (all the way to the telomere), interstitial, or part of a more complex chromosomal rearrangement. The molecular diagnosis is made by targeted FISH analysis for the 1p36 chromosomal region, but it will also be detected by array analysis. About one-fourth of all cases have deletions greater than 5 Mb. Those deletions would also be seen by standard chromosome analysis and light microscopy.

Deletion 4p (Wolf-Hirschhorn Syndrome)

The partial monosomy of the short arm of chromosome 4 (i.e., terminal deletion 4p16.3) results in a characteristic mental retardation syndrome with pre- and postnatal **growth retardation**, **microcephaly**, and typical **facial dysmorphisms**, including high forehead; hypertelorism with downward-slanting palpebral fissures; strabismus; broad nose with an elevated, prominent root (referred to as "greek helmet" facies); short philtrum; down-turning corners of the mouth; micrognathia; and low-set, dysplastic ears that occasionally have preauricular tags (■ Fig. 19.15). Occasionally there are anomalies of the eyes (e.g., iris coloboma). Accompanying deformities include cleft lip/cleft palate, occasional cardiac defects, central nervous system (CNS) anomalies, and urogenital malformations. About one-third of the patients with Wolf-Hirschhorn syndrome die within the first year. Most of the surviving children have severe to

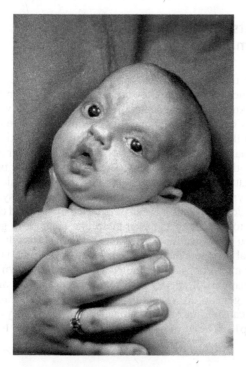

■ **Figure 19.15. Wolf-Hirschhorn Syndrome.** A high forehead, hypertelorism, downslanting palpebral fissures, a broad nasal root, and a dysplastic ear. (Courtesy of G. Tariverdian, Institut für Humangenetik Heidelberg.)

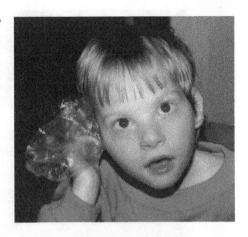

Figure 19.16. Cri-du-Chat Syndrome. A 5-year-old boy shows mild facial dysmorphism with hypertelorism, a broad root of the nose, and strabismus.

profound intellectual disability and epilepsy. In the majority of cases, the deletion is **visible by light microscopy**. Most of the cases are **de novo deletions** (85% to 90%), the majority of which occur on the paternal chromosome 4. In 10% to 15% of the cases, one of the parents has a balanced translocation involving the short arm of chromosome 4.

Deletion 5p (Cri-du-Chat Syndrome)

A partial deletion of the short arm of chromosome 5 results in cri-du-chat syndrome. The critical region is 5p15.2. A laryngeal defect, which also results in congenital stridor, causes infants to have **catlike, wailing, high-pitched cries** in the first months after birth that, over the course of the first year, eventually resolve. At birth, most of the children are growth delayed and have muscular hypotonia. The typical facial dysmorphism includes **microcephaly, a round face, hypertelorism** with a broad nasal root, epicanthal folds and downslanting palpebral fissures, a high-arched palate, and low-set, slightly dysplastic ears (Fig. 19.16). Most patients have severe to profound intellectual disability; the average IQ in adulthood is near 35. **De novo deletions** are the cause of **85% to 90%** of the cases of cri-du-chat syndrome, most of which are **visible by light microscopy**. Parental FISH with probes from the deleted region is indicated to evaluate for rearrangements, which would confer an increased recurrence risk in future pregnancies.

Important

Cytogenetic Commonalities of Wolf-Hirschhorn Syndrome and Cri-du-Chat Syndrome
— In most cases, the deletions are visible under the light microscope.
— Deletions are on the short arm of the chromosome (Wolf-Hirschhorn syndrome: 4p, cri-du-chat syndrome: 5p).
— Approximately 85% to 90% are de novo deletions, and 10% to 15% are translocations.
— Most de novo deletions are of paternal origin.

Williams Syndrome (Microdeletion Syndrome 7q11.23)

This is a clinically characteristic microdeletion syndrome, with vascular anomalies, typical facial features, and a friendly, outgoing personality. The specific vascular defect seen in Williams syndrome is **supravalvular aortic stenosis**, occurring in 50% of the patients. In 27% of patients, there is a pulmonic valvular stenosis. Newborns with Williams syndrome frequently have muscular hypotonia and intermittent hypercalcemia. The **characteristic facies** of patients with Williams syndrome has been described as "elfin-like," yet this is now viewed as derogatory by most parents (Fig. 19.17). The palpebral fissures are short, with telecanthus and periorbital fullness of subcutaneous tissues. The midface is hypoplastic and the nose short, sometimes with a depressed bridge and anteverted nares. Cheeks and lips are full, the philtrum is long, and the mouth is relatively large and often kept open. Small and widely spaced teeth are frequently

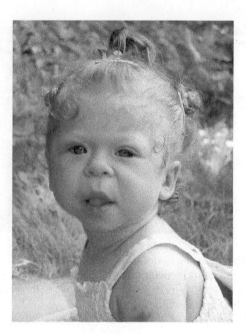

Figure 19.17. Williams Syndrome. Typical facial features in a 13-month-old girl include short palpebral fissures, full periorbital region, hypoplastic midface, anteverted nares, and a long, prominent philtrum.

seen. In patients with blue or lightly pigmented eyes, a "**stellate iris**" (or starburst appearance) is evident. With increasing age the facial features may coarsen. There is mild microcephaly and relative short stature.

The personality of individuals with Williams syndrome is quite specific, and is nearly always friendly and outgoing, sometimes to a fault, as socially appropriate physical distances are not maintained. They are verbally very expressive, yet what they say often lacks content (also called "**cocktail party behavior**"). Additionally, persons with Williams syndrome have extremely poor visuospatial abilities and are unable to draw simple figures. Because of the friendly behavior and verbal strengths, the intellectual abilities of an individual with Williams syndrome is often overestimated when compared to formal evaluations. The average IQ of an adult with Williams syndrome is 56, with a range of 40 to 80. Additional characteristics are a hoarse voice, sensitivity to loud noise, and love of music. Williams syndrome is caused by a **microdeletion of region 7q11.23**. Diagnosis is made by FISH of the respective region (Fig. 19.18) or array analysis. In most cases, there is a 1.5 Mb deletion. More than 20 genes in this region have been identified, among them *ELN* (coding for **elastin**) and *LMK1* (coding for LIM kinase 1).

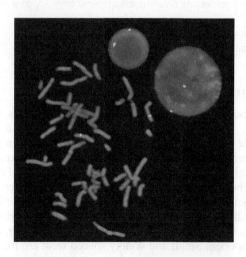

Figure 19.18. Williams Syndrome. Control probes of chromosome 7 (green) reveal two signals each on both chromosomes in the interphase nuclei; the probe for the Williams region (red), however, is only present once. (Courtesy of A. Jauch, Institut für Humangenetik Heidelberg.)

Smith-Magenis Syndrome

Once described purely as a contiguous gene deletion syndrome due to a cytogenetically visible deletion of 17p11.2, the cardinal features of Smith-Magenis syndrome (SMS) are now known to be due to haploinsufficiency of a single gene, *RAI1*, which maps within the critical region. The incidence of SMS has been reported to be 1 in 25,000 births. To date, more than 90% of patients identified as having SMS harbor a microdeletion, while the remainder have a heterozygous mutation of *RAI1*. Newborns and infants with SMS are usually hypotonic and may have congenital cardiovascular disease (when severe, this may involve the right side of the heart, e.g., tetralogy of Fallot), cleft lip/palate, and renal anomalies. Many infants with SMS have feeding problems and need to be awakened to feed due to hypersomnolence. Facial features common to persons with SMS include brachycephaly, synophrys, midfacial hypoplasia, and prognathism (in older children and adults; ◘ Fig. 19.19). While the physical features of SMS are not particularly indicative of this condition, the negative behaviors, sleep disturbances, and **behavioral profile** are very characteristic. The most frequent neurobehavioral abnormality is the sleep disturbance, which is characterized by frequent and prolonged nocturnal awakenings and excessive daytime sleepiness associated with an inversion of the circadian rhythm of melatonin. During their waking hours, children with SMS are attention seeking and adult oriented, and they can precipitously exhibit aggressiveness, self-injurious behavior, and tantrums with the slightest provocation. The vast majority of individuals with SMS have intellectual disability. Two stereotypic behaviors, the so-called "**self-hugging**" and finger lick and page flipping ("**lick and flip**"), are highly associated with SMS. Adolescents and adults with SMS should be monitored closely and treated for hearing impairment, hypercholesterolemia, obesity, and scoliosis.

◘ **Figure 19.19. Teenager with Smith-Magenis Syndrome.** Characteristic facial features include a broad, square-shaped face that is often referred to as "coarse"; prominent forehead; midface hypoplasia; and prognathia. The latter becomes more prominent with increasing age. (Photo courtesy of Rick Guidotti, www.positiveexposure.org.)

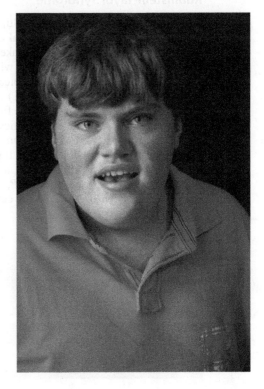

Potocki-Lupski Syndrome (Microduplication Syndrome 17p11.2)

Potocki-Lupski syndrome (PTLS) was the first **microduplication syndrome** described, and it shares the same mechanism and genomic region as SMS. Although SMS and PTLS are both due to abnormal dosage of *RAI1* within the 17p11.2 region, the clinical features of each condition are distinct. Infants with PTLS often have severe feeding difficulty and failure to thrive, hypotonia, and developmental delay. Cardiovascular abnormalities in PTLS usually involve the left side of the heart, including hypoplastic left heart, bicuspid aortic valve, and an aortopathy associated with aortic dilatation. Individuals with PTLS do not have subjective sleep disturbances, yet exhibit obstructive and/or central apnea on polysomnography. Hyperactivity is very common in young children with PTLS, as is verbal apraxia and autistic spectrum disorder. The majority of individuals have mild to moderate intellectual disability. Most individuals with PTLS are **not dysmorphic**; however, they share characteristic facial features, such as triangular facies, gently downslanting palpebral fissures, and micrognathia (in childhood). While the SMS microdeletion can be visualized by routine cytogenetic studies and FISH analysis, the PTLS microduplication is often overlooked by these methods; hence, array analysis is critical in the detection. Most individuals have nonaffected parents; however, parent-to-child transmission has occurred.

Deletion 22q11 (Velocardiofacial Syndrome, DiGeorge Syndrome, and Others)

With an estimated incidence of 1 in 2,000, deletion 22q11 is one of the most frequent known microdeletion/multiple congenital anomaly syndromes in humans. It also is one of the most frequent causes of congenital syndromic cardiac defects, especially of the outflow side of the heart. A detailed description is found in Section 21.1.

19.3   Multiple Congenital Anomalies Due to Single Gene Defects

Rubinstein-Taybi Syndrome

Rubinstein-Taybi syndrome is a multiple congenital anomaly syndrome, with **microcephaly**, postnatal **short stature**, and **typical craniofacial anomalies**, including hypotelorism with downslanting palpebral fissures, beaked nose with the columella extending below the nares, short philtrum, hypoplastic maxilla with high-arched palate, micrognathia, and low-set dysplastic ears (◻ Fig. 19.20). Very typical features are **broadened terminal phalanxes of the thumbs and big toes** (◻ Fig. 19.21) and malposition of the first metacarpal, resulting in a thumb that protrudes at a right angle from the hand. Bone maturity is delayed, cardiac defects are not infrequent, and there is significant developmental delay and cognitive impairment. For a long time Rubinstein-Taybi syndrome was considered a *contiguous gene syndrome*, as some patients harbored microdeletions of 16p13.3. However, only 10% of the patients have detectable deletions of 16p13.3 by FISH, and the majority (30% to 50%) harbor a heterozygous **mutation** of a single gene (*CREBBP*, *cyclic AMP regulated enhancer binding protein*) within this region. Another 10% to 20% are caused by exonic or single-gene deletions of *CREBBP*. A

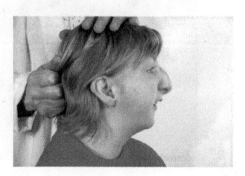

◻ **Figure 19.20. Rubinstein-Taybi Syndrome.**
Typical profile. (Courtesy of G. Tariverdian, Institut für Humangenetik Heidelberg.)

Figure 19.21. Rubinstein-Taybi Syndrome. Broad, malpositioned thumb.

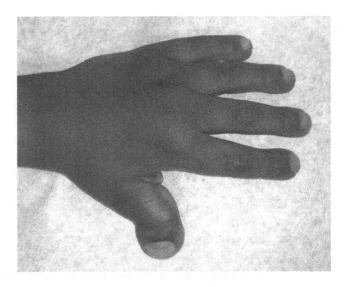

small percentage of cases of Rubinstein-Taybi syndrome are caused by mutations or deletions of yet another gene, *EP300*.

Smith-Lemli-Opitz Syndrome

Smith-Lemli-Opitz syndrome (SLOS) represents the most common disorder of cholesterol biosynthesis, resulting from deficiency of the enzyme 7-dehydrocholesterol reductase. Patients with SLOS present with pre- and postnatal growth retardation, microcephaly, and moderate to severe intellectual disability. Multiple congenital anomalies include midline defects, such as brain malformations, cleft palate, and cardiac and urogenital malformations (e.g., hypospadias and cryptorchidism). An important diagnostic clue is **syndactyly of the second and third toes** (Fig. 19.22).

Infants with SLOS frequently have feeding problems due to a combination of hypotonia, oromotor dysfunction, and gastrointestinal problems, including gastroesophageal reflux and dysmotility. Behavioral abnormalities in patients with SLOS include sensory hypersensitivity, irritability, self-injurious behavior, and autism spectrum behaviors. Cholesterol supplementation may have a positive effect on behavior and course of the disease, but it does not prevent severe intellectual disability. Furthermore, the efficacy of treatment has not been conclusively proven.

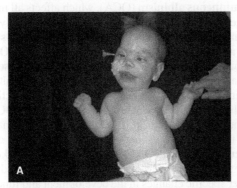
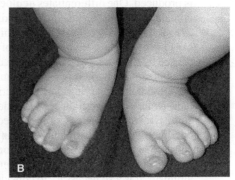

Figure 19.22. Smith-Lemli-Opitz Syndrome (SLOS). A. Affected children usually have microcephaly with a prominent forehead, a small nose with anteverted nares, and micrognathia. **B.** An important diagnostic clue is syndactyly of the second and third toes.

20 Skin and Connective Tissue

LEARNING OBJECTIVES

1 Name at least one genetic skin disorder for each of the following modes of inheritance: autosomal dominant, autosomal recessive, X linked, semidominant, and multifactorial.

2 Give an example of the clinical presentation of patients with Ehlers-Danlos syndrome: classic type, hypermobility type, and vascular type.

3 Name the two major criteria for the clinical diagnosis of Marfan syndrome and four systemic manifestations, according to the revised Ghent criteria.

4 Formulate a "plan of care" for an 18-year-old patient who is newly diagnosed with Marfan syndrome.

As the largest human organ, the skin is critically important in every clinical genetic examination. Skin changes can provide valuable evidence for numerous genetic diseases. Of special importance is the pigmentation of the skin (hyperpigmentation or hypopigmentation); also important are its texture and elasticity. The distribution of skin changes can indicate when, during embryonic development, a gene mutation occurred or can point to an underlying hereditary mechanism (e.g., X inactivation and lyonization).

> **Important**
>
> Skin changes should always direct attention to other organs of ectodermal origin, including hair, teeth, nails, and sweat glands.

Finally, there are also neurocutaneous syndromes or hamartoses, which are a heterogeneous group of genetic diseases that usually manifest themselves as dysplasias of the neuroectodermal tissue (Section 32.6).

20.1 Congenital Skin Disorders

Albinism

The term *albinism* includes a range of genetic **disorders of melanin synthesis**. In these disorders, the number, distribution, and structure of melanocytes in the skin, the hair follicles, and the eye are normal, as are the melanosomes within the melanocytes. The only difference is that less melanin is produced. One differentiates **oculocutaneous albinism** (OCA), which affects all melanocyte-containing organs (e.g., skin, hair, and eyes), from **ocular albinism** (OA), which only affects the eye. The cumulative incidence of albinism is approximately 1 in 10,000 individuals.

One of the most frequent forms of albinism is oculocutaneous albinism type 1 (**OCA1**). It is caused by mutations of the *TYR* gene on chromosome 11, which codes for **tyrosinase**. This type of albinism is inherited in an autosomal recessive manner. Different mutations result in clinical manifestations of varying clinical severity. Patients with **OCA1A** have no tyrosinase activity. White hair, white skin, and light blue to reddish eyes are evident at birth. Patients with **OCA1B** have some tyrosinase activity. Oculocutaneous albinism type 2 (**OCA2**) is also an autosomal recessive condition. It is caused by mutations in the *OCA2* gene, which codes for "P protein," on chromosome 15. The most frequent type of **ocular albinism (OA1)** is inherited in an X-linked manner.

Cutaneous and ocular hypopigmentation are not sufficient to establish a formal diagnosis of albinism. It is also necessary to consider specific changes in the development and function of the eyes and optic nerves, as melanin is crucial for the embryonic development of the entire optical system. Besides hypopigmentation, the chief symptoms of albinism are **nystagmus, reduced visual acuity** (as a result of foveal hypoplasia), strabismus, and reduced spatial visual acuity (caused by reduced depth perception resulting from abnormal connections between the retina and the visual cortex). Cognitive impairment, intellectual disability, and psychomotor retardation are not features of albinism and, if present, should instigate a diagnostic evaluation for other etiologies.

The reduced melanin content of the skin results in strong light sensitivity and increased risk of severe, recurrent sunburn and subsequent skin cancer. Therefore, protecting the skin and eyes from light is of utmost importance for therapy and prophylaxis.

■■■ **Association with Prader-Willi or Angelman Syndrome**
The *OCA2* gene is located on the long arm of chromosome 15 and is haploinsufficient in individuals with Prader-Willi syndrome and Angelman syndrome, diseases caused by the deletion of 15q11-q13. **Hypopigmentation** of the skin is one of the typical symptoms in these cases. There are also case reports of individuals with true oculocutaneous albinism type 2, in addition to Prader-Willi syndrome or Angelman syndrome. In most of these cases, there is a deletion on one allele, while the other allele has a mutation in the *OCA2* gene.

Vitiligo

Vitiligo is a rather frequently **acquired** loss of skin pigmentation. It tends to occur in families; men and women are equally affected. Details of heredity are still unknown, but single nucleotide polymorphisms (SNPs) in the gene *NALP1*, which codes for NACHT leucine-rich protein 1, a regulator of the innate immune system, have been associated with certain types of vitiligo. SNPs in and around *NALP1* show an association with vitiligo and several epidemiologically associated autoimmune and autoinflammatory diseases, implicating the innate immune system in the pathogenesis of these disorders.

Incontinentia Pigmenti

Incontinentia pigmenti, also called Bloch-Sulzberger syndrome, is a rare, X-linked dermatosis caused by mutations in the *NEMO* gene. Mutations in this gene are typically lethal in the hemizygous state. It is described in Section 4.4 as an example of an X-chromosomal disorder that exemplifies the mechanism of lyonization.

Xeroderma Pigmentosum

This is a rare **autosomal recessive** inherited disorder characterized by extreme **photosensitivity**. It can be caused by mutations in various genes, whereby the respective gene products are involved in excision repair after ultraviolet radiation–induced DNA damage. Affected children develop severe burns after sun exposure, leading to a chronic sun damage of the skin (■ Fig. 20.1). **Skin cancer** develops during midchildhood, primarily basal cell carcinomas or squamous cell carcinomas. Approximately 97% of these tumors occur on the face, scalp, or neck of patients, which points to the crucial pathogenetic role of sun exposure. Melanomas are seen in only 5% of patients. Most patients manifest progressive ophthalmologic symptoms (e.g., photophobia, conjunctivitis, telangiectasias of conjunctiva, and palpebrae), including ophthalmologic neoplasms.

Ichthyoses

Ichthyoses are heritable dermatoses characterized by a dysfunction of epidermal differentiation with excessive keratin production (■ Fig. 20.2). The autosomal dominant **ichthyosis vulgaris** represents the most common type. In contrast to other ichthyoses, neonates with ichthyosis vulgaris are asymptomatic. Only after the first 3 months of life does the skin become increasingly dry, with the formation of white to dirty gray adherent scales typically on the extensor surface of the extremities. Ichthyosis vulgaris is caused by mutations in the *FLG* gene, which codes for filaggrin, a protein that facilitates terminal differentiation of the epidermis and the formation of the skin barrier. Ichthyosis vulgaris is **semidominant**; that is, heterozygotes have either no discernible phenotype or mild ichthyosis, whereas homozygotes or compound heterozygotes have marked ichthyosis and a histological skin barrier defect.

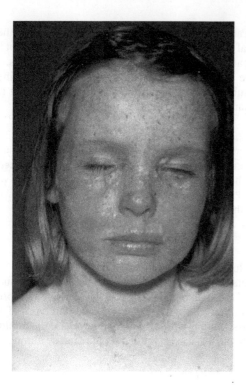

Figure 20.1. Xeroderma Pigmentosum. Unprotected sun exposure has severely damaged the face of an 8-year-old girl. (Courtesy of V. Voigtländer, Klinikum Ludwigshafen.)

On average, 1 in every 6,000 boys is affected by the **X-linked** ichthyosis. This differs from the autosomal dominant type by occurring earlier and by more pronounced ichthyotic scaling. The palms of the hands and the soles of the feet are unaffected (in contrast to the autosomal dominant type). The disease is caused by a lack of steroid sulfatase. In most cases there is a complete loss of the gene due to a deletion of a portion of the short arm of the X chromosome.

Epidermolysis Bullosa

The term *epidermolysis bullosa* covers a heterogeneous group of inherited (mechanobullous) or acquired (autoimmune) genodermatoses, where slight trauma or mechanical stress can result in the formation of skin blisters (Koebner phenomenon; Fig. 20.3). The three major **intraepidermal types** of epidermolysis bullosa are caused by mutations in genes that code for proteins of the **keratin** family: epidermolysis bullosa simplex (EBS), epidermolysis bullosa herpetiformis (EBH), and epidermolytic hyperkeratosis (EH). These types of epidermolysis bullosa do not form scars. The major **scarring (dermolytic) type** is also called epidermolysis bullosa dystrophica (EBD). This is caused by **mutations of collagen type 7**, a major component of the fibrillar anchors of the basement membrane. In **junctional epidermolysis bullosa**, separation

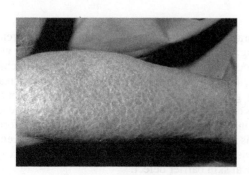

Figure 20.2. X-Linked Ichthyosis. Hyperkeratosis with dirty gray adherent scales. (With permission of V. Voigtländer, Klinikum Ludwigshafen.)

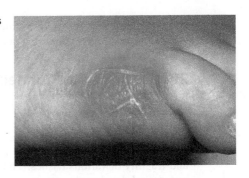

Figure 20.3. Koebner Phenomenon in Epidermolysis Bullosa Simplex. (Courtesy of V. Voigtländer, Klinikum Ludwigshafen.)

occurs above the basement membrane of the dermis, resulting in nonscarring blistering. This is caused by mutations in genes whose gene products are part of the hemidesmosomes or the lamina rara, **laminin 5**, and **type 17 collagen**.

Psoriasis

Psoriasis is one of the most frequent skin diseases, occurring in approximately **2% of the population**. It is a chronic skin disorder, typically characterized by erythematous plaques with a silver scale, although other presentations occur. It occurs mostly on the extensor surface of the extremities, especially the joints and elbows, but it can also present on the scalp and the lower back. Psoriasis is a multifactorial disease. Studies of families and twins have shown a strong genetic component. The concordance rate for identical twins is 65% to 70%; the concordance rate for fraternal twins is 15% to 20%. First-degree relatives have an 8% to 23% risk of also developing psoriasis. Several **psoriasis susceptibility gene loci** have been identified, and some of these loci are identical with the genetic linkage of atopic dermatitis (eczema). The predisposition for psoriasis is also influenced by polymorphisms of various cytokine alleles. Among the environmental trigger factors for psoriasis are streptococcal infections, stress, and medications (e.g., lithium and beta-blockers).

Telangiectatic Malformations

Telangiectasias are defined as dilations of the capillaries in skin and mucous membranes that, in contrast to petechiae, blanch upon applying pressure (diascopy). They are mostly acquired, though they are also seen in several genetic disorders, including ataxia telangiectasia (Louis-Bar syndrome; Section 31.1.2), hereditary hemorrhagic telangiectasia (Osler-Weber-Rendu syndrome; Fig. 20.4), and Sturge-Weber syndrome. Among the telangiectatic malformations

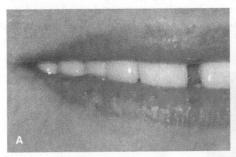
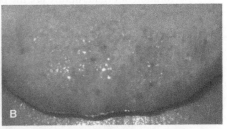

Figure 20.4. Telangiectases in Hereditary Hemorrhagic Telangiectasia (HHT). Telangiectasias of **(A)** the lips and **(B)** the mucous membranes (here the tongue) are typical in the autosomal HHT, which frequently presents with nosebleeds and possibly severe gastrointestinal, pulmonary, or cerebral hemorrhages. Life-threatening lung hemorrhages, resulting from arteriovenous malformations, are a serious complication in pregnancy. HHT is caused by mutations in genes involved in the transforming growth factor-β (TGF-β) signaling cascade (e.g., *ENG*, *ALK1*, and *SMAD4*).

is **nevus flammeus** (port-wine stain), mostly present at birth; only in certain configurations, such as a stork-bite mark on the neck, is a large nevus reversible.

20.2   Congenital Connective Tissue Disorders

Ehlers-Danlos Syndrome

Ehlers-Danlos syndrome includes a group of genetically, biochemically, and clinically heterogeneous hereditary connective tissue disorders, with hyperextensibility of joints and skin and fragility of various tissues. The estimated prevalence is 1 in 5,000. Inheritance is usually **autosomal dominant**.

■■■ What Is Hyperextensibility?
The definition of "hyperextensibility of the joints" results from five or more features of the Beighton and Wolf scale (maximum of nine total features):
— Passive dorsiflexion of the fifth finger beyond 90 degrees: 1 point per hand
— Passive apposition of the thumb to the flexor surface of the forearm: 1 point per hand
— Hyperextension of the elbow greater than 10 degrees: 1 point per elbow
— Hyperextension of the knee greater than 10 degrees: 1 point per knee
— Ability to place the palms on the floor with knees fully extended: 1 point

Ehlers-Danlos Syndrome, Classic Type (Previously Types I and II). The best-known characteristics of classic Ehlers-Danlos syndrome (EDS) are skin hyperextensibility and hypermobility of joints (◻ Fig. 20.5). The skin is fragile, bruises and lacerates easily, and heals poorly; scars appear widened and atrophic. In addition to joint hypermobility, there are frequent dislocations/subluxations of the patella, digits, hip, shoulder, radius, and clavicle, which usually resolve spontaneously and are easily managed by the affected individual. The "Gorlin sign" (tip of the tongue can touch the nose) is nonspecific. The typical fragility of connective tissues results in frequent hiatal hernias, rectal prolapse, bladder diverticula, uterine prolapse, and cervical insufficiency in women. There is a significant risk for dilatation of the ascending aorta (present in up to 25% of individuals with EDS classic type), with possible aortic rupture. A majority of the cases result from **defects of collagen V**, which is caused by mutations in the *COL5A1* and *COL5A2* genes.

Ehlers-Danlos Syndrome, Hypermobility Type (Previously Type III). This is considered the least severe type of EDS. In contrast to other types, it is not characterized by skin fragility and abnormal scarring. The main characteristics are hypermobility of the small and large joints as well as a velvety, mildly hyperelastic skin. A subset of cases of EDS, hypermobility type, is caused by haploinsufficiency of tenascin X, an extracellular matrix glycoprotein, encoded by *TNXB*.

Ehlers-Danlos Syndrome, Vascular Type (Previously Type IV). The skin in this type of EDS is not elastic but very tight, thin, and fragile. Vascular rupture or dissection and gastrointestinal perforation or organ rupture are the presenting symptoms in 70% of adults with this condition. Neonates may present with congenital dislocation of the hips. There is easy bruising. The veins

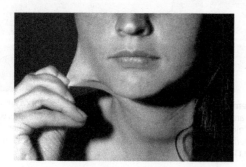

◻ **Figure 20.5. Ehlers-Danlos Syndrome.** (Courtesy of V. Voigtländer, Klinikum Ludwigshafen.)

can readily be seen under the thin, translucent skin. Scarring is normal, and hyperextensibility is limited to small joints. The average life expectancy is 48 years. The disorder is caused by deficiencies in the synthesis, structure, or secretion of **collagen III**.

Marfan Syndrome

It has been more than 100 years since Dr. Antoine Marfan described the first case of this disease, which he named "**dolichostenomelia**" (long and slender limbs). Diagnosis is typically made based on clinical criteria; however, molecular analysis may be helpful when features or family history is equivocal.

Case History

Nine-year-old Dennis is brought to the clinic by his parents for suspicion of Marfan syndrome (MFS). Pregnancy and birth were uncomplicated. Dennis walked at 11 to 12 months; he did not speak until age 2½ years. He had muscular hypotonia and was noted to be above average height (97th percentile). He is now in the third grade of elementary school, in all regular classes, and is doing well. When he was 7, he had an episode of palpitations; a cardiological examination showed dilatation of the ascending aorta and mitral valve prolapse. An ophthalmological examination revealed a subluxation of both lenses. Dennis was subsequently referred to the genetics clinic for further evaluation. The detailed family history is unremarkable. The physical examination shows Dennis as a friendly boy with normal development for his age. Height (approximately 4 feet 10 inches) and arm span (approximately 4 feet 11 inches) are above normal; their proportion, however, is within normal range (less than 1.05). He is noted to have arachnodactyly, and the wrist and thumb sign are positive. In addition, there is hypermobility of the joints. Dennis has a high-arched palate and mild retrognathia. There is a mild pectus excavatum, but no scoliosis. There are no other pertinent positives on physical examination. A clinical diagnosis of MFS is made, as both ectopia lentis and aortic dilatation (albeit mild) are present in addition to systemic manifestations. Both parents are clinically unaffected. You explain that Dennis's MFS is likely the result of a de novo mutation and refer Dennis for cardiological and ophthalmological follow-up.

Epidemiology

The incidence of MFS is **1 to 2 per 10,000** individuals, with no gender preference. Inheritance is **autosomal dominant**; approximately 25% of cases are caused by de novo mutations. Most of those originate from the paternal germ line, with a higher incidence in advanced paternal age, a phenomenon that has been reported for several autosomal dominant diseases (e.g., also for achondroplasia).

Clinical Features and Diagnostic Criteria

Diagnosing MFS involves the evaluation of clinical criteria, which have been recently revised (Ghent nosology). There are two cardinal features, aortic root aneurysm and ectopia lentis. In the absence of any family history, the presence of these two manifestations is regarded as sufficient for the unequivocal diagnosis of MFS. In the absence of either of these, the presence of a confirmed pathogenic mutation in the *FBN* gene or a combination of systemic manifestations (using a scoring system) is required.

One of the two key diagnostic criteria in the revised Ghent nosology is **aortic root aneurysm or dissection**. Echocardiographically, the aneurysm is defined as significant dilatation of the aortic root at the level of the sinuses of Valsalva (standardized "Z score" greater than or equal to 2). Other vascular anomalies, such as mitral valve prolapse or pulmonary artery dilation, may be present but are not regarded as sufficiently specific for the diagnosis of MFS. Severe cardiovascular complications, such as ruptured aortic aneurysm (which may be in the thoracic or abdominal aorta) or left-sided heart failure due to chronic aortic valve failure, are the major causes of death in MFS.

The other key diagnostic criterion of MFS is **subluxation of the lens** (ectopia lentis), which typically occurs in the upward direction (Fig. 20.6). This is in contrast to homocystinuria and traumatic events (in healthy individuals), where the lens usually luxates downward. MFS patients may also have an abnormally flat cornea and increased axial length of the globe, causing **myopia**.

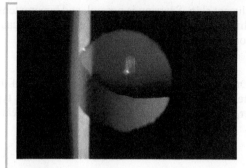

Figure 20.6. Subluxation of the Lens in Marfan Syndrome (MFS). In MFS, the zonular suspension of the crystalline lens is weakened or missing in some meridians. This perturbs the tension in the normally symmetric suspension, thus allowing the lens to dislocate in the direction of the remaining intact elastic zonular fibers. In this slit-lamp photograph, the partially dilated iris is illuminated by the slit beam, and the inferior rim of the lens is seen in retroillumination. The lens of the right eye is dislocated upward and inward toward the 2 o'clock meridian. (Courtesy of R. Lewis, Baylor College of Medicine, Houston.)

Typical symptoms and signs in other organ systems are of diagnostic value in patients with only one of the two cardinal manifestations. The **revised Ghent nosology** includes a scoring system (□ Table 20.1), with a possible maximum of 20 points; a score of 7 or more indicates systemic involvement.

Changes in the skeletal system are especially prominent in MFS. **Tall stature** in itself is not a diagnostic criterion; essential are excessively long arms and legs in proportion to the torso. This is measured by the ratio of arm span to height, which is increased in MFS (greater than 1.05 in adults), or the upper-to-lower segment ratio (less than 0.85 in adults). **Arachnodactyly** is measured by the wrist and thumb sign (□ Fig. 20.7). Additional skeletal signs are pectus carinatum (□ Fig. 20.8), severe forms of pectus excavatum, scoliosis (greater than 20 degrees), protrusio acetabuli, and pes planus caused by medial displacement of the medial malleolus.

Important	

- **Wrist (Walker-Murdoch) sign**: Overlapping of the complete distal phalanx of the thumb and fifth finger when wrapped around the opposite wrist.
- **Thumb (Steinberg) sign**: Extension of the entire distal phalanx of the thumb beyond the ulnar border of the hand when opposed across the palm.

Other clinical features of MFS include **pneumothorax**, which occurs through rupture of apical blebs, atrophic striae of the skin, and a specific **lumbosacral dural ectasia** that may cause

Table 20.1. Systemic Features of Marfan Syndrome

Clinical Feature	Score
Wrist AND thumb sign (less specific: wrist OR thumb sign)	3 (1)
Pectus carinatum deformity (less specific: pectus excavatum or chest asymmetry)	2 (1)
Hindfoot deformity (less specific: pes planus)	2 (1)
Pneumothorax	2
Dural ectasia	2
Protrusion acetabuli	2
Reduced upper-to-lower segment ratio (age-dependent <1 to <0.85), AND Increased arm span-to-height ratio (in adults >1.05), AND No severe scoliosis	1
Scoliosis or thoracolumbar kyphosis	1
Reduced elbow extension	1
Typical facial features	1
Skin striae	1
Myopia >3 diopters	1
Mitral valve prolapse	1

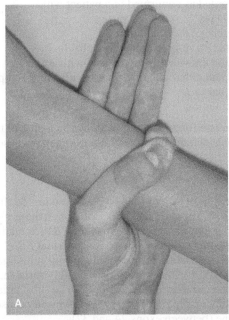
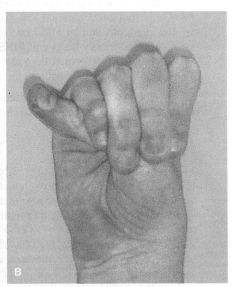

Figure 20.7. Typical signs of Marfan syndrome in a 13-year-old boy. **A.** Wrist (Walker-Murdoch) sign. **B.** Thumb (Steinberg) sign.

lower back pain, genital and rectal pain, weakness, and numbness in the lower extremities. Dural ectasia is identified through imaging techniques (computed tomography or magnetic resonance imaging). Typical **facial features** include dolichocephaly, enophthalmos, downslanting palpebral fissures, malar hypoplasia, and retrognathia (see Fig. 20.8).

Figure 20.8. Typical facial features of Marfan syndrome and pectus carinatum. (Courtesy of G. Tariverdian, Department of Human Genetics, Heidelberg.)

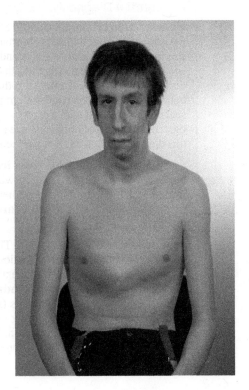

The diagnosis of MFS may be regarded as confirmed in a patient with:

- Aortic root aneurysm and ectopia lentis
- Aortic root aneurysm and a pathogenic *FBN1* mutation
- Aortic root aneurysm and a systemic score greater than or equal to 7
- Ectopia lentis and an *FBN1* mutation known to be associated with aortic root aneurysms
- Confirmed family history of MFS and either an aortic root aneurysm or ectopia lentis, or a systemic score greater than or equal to 7
- A familial confirmed pathogenic mutation

Ectopia lentis without aortic root aneurysm (or a typical mutation), regardless of the systemic score, is denoted *ectopia lentis syndrome*, which may be caused by mutations in several genes (including *FBN1*).

Etiology and Genetics

MFS is caused by mutations in the **fibrillin-1** (*FBN1*) gene on chromosome 15q. In about one-fourth of cases this is a de novo mutation. Approximately 70% of all mutations are *missense*, yet deletions of *FBN1* also cause disease. While the mechanism of *FBN1* mutations in MFS was thought to be mechanical in nature, recent findings indicate abnormal *FBN1* upregulates transforming growth factor-β (**TGF-β**), causing perturbations in multiple organ systems. Penetrance of MFS is very high (nearly 100%), but expressivity is highly variable. Genotype–phenotype correlation is incomplete, and intrafamilial variability can be substantial; however, a particularly severe phenotype (sometimes called *neonatal form*) is typically caused by mutations in the central segments of the gene (between exons 24 and 32).

Fibrillin-1. Fibrillin-1 is a protein of the extracellular matrix and a building block for microfibrils. Microfibrils not only serve structural functions but also regulate the matrix sequestration and activation of the growth factor TGF-β. A dysregulation of the TGF-β signaling pathway has been observed in the developing lung, the mitral valve, skeletal muscle, and the ascending aorta. In a mouse model of MFS, TGF-β antagonism has been shown to attenuate or prevent several of the symptoms and complications of the disorder.

Differential Diagnosis

Homocystinuria is an autosomal recessive metabolic disorder caused by a lack of cystathionine-β-synthetase. It has numerous Marfan-like symptoms, such as ectopic lens (typically downward), severe myopia, tall stature with slender limbs, chest deformities, scoliosis, mitral valve prolapse, and hernias. Additional symptoms that differentiate homocystinuria from MFS include intellectual disability, seizures, and, often, life-threatening, recurrent thromboembolic events. Approximately half of the patients respond well to pyridoxine (vitamin B_6) therapy, and the remaining can be successfully treated with a protein- and methionine-restricted diet and betaine, which promotes the remethylation of homocysteine to methionine. It is therefore especially important to exclude this diagnosis when MFS is suspected.

Ectopia Lentis. Familial **ectopia lentis syndrome** without aortic disease may be caused by mutations in the *FBN1* gene, in which case cardiovascular follow-up should be maintained throughout life. Mutations in other genes with autosomal recessive inheritance have been reported. Patients with **Weill-Marchesani syndrome** show lens dislocation, short stature, brachydactyly, and joint stiffness.

Cardiovascular Manifestations. The **MASS phenotype** is characterized by myopia, mitral valve prolapse, mild aortic dilatation (Z score less than 2), and skeletal and skin abnormalities (systemic score less than 5) in the absence of ectopia lentis; it may be caused by *FBN1* mutations. **Mitral valve prolapse syndrome** (MVPS), without aortic dilatation or ectopia lentis but with limited systemic features (score less than 5), is common and appears to be linked to several genetic loci. **Loeys-Dietz syndrome** is characterized by aortic aneurysm/dissection in conjunction with hypertelorism, broad or bifid uvula, cleft palate, and/or arterial tortuosity; it is caused by mutations in one of two genes coding for subunits of the TGF-β receptor.

Affected patients are not usually very tall but may show other morphological abnormalities and often have a more severe disease course (e.g., high risk of complications during pregnancy). Other differential diagnoses include **Ehlers-Danlos syndrome, vascular type** (Section 20.2); **bicuspid aortic valve** syndrome that may be associated with aortic aneurysms; and **familial thoracic aortic aneurysm and dissection syndrome**, which may be caused by mutations in several genes.

Systemic Manifestations. Patients with **Shprintzen-Goldberg syndrome** may have skeletal and facial features of MFS that are associated with craniosynostosis and intellectual disability, but they do not have aortic root dilatation. **Congenital contractural arachnodactyly** (Beals syndrome) is characterized by a Marfan-like habitus and arachnodactyly, in addition to congenital contractures of major joints and typical "crumpled" ears; there is little or no aortic root dilatation. The condition is caused by mutations in the fibrillin-2 gene *FBN2*.

Clinical Management

During childhood and adolescence special attention should be paid to the prevention of severe scoliosis. It is recommended that the child be seen and followed by a pediatric orthopedic surgeon. Frequent eye involvement (severe myopia and lenticular subluxation) also necessitates regular ophthalmic examinations.

Cardiovascular complications can occur at any age. Aortic root dilatation is usually progressive, and echocardiography is recommended at least annually to monitor the status of the ascending aorta. More frequent examinations are necessary when the aortic root diameter exceeds 1.8 inches (4.5 cm) or shows rapid change. Subacute bacterial endocarditis prophylaxis is indicated for dental work and all procedures expected to contaminate the bloodstream with bacteria.

Treatment with beta-blockers without intrinsic sympathomimetic activity (e.g., metoprolol and atenolol) results in a reduction of aortic root diameter and the associated complications (especially aortic dissection). It has, therefore, been the standard therapy for every patient with MFS. Angiotensin receptor blockers (ARBs) may prevent dilatation of the aorta in MFS and are under investigation. Afterload reducing agents (e.g., angiotensin-converting enzyme [ACE] inhibitors) are used as adjunctive therapy to reduce volume overload in patients with significant valve dysfunction.

Contact sports (e.g., football, soccer, basketball, and boxing) are to be avoided. Individuals with MFS can and should remain active, with isometric aerobic activities performed in moderation.

21 Cardiovascular System and Hematology

LEARNING OBJECTIVES

1 Name chromosomal aberrations and their typically associated congenital heart defects.

2 Explain the term *heterozygote advantage* using disorders of hemoglobin synthesis as an example.

3 Develop a list of hematological and genetic tests that should be ordered for
   a. A male neonate with prolonged oozing after circumcision
   b. A neonate with perinatal thrombosis of the vena cava

21.1 Congenital Heart Defects

Approximately **7 to 8 of every 1,000** neonates are born with a congenital heart defect. This number does not include patent ductus arteriosus or bicuspid aortic valve and mitral valve prolapse (which are mostly asymptomatic during childhood). In 2 to 3 of every 1,000 neonates the abnormality requires surgical intervention during the first year. There is no gender preference for the total prevalence of congenital heart defects. Individual defects, however, tend to be sex specific; obstructive defects of the left heart and transposition of the great arteries are more frequent in boys, while persistent ductus arteriosus, atrial septal defects, and pulmonary stenosis occur more frequently in girls.

Ventricular septal defect (VSD) is by far the most frequent cardiac defect. The relative frequency of the various congenital cardiac abnormalities is listed in ◘ Table 21.1.

Epidemiological studies have shown a 2% to 5% **global recurrence risk** of isolated cardiac defects within a family. This statistic refers to a mostly polygenic and multifactorial genesis. Frequently familial recurrence does not involve the same cardiac malformation. Even with the same abnormality, expressivity and clinical severity can differ significantly. The recurrence risk for different cardiac defects is quite variable. Obstructions in the left heart have an especially high recurrence risk: 8% for a hypoplastic left heart syndrome (HLHS) and more than 6% for coarctation of the aorta. At 6%, the risk of **women** transmitting a cardiac defect to their own children is nearly twice as high as that of affected men. ◘ Table 21.2 lists empirical recurrence risks in various scenarios.

Etiology of Cardiac Defects. Today's estimates for risk of cardiac defects are based on the assumption that approximately 80% of all congenital cardiovascular abnormalities are multifactorial. At this time, only one in five cardiac defects has a clearly identified pathogenetic cause. About 15% to 20% of congenital cardiac defects are caused by chromosomal aberrations (including copy number variants). Approximately 3% to 5% are caused by single-gene defects and 1% to 2% by teratogenic exposures during pregnancy. The evaluation of a congenital heart defect should therefore always include a detailed family history, a detailed history of possible infections during pregnancy, and a detailed history of teratogenic exposures (alcohol, drugs, medications, and chemical substances). Poorly controlled maternal metabolic diseases, such as diabetes mellitus or phenylketonuria, have been associated with childhood cardiac defects. A list of various teratogens is presented in ◘ Table 21.3.

Isolated Finding or Part of a Genetic Syndrome? Additional extracardiac malformations are seen in up to 25% of all patients with congenital heart defects. The most frequent underlying cause for additional congenital malformations is trisomy 21. Approximately 45% of patients with Down syndrome have a cardiac defect, with atrioventricular defects being the most typical and frequent (Section 19.1). Microdeletion syndrome 22q11 (see below) is typically associated with conotruncal cardiac defects (e.g., abnormalities of the aortic arch, tetralogy of Fallot [TOF], pulmonary atresia with VSD, double outlet right ventricle [DORV], or dextro-transposition

Table 21.1. Relative Frequency of Congenital Heart Defects

Cardiac Defect	Abbreviation	Relative Frequency (%)
Ventricular septal defect	VSD	30–45
Pulmonary stenosis	PaVS	5–13
Atrial septal defect	ASD	5–11
Persistent ductus arteriosus	PDA	5–10
Aortic valve stenosis	AoVS	4–8
Coarctation of the aorta	CoA	4–7
d-Transposition of the great arteries	d-TGA	3–7
Tetralogy of Fallot	TOF	3–5
Hypoplastic left heart syndrome	HLHS	1–4

Adapted from von Bernuth, 2003.

Table 21.2. Recurrence Risk for Congenital Heart Defects

	Empirical Recurrence Risk (%)
Healthy parents, one affected child	1–3
Affected father	2–3
Affected mother	5–6
Two affected children or one affected parent + one affected child	10
More than two affected first-degree relatives	50

Table 21.3. Association of Some Teratogens with Congenital Heart Defects

Teratogen	Risk for Congenital Cardiac Defects (%)	Most Frequent Cardiac Defects
Rubella infection	35	Peripheral pulmonary artery stenosis, PDA, VSD, ASD
Maternal diabetes mellitus	3–5	Conotruncal cardiac defects
Maternal PKU	25–50	TOF
Maternal systemic lupus erythematosus	20–40	Conduction defects
Maternal alcohol abuse	25–30	VSD, ASD
Retinoic acid	10–20	Conotruncal cardiac defects
Lithium	???	Ebstein anomaly

PKU, phenylketonuria.
Adapted from Burn and Goodship, 2002.

Table 21.4. Syndromic Disorders with Congenital Heart Defects

Disorder	Frequency of Congenital Heart Defects (%)	Typical Cardiac Defects
Numerical Chromosome Abnormalities		
Down syndrome (trisomy 21)	45	AV canal (40%)
Edwards syndrome (trisomy 18)	80–90	Septal and valvular defects (especially multiple valvular defects)
Pätau syndrome (trisomy 13)	80–90	Septal and valvular defects
Turner syndrome (monosomy X)	25	Coarctation of the aorta (10%)
Microdeletion Syndromes		
DiGeorge syndrome/VCFS (microdeletion 22q11)	85	VSD (62%), DORV (52%), TOF (21%)
Williams syndrome (microdeletion 7q11)	60	Supravalvular aortic stenosis (50%–75%), peripheral pulmonary stenosis
Syndromes with Mutation/Deletion of Individual Genes		
Noonan syndrome	50–80	Pulmonary valve stenosis (20%–50%)
Alagille syndrome	>90	Peripheral pulmonary stenosis (60%–70%), TOF (7%–15%)
Holt-Oram syndrome	70–80	ASD, VSD

Adapted from Kreuder, 2004.

of the great arteries [d-TGA]). The presence of such a cardiac defect in the context of the respective clinical picture warrants additional testing by DNA array (or targeted fluorescence in situ hybridization [FISH] analysis if the suspicion for a specific syndrome is high). In cases of supraventricular aortic stenosis or peripheral pulmonary stenosis, 7q11 microdeletion (i.e., Williams syndrome) should be considered in the differential diagnosis. ■ Table 21.4 lists syndromic disorders with associated congenital heart defects.

> **Important**
>
> Supraventricular aortic stenosis in a newborn—think Williams syndrome!

> **Important**
>
> The differential diagnosis in a newborn with excessive nuchal skin/webbed neck includes Turner syndrome and Noonan syndrome. Note that patients with Noonan syndrome frequently have **right-sided** heart defects (e.g., pulmonary valve stenosis), whereas patients with Turner syndrome more typically have **left-sided** heart defects (e.g., bicuspid aortic valve, coarctation of the aorta).

Noonan Syndrome. Noonan syndrome is an autosomal dominant condition, which is characterized by short stature, distinctive craniofacial features (■ Figs. 21.1 and 21.2), congenital cardiovascular disease, and other more variable clinical findings such as developmental delay and intellectual disability, bleeding diathesis, lymphatic abnormalities, and genitourinary abnormalities. Although Noonan syndrome occurs in 1 in 1,000 to 1 in 2,500 persons, individuals with Noonan syndrome may escape diagnosis if the features are only mildly expressed. The genes implicated in Noonan syndrome and other clinically related conditions function in a complex signal transduction pathway (Ras/MAPK [mitogen-activated protein kinase]). While clinical testing is available for many of these genes (including *PTPN11, KRAS, SOS,* and *RAF1*), mutations are detected in approximately 60% of individuals with an established clinical diagnosis of Noonan syndrome. Mutation analysis is helpful, however, as once a mutation is established in an individual, other at-risk family members can be tested and treated appropriately if necessary.

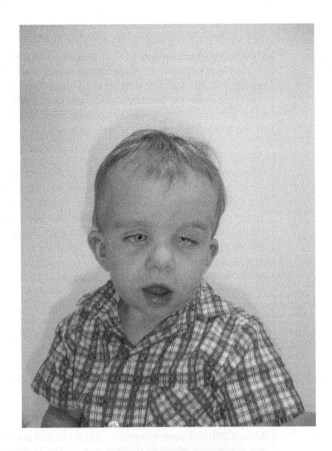

Figure 21.1. Noonan Syndrome in an 18-Month-Old Boy. Facial features include hypertelorism and telecanthus, ptosis, and downslanting palpebral fissures. Noonan syndrome should be considered in the differential diagnosis of all children with short stature, heart defects, and the respective facial features.

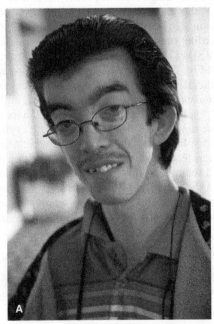
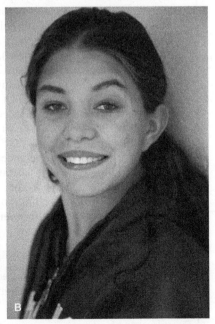

Figure 21.2. A, B. Noonan Syndrome in Two Adults. Note the facial features including mild hypertelorism, ptosis (more pronounced in the individual on the left), and low-set and posteriorly rotated ears. Facial features of Noonan syndrome change with age and tend to be more subtle in adulthood. (Photos courtesy of Rick Guidotti, www.positiveexposure.org.)

III

22q11.2 Deletion Syndrome (Velocardiofacial Syndrome, Shprintzen Syndrome, DiGeorge Syndrome)

DiGeorge syndrome was first described in 1968 as a combination of hypoparathyroidism and thymus hypoplasia. **Shprintzen syndrome**, also called **velocardiofacial syndrome**, was reported in 1978 and described individuals with a combination of cleft palate, cardiac defects, and typical facies. Interestingly, both syndromes are merely different manifestations of the same genetic defect, a classic microdeletion syndrome that results in a developmental disorder of the third and fourth branchial arches.

Case History

Julia, age 5 years, is brought to the genetics clinic after DNA array analysis revealed a diagnosis of microdeletion 22q11. The parents report that Julia was small for gestational age, with symmetric growth retardation at birth. Additional anomalies noted at birth included a cleft palate and a clinically insignificant cardiac defect (perimembranous VSD). The cleft palate was surgically repaired at 2 years. Growth continued to be slightly below the third percentile. A well-child visit at the age of 3 years documented mild muscular hypotonia and hyperextensible joints. Motor development was normal, while speech development was delayed. A chromosome analysis was normal at the time. Julia has a new pediatrician and, given the combination of heart defects, cleft palate, and typical facial features, he suspected 22q11.2 deletion syndrome; this was confirmed by DNA array analysis. You discuss the diagnosis of 22q11.2 deletion syndrome with Julia's parents and provide anticipatory guidance. Both parents are clinically examined with regard to possible signs of the microdeletion, and genetic testing is offered. Given Julia's short stature, you refer her to a pediatric endocrinologist for growth hormone therapy. An evaluation by a speech pathologist is initiated.

Epidemiology

The 22q11.2 deletion syndrome is one of the most common microdeletion syndromes. Incidence is approximately 1 in every 2,000 individuals.

Clinical Features

Almost 200 different symptoms and findings have been described in patients with 22q11.2 deletion syndrome. None of these symptoms or findings is pathognomonic, and none is obligatory, but there are some "cardinal symptoms" that make the respective diagnosis very likely.

Up to 80% of patients with deletion 22q11 have a congenital **heart defect**, typically a **"conotruncal"** defect affecting cardiac outflow. The most frequent defects are tetralogy of Fallot (23% of all patients), VSDs (15%), and interrupted aortic arch (10%). The other typical defect is **cleft palate** (◻ Fig. 21.3); sometimes there is also laryngomalacia. Shprintzen syndrome or velocardiofacial syndrome (VCFS) has typical facial features, including a long, oval face with an unusual nose (prominent nasal root, bulbous nasal tip, and hypoplastic alae nasi); "hooded" eyelids; and abnormally shaped ears (overfolded or squared-off helix) (◻ Fig. 21.4). Some newborns show an asymmetric crying face. About 70% to 80% of patients with VCFS display muscular hypotonia, which, in combination with velopharyngeal incompetence, can lead to severe feeding difficulties during infancy and early childhood. Other associated features include hypernasal speech and obstructive sleep apnea. DiGeorge syndrome, on the other hand, includes hypoparathyroidism with hypocalcemia (60%), as well as more severe symptoms such as tetany and seizures (20%). Thymic hypoplasia can result in an increased susceptibility to infection—impaired T-cell production is the primary defect.

> **Important**
>
> The combination of heart defects (especially conotruncal) and cleft palate in a newborn should prompt a DNA array analysis for 22q11.2 deletion.

Development

Almost all children with microdeletion 22q11 have some degree of developmental delay. The average IQ of individuals with 22q11.2 deletion syndrome is 75 to 80, but only 30% fall into

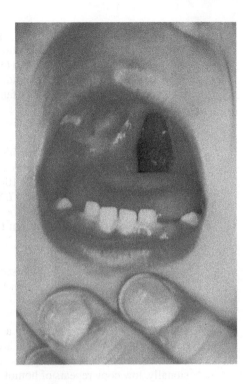

Figure 21.3. Cleft Palate. (Courtesy of HJ Müller, Department of Medical Genetics, University Children's Hospital Basel, Switzerland.)

the intellectual disability range since two-thirds are only mildly affected. Verbal IQ scores are significantly higher than performance IQ scores.

Neurobehavioral and neuropsychiatric problems include attention deficit disorder, anxiety, perseveration, and autism spectrum disorder. The incidence of schizophrenia, depression, and bipolar disorder is increased as compared to the general population.

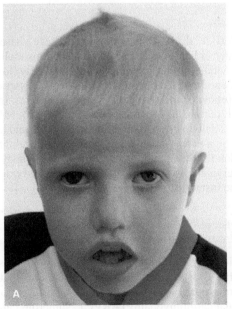
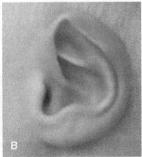

Figure 21.4. 22q11.2 Deletion Syndrome. A. Boy with oval face, long midface, and typical prominent nose. **B.** Overfolded helix.

Etiology

This disorder is caused by a deletion on the long arm of chromosome 22 (22q11.21-q11.23). The typical deletion is **1.5 to 3 Mb large** (3 Mb in almost 90% of cases). It usually encompasses 25 to 30 genes. Some of the candidate genes for VCFS-associated symptoms include *TBX1*, a transcription factor of the T-Box family (cardiac defects), and *COMT*, coding for catechol-*O*-methyltransferase (psychiatric phenotypes).

In 15% of patients, a deletion is visible under the light microscope. The "gold standard" for securing a diagnosis of 22q11.2 deletion syndrome is **DNA array analysis**; however, once a diagnosis is established in an individual, the parents can have a FISH analysis to evaluate whether either one of them has the deletion. Some patients with a clinical diagnosis of VCFS will be found to have a microdeletion of 10p13-p14. This region has been named "VCFS2." Recently, patients with point mutations in *TBX1* have been described with a VCFS-like phenotype.

In **90%** of cases the deletion occurs **de novo**. The remaining 10% are inherited deletions. Inheritance is **autosomal dominant**. Intrafamilial variability, however, is considerable.

> **Important**
>
> When 22q11.2 deletion is diagnosed, consideration should be given to testing first-degree family members, since the deletion can be oligosymptomatic and the only symptoms in some affected adults may be some mild learning problems or mild psychiatric phenotypes.

Chromosomal region 22q11.2 is a so-called "recombination hotspot," which explains why deletions and duplications of this area are so frequently seen. The "critical" region is flanked on both sides by low copy repeats. There are several such regions on chromosome 22. Occasionally, low copy repeats of homologous (i.e., sequence identical) but nonallelic (i.e., not the exact same segment on the other allele of chromosome 22) sequences align during prophase of meiosis. When recombination occurs (in this case **nonallelic homologous recombination [NAHR]**), this leads to the loss of interspersed segments on one allele (causing 22q11.2 deletion) and the gain (22q11.2 duplication) on the other. In rare cases, low copy repeats (flanking the 22q11.2 critical region) of the **same allele** lead to the formation of **intra**chromosomal loops and the region between them (22q11.21-q11.23) is lost. This would represent a case of **intrachromosomal recombination**.

Treatment and Management

All neonates diagnosed with 22q11.2 deletion syndrome should have a baseline ionized calcium test to evaluate for hypoparathyroidism. Other baseline evaluations include measurement of lymphocyte count, renal ultrasound, echocardiogram, chest radiography (to evaluate for thoracic vertebral anomalies), and evaluation of feeding and swallowing (to assess for velopharyngeal insufficiency, submucous cleft palate, and oral pharyngeal dysphagia). Infants with lymphocyte abnormalities should not receive live vaccines (e.g., oral polio, MMR). By the age of 1 year, all children with 22q11.2 deletion should have a formal speech and language assessment. Evaluation and reassessment by a developmental pediatrician or developmental psychologist are essential to formulate a plan for therapeutic intervention from infancy through school-age years. By the age of 4 years, cervical spine films (including flexion and extension views) should be examined for cervical spine instability.

21.2   Cardiomyopathies

The World Health Organization (WHO) defines cardiomyopathies as disorders of the myocardium associated with cardiac dysfunction. They are classified as dilated cardiomyopathy (DCM), hypertrophic cardiomyopathy (HCM), restrictive cardiomyopathy (RCM), and arrhythmogenic right ventricular cardiomyopathy (ARVC). Numerous cardiomyopathies have familial occurrence. A detailed family history, therefore, is imperative in the evaluation of all cases of cardiomyopathy.

Hypertrophic Cardiomyopathy

Hypertrophic cardiomyopathy is defined by myocardial hypertrophy that is often asymmetric and frequently involves the interventricular septum. Patients typically have preserved systolic function but decreased ventricular compliance, leading to diastolic dysfunction. HCM occurs in 0.2% of the population and is one of the most frequent causes of sudden death in **young competitive athletes** (the disorder accounts for one-third of all such cases). More than half of the cases of HCM are familial. Inheritance mostly is autosomal dominant with incomplete penetrance. A great number of mutations in as many as 12 different genes, encoding different components of the sarcomere, have been identified as causative for HCM thus far. The most frequent causes are mutations in the genes for **β-myosin heavy chain** (40%), **myosin binding protein C** (40%), and **troponin T** (5%) or **troponin I** (5%).

Common symptoms include shortness of breath (especially with exertion), palpitations, chest pain, and orthostasis. The main complication with hypertrophic cardiomyopathies is sudden cardiac death, which occurs most frequently between the ages of 14 and 30 years. Young men in families with a history of sudden cardiac death are at high risk and should undergo evaluation with an echocardiogram.

HCM in **neonates and infants** is extremely rare. In such cases, the possible causes might be metabolic diseases (e.g., glycogen storage disease type II [Pompe disease], fatty acid oxidation disorders, mitochondrial disorders) as well as other monogenic disorders (especially Noonan syndrome).

Dilated Cardiomyopathy

Dilated cardiomyopathy is defined as ventricular enlargement and systolic dysfunction with normal left ventricular wall thickness. The prevalence of 0.04% (1 in every 2,500 individuals) is considerably less than in HCM. DCM can be idiopathic (isolated occurrence of cardiomyopathy) or part of a more complex, systemic disorder (muscular, neuromuscular, metabolic, or other disorders). Examples of the latter include muscular dystrophies (e.g., Duchenne, Becker, Emery-Dreifuss, and limb-girdle type), Friedreich ataxia, congenital disorders of glycosylation, and mitochondrial disorders.

About 20% to 50% of the cases of **idiopathic dilated cardiomyopathy** are familial with mostly autosomal dominant inheritance. Mutations in more than 20 different genes have been identified as causing idiopathic DCM. Those include *LMNA* (coding for **lamin A/C**; 7% to 8%), *MYH7* (coding for **myosin 7**; 5% to 8%), and the genes for desmin, α-actin, titin, and δ-sarcoglycan.

21.3 Heritable Arrhythmogenic Disorders

Long QT Syndrome

Long QT syndrome (LQTS) is characterized by a lengthening of the frequency-corrected QT time (QTc), frequently accompanied by changes in T-wave morphology. QTc greater than 480 ms means an increased risk for ventricular tachycardias, especially **torsades de pointes tachycardia**. This can manifest itself as syncope or chest pain or directly as sudden cardiac death.

Acquired and congenital forms of LQTS can be differentiated. Mutations in more than 10 different genes have, thus far, been associated with **congenital types of long QT syndrome**. The idiopathic (nonsyndromic) form of congenital LQTS is called **Romano-Ward syndrome**. More than 95% of the cases have loss-of-function mutations in genes that encode for different subunits of two **potassium channels (IKs and IKr)** that control the action potential of the cardiac conduction system in the Purkinje fibers. It is interesting to note that there is also a short QT syndrome that is caused by gain-of-function mutations in these genes, which can also lead to sudden cardiac death. In many cases a long QT syndrome is acquired through **medications** that inhibit transmembrane transport of potassium ions. Some of these patients have been found to have predisposing mutations in one of the genes that cause the inheritable long QT syndrome. As with other diseases, this disorder also involves a spectrum of genetic and nongenetic factors whose combinations determine the actual clinical picture.

The differential diagnosis of LQTS includes Timothy syndrome (LQTS with syndactyly), Jervell and Lange-Nielsen syndrome (LQTS and sensorineural hearing loss), and Andersen-Tawil syndrome (LQTS and periodic paralysis).

21.4   Blood Groups

Blood groups are heritable structural qualities of blood components that show genetic variability within a population and are identified by specific antibodies. The most important blood group antigens are glycosylated lipids or proteins on the surface of erythrocytes.

The ABO System

In 1901 Karl Landsteiner was the first to describe the ABO system; in 1930 he was awarded the Nobel Prize in medicine for his work. The blood groups of the ABO system represent the most important blood group features for blood transfusions. They are determined by the ABO gene on chromosome 9. As described in Section 4.2, blood groups A and B are **codominant** among themselves but **dominant** over blood group O. Accordingly, there are four major phenotypes: blood group A (genotype AA or AO), blood group B (genotype BB or BO), blood group O (genotype OO), and blood group AB (genotype AB).

A specific characteristic of the ABO system is that individuals without antigen A or B always form antibodies against the missing antigen. This is probably due to naturally occurring intestinal bacteria, which have similar surface antigens. Beginning from the ages of 3 to 6 months, all carriers of blood group A have antibodies for group B in their serum, all carriers of blood group B have antibodies for group A, and all carriers of blood group O have antibodies for groups A and B. Individuals with blood group AB have antibodies for neither A nor B in their serum.

The basic technique in identification of ABO blood groups is the agglutination test with test sera (anti-A and anti-B; ◨ Fig. 21.5). ◨ Table 21.5 lists the frequency of ABO blood groups in the United States.

The Rhesus System

The erythrocytic Rhesus system consists of a total of five antigens: C, D, E, c, and e. It is coded by two homologous neighboring genes on chromosome 1p36. The commonly used terms Rhesus positive (Rh+) and Rhesus negative (Rh−) refer to the D antigen only. Rhesus positive individuals have at least one functional copy of the *RHD* gene, while Rhesus negative individuals are homozygous for a deletion of this gene. C/c or E/e refers to different epitopes of the protein coded by the *RHCE* gene, with each case based on two different, codominant alleles. There also is a rare null mutation of the *RHCE* gene that causes chronic hemolytic anemia when homozygous in combination with a homozygous *RHD* deletion.

◨ **Figure 21.5. Determination of Blood Groups.**

Blood group	Test sera		
	Anti-A	Anti-B	Anti-A and Anti-B
A	●	○	●
B	○	●	●
AB	●	●	●
0	○	○	○

 ○ = No agglutination   ● = Agglutination

Table 21.5. Frequency of Blood Groups of the ABO System

Blood Group Types	Frequency in United States (%)
A	41
O	45
B	10
AB	4

The percentage of Rhesus negative individuals varies greatly between different ethnic groups. Approximately 16% of Europeans are Rhesus negative, while this is true for only 7% of African American and 1% of Native Americans. Rhesus negative individuals only form antibodies against Rhesus antigen when the immune system is exposed to it. This can happen in blood transfusions or in women during pregnancy with a Rhesus positive child, especially during invasive procedures (e.g., amniocentesis) and during delivery.

21.5 Anemias

Hereditary Spherocytosis

With a prevalence of 1 in 5,000, hereditary spherocytosis is the most frequent congenital hemolytic anemia in central Europe. In at least 75% of cases, the spherocytosis is inherited as autosomal dominant, and there is one affected parent. The remaining 25% are either inherited as autosomal dominant with incomplete penetrance, inherited as autosomal recessive, or caused by new mutations.

Hereditary spherocytosis is caused by genetic defects of structural proteins of the erythrocytic membrane, mostly **spectrin** or **ankyrin**. Typical presentation is anemia and/or jaundice in early infancy. Occasional crises with jaundice, fever, and upper abdominal pain occur during adulthood. There is an increased incidence of pigmented (bilirubin) gallstones. Recurring hemolytic crises may be treated with splenectomy, but only in children older than 5 years.

Sickle Cell Anemia

Case History

Darius is a 3-year-old boy who moved to the United States with his parents from the Republic of Benin in West Africa 1 year ago. Only 2 months after moving to Chicago, Darius was admitted to the hospital with nausea and vomiting. Following a febrile illness, his condition worsened and his mother noticed a large abdominal tumor at the time. In the emergency room, Darius was found to have a spleen palpable 8 cm below the costal margin, and spleen size was determined to be 20 × 15 × 8 cm on ultrasound, which is markedly enlarged. His complete blood count (CBC) was significant for anemia with a hemoglobin of 6.2 g/dL and a hematocrit of 18.8%. Sickle cells were seen on a peripheral blood smear, and the diagnosis of sickle cell anemia was subsequently confirmed by hemoglobin electrophoresis. Darius was treated for splenic sequestration crisis with red blood cell transfusions, and he recovered within 2 days. Targeted mutation analysis of the *HBB* gene found it homozygous for HbS. Darius has since been followed by a pediatric hematologist. He was started on hydroxyurea, penicillin V, and folic acid, and he has been doing fairly well with no additional hospitalizations for his sickle cell anemia (HbSS).

Epidemiology

Sickle cell anemia is the most frequent hemoglobinopathy and one of the most frequent autosomal recessive heritable diseases worldwide. In equatorial Africa, 20% to 40% of the population are heterozygous carriers. An estimated 15 million Africans are affected by sickle cell disease. Among African Americans in the United States, the prevalence of sickle cell trait (HbAS) is 8% to 10%, which leads to an incidence of sickle cell anemia (HbSS) of approximately 1 in 1,100.

III

Clinical Features

Heterozygous carriers are mostly asymptomatic, although rhabdomyolysis, renal failure, and even death can occur under extreme conditions of environmental or physical stress in persons with sickle cell trait. Sickle cell disease (HbSS) symptoms typically first manifest 3 to 6 months after birth, when HbF is increasingly substituted by HbS. The clinical features are related to chronic hemolytic anemia and painful vascular occlusive crises with organ infarcts (e.g., spleen, kidneys, brain, lungs, bones).

Dactylitis is frequently seen as the first manifesting feature in infants with sickle cell disease and is defined as a painful swelling of the hands and feet. **Splenic sequestration crisis** (typically seen between 6 months and 3 years of age) is characterized by acute enlargement of the spleen and a decrease in the hemoglobin concentration by 2 g/dL or more. Clinical symptoms include abdominal pain, nausea, and vomiting. Vaso-occlusive crises involving the lungs manifest as **acute chest syndrome** (ACS) with respiratory symptoms and hypoxemia, either with or without fever. New pulmonary infiltrates are seen on chest radiography. ACS can progress rapidly, within hours or days, to requiring intubation and mechanical ventilation. Lastly, **strokes** are among the most catastrophic manifestations of sickle cell disease.

Pathogenesis and Genetics

In adults, hemoglobin is a tetramer of two α-globin chains and two β-globin chains coded by different genes. Sickle cell hemoglobin HbS occurs through a point mutation in the sixth codon of the *HBB* gene coding for the β-chain. A base switch from GAG to GTG (at the nucleotide level, called mutation c.17A>T) results in an amino acid substitution from glutamic acid to valine (at the protein level, called mutation p.E6V). HbS is a tetramer of two normal α-chains and two abnormal β-chains. The serum hemoglobin of homozygous HbSS patients consists of 80% HbS and 20% HbF (αα/γγ). In the deoxygenated state, HbS clots and erythrocytes take on a sickle shape, lose their flexibility, are sequestered in the spleen and liver, and disintegrate. They obstruct capillaries and small arterioles, which leads to organ infarcts. Among the most affected organs is the spleen—by midchildhood basically all individuals with sickle cell disease are functionally asplenic ("autosplenectomy").

> **Important**
>
> Sickle cell anemia is caused by a specific amino acid substitution of Glu to Val at position 6 of hemoglobin's β-chain. In contrast to other mutations in the *HBB* gene, which result in functional loss and β-thalassemia, this mutation causes clotting during the deoxygenated state of the hemoglobin, resulting in the typical altered shape of the erythrocytes.

Sickle hemoglobin C disease (**HbSC**) is caused by coinheritance of HbS with another abnormal globin β-chain variant.

Diagnosis

Because of the high morbidity and mortality of sickle cell disease, all 50 US states offer newborn screening for this condition. The vast majority of newborn screening programs perform **isoelectric focusing** of an eluate of dried blood spots, demonstrating significant amounts of HbS. Other diagnostic tests for sickle cell disease include high-performance liquid chromatography, cellulose acetate electrophoresis, and targeted mutation analysis of the *HBB* gene.

Therapy

HbSS patients can only be cured by allogeneic bone marrow transplants or stem cell transplants. Ongoing education is important to decrease morbidity and mortality. Patients with sickle cell disease and sickle cell trait should maintain good hydration, try to avoid hypoxemia and extreme climates, and monitor themselves for signs and symptoms of acute decompensation requiring medical intervention. Because of autosplenectomy in persons with sickle cell disease, individuals should be immunized against pneumococci and *Haemophilus influenza*.

Hydroxyurea is used to decrease the number of pain crises and episodes of acute chest syndrome via vasodilatation and the induction of HbF synthesis, resulting in decreased sickling.

Prophylaxis with penicillin V prevents 80% of life-threatening episodes of *Streptococcus pneumoniae* sepsis during childhood. Use of **folic acid** should be considered to help increase red blood cell turnover.

Various complications of sickle cell disease might require specific treatments, including aggressive hydration and optimal analgesia for pain crises; oxygen, antibiotics, transfusion, or exchange transfusion for acute chest syndrome; and consideration of splenectomy in splenic sequestration crisis.

■■■ Sickle Cell Anemia and Malaria

Heterozygous carriers for sickle cell anemia manifest a certain resistance against *Malaria tropica* (by infection with *Plasmodium falciparum*). In areas where malaria is endemic, this presents a selection advantage, thus explaining the high allele frequencies of the sickle cell allele in equatorial Africa and other areas where malaria occurs.

Thalassemias

As the name implies (Greek, *thalassa* or *thalatta,* "sea"), **thalassemia** is especially prevalent in the Mediterranean as well as in other subtropical and tropical countries. Thalassemias are so frequent in these areas because their heterozygote state provides carriers with partial resistance to malaria (as with glucose-6-phosphate dehydrogenase [G6PD] deficiency or sickle cell anemia). This represents a selection advantage for heterozygotes in endemic regions. Increasing migration and mobility, however, have made thalassemias a worldwide phenomenon.

Thalassemias are **quantitative disturbances in hemoglobin synthesis** (in contrast to qualitative disturbances such as sickle cell anemia). These disturbances result from defects in the regulation of synthesis of hemoglobin's globin chains; in **α-thalassemia** this affects the α-chain of the globin, while in **β-thalassemia** the synthesis of the β-chain is diminished.

Case History

Chariklía, a newborn female of Greek ancestry, had a hemoglobin analysis done since both parents were diagnosed with heterozygous β-thalassemia. She was subsequently diagnosed with homozygous thalassemia major. Until school age, Chariklía remained asymptomatic; with Hb values of 8 to 9 g/dL, she did not need a transfusion, and her physical development was normal. At the age of 8 years, however, Chariklía was seen in the hematology clinic because she had been suffering from worsening anemia as well as hepatosplenomegaly and jaundice. The CBC was significant for hypochromic, microcytic anemia (hemoglobin [Hb] 6.9 g/dL, hematocrit [Hct] 22%, mean corpuscular volume [MCV] 61 fl, mean corpuscular hemoglobin [MCH] 19.4 pg). The blood smear revealed typical poikilocytosis and anisocytosis of the erythrocytes. Leukopenia (3,000/μL) and thrombocytopenia (105,000/μL) were indicators of hypersplenism. The hemoglobin analysis revealed clearly elevated concentrations of HbA2 ($\alpha\alpha/\delta\delta$ 5%) and HbF ($\alpha\alpha/\gamma\gamma$ 37%). An echocardiogram showed normal heart function and heart morphology. Radiography revealed typical bone changes caused by increased hematopoiesis in the skull and long bones. Chariklía has been scheduled for splenectomy. Molecular genetic tests revealed compound heterozygosity for two different mutations, one of which was associated with some residual function. It is interesting to note that Chariklía also had a heterozygous deletion of one of the two α-globin genes (three functioning gene copies, carrier status for α-thalassemia). The resulting reduced synthesis of excessive α-globin chains possibly contributed to the favorable phenotype of thalassemia intermedia (modified case history published by Kulozik et al. [1993] *Ann Hematol* 66:51–54.)

α-Thalassemia

α-Thalassemias are relatively rare in Western countries. They mostly occur in Southeast Asia, Southern China, and the Middle East.

In order to understand α-thalassemia, one has to realize that α-globin is coded **by two homologous genes** (*HBA1* and *HBA2*), meaning that there are a total of four gene copies of α-globin. Both genes are positioned one after the other on chromosome 16p13.3 and, thus, are normally inherited as a pair. The severity of the clinical phenotype depends on how many of these four gene copies are missing or altered through mutation:

- If only one gene copy is missing, this results in **thalassemia minima**, which is clinically asymptomatic.

II

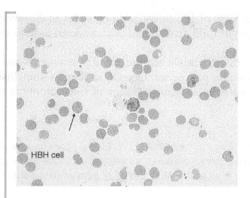

Figure 21.6. HbH Disease. HbH cells in a blood smear stained with brilliant cresyl blue. (Courtesy of A. Kulozik, Universitäts-Kinderklinik Heidelberg.)

HBH cell

— If two gene copies are missing (genotype either $-\alpha/-\alpha$ or $--/\alpha\alpha$, this results in **thalassemia minor**. Affected individuals are often clinically asymptomatic but have laboratory anomalies (mild microcytic anemia, mild poikilocytosis, and anisocytosis).

— Absence of three gene copies is called **HbH disease** ($--/-\alpha$). This leads to the formation of HbH ($\beta\beta/\beta\beta$) that precipitates and forms intraerythrocytic inclusion bodies (Fig. 21.6). Clinically these patients manifest variable degrees of hemolytic anemia, splenomegaly, and occasionally hepatomegaly.

— Functional loss of all four gene copies results in the most severe form of α-thalassemia, **Hb-Bart disease**. It causes hydrops fetalis (Fig. 21.7) and is not compatible with life. The few patients who are born alive usually die within a few days. This disorder is characterized by the formation of Hb-Bart, a hemoglobin that is exclusively made up of γ-globins ($\gamma\gamma/\gamma\gamma$). It has high oxygen affinity and causes severe hypoxia of the peripheral tissues.

β-Thalassemia

β-Thalassemias are far more frequent than α-thalassemias. In the **Mediterranean** they belong to the most frequent causes of microcytic anemia. Since there is only one gene and two gene copies for β-globulin, there are only two types of β-thalassemia: **thalassemia minor** (with heterozygosity, $-/\beta$) and **thalassemia major** (with homozygosity for a mutation of the β-globulin $-/-$).

Patients with β-thalassemia minor are clinically asymptomatic or have only mild symptoms. Sometimes there is slight splenomegaly in addition to mild anemia. Laboratory tests typically show mild microcytic anemia (Hb 10 to 11 g/dl, decreased MCV and MCH); HbA_2 ($\alpha\alpha/\delta\delta$) is always elevated. The blood smear may reveal anisocytosis, poikilocytosis, and target cells. The important differential diagnosis of iron-deficient anemia can be excluded easily since thalassemia minor usually has a normal or even elevated iron level in the serum. In contrast to spherocytosis, the osmotic resistance of the erythrocytes in thalassemia minor is increased (while decreased in spherocytosis). Thalassemia minor normally does not require therapy.

β-Thalassemia major is a serious disease. Affected children are asymptomatic at birth, since HbF ($\alpha\alpha/\gamma\gamma$) contains no β-globin. At the age of 3 to 6 months, the infant develops progressive

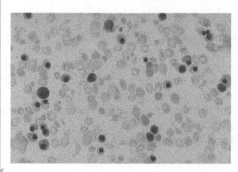

Figure 21.7. Hb-Bart Hydrops Fetalis. Peripheral blood picture. (Courtesy of A. Kulozik, Universitäts-Kinderklinik Heidelberg.)

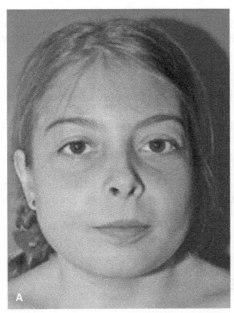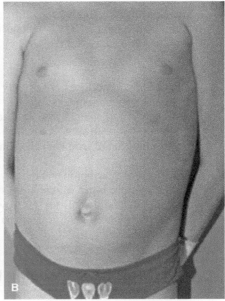

◻ **Figure 21.8. β-Thalassemia Intermedia in a 13-Year-Old Girl. A.** Typical thalassemic facies with enlargement of cheek bones and maxilla. **B.** Distinct abdominal swelling from hepatosplenomegaly. (Courtesy of A. Kulozik, Universitäts-Kinderklinik Heidelberg.)

hepatosplenomegaly and severe microcytic anemia with anisocytosis and poikilocytosis, poly-chromasia, and dacryocytosis (teardrop erythrocytes). The excessive α-chains tend to aggregate and form insoluble inclusion bodies in the erythrocytic precursor cells of the bone marrow.

Hepatosplenomegaly with thalassemia major is the result of extramedullary hemopoiesis. Intramedullary hemopoiesis is significantly increased as well, which results in bone changes. Among these are typical facial changes such as enlargement of facial bones (thalassemic facies; ◻ Fig. 21.8), pathological fractures, growth defects, and typical radiological symptoms (e.g., so-called "hair-on-end" appearance; ◻ Fig. 21.9). Excessive intestinal iron absorption can result in hemosiderosis with subsequent pathology in the heart, pancreas, liver, and other organs.

Etiology

α-Thalassemia is mostly caused by **deletions** in the region of the two α-globin genes that result from incorrect chromosomal pairing. Very large deletions contain both α-globin genes and are responsible for the severe forms of α-thalassemia. Point mutations as causes for α-thalassemia

◻ **Figure 21.9. β-Thalassemia Major.** "Hair-on-end" appearance of the skull. (Courtesy of A. Kulozik, Universitäts-Kinderklinik Heidelberg.)

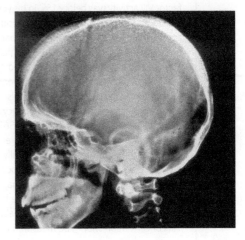

are relatively rare. **β-Thalassemia**, on the other hand, is rarely caused by larger deletions. More than 700 different *HBB* variants have been described, mostly caused by **point mutations** or small insertions/deletions.

Therapy

Thalassemia minor does not usually require therapy. **Symptomatic** treatment of thalassemia major has two components:

- Treatment of anemia with **packed red blood cells** (usually every 4 weeks with the goal of maintaining Hb above 10 g/dL)
- **Elimination of iron** with chelating agents such as deferoxamine (beginning at age 3 years)

With consistent symptomatic therapy the average life expectancy today is more than 40 years.

Allogeneic bone marrow or stem cell transplants represent a causal and curative approach to therapy. Bone marrow transplants from human leukocyte antigen (HLA)-identical donors have a greater than 90% success rate. Gene therapeutic approaches are being tested.

21.6   Heritable Bleeding Disorders

Hemophilias

Within the large group of blood coagulation disorders, the term *hemophilia* is applied to two X-chromosomal heritable diseases: **factor VIII deficiency** (**hemophilia A**) and **factor IX deficiency** (**hemophilia B**).

Important

Blood clotting factor VIII has two functional subunits:
- Factor VIII = antihemophilic globin, encoded by an X-chromosomal gene
- VWF = von Willebrand factor, carrier protein of factor VIII, encoded by an autosomal gene

A deficiency in factor VIII results in hemophilia A, while a deficiency in VWF results in von Willebrand disease.

Hemophilia A

Case History

Mrs. Landau is 26 years old and pregnant for the first time. Her deceased father had hemophilia A; she comes for genetic counseling to inform herself about the risks. Her father began having frequent bruises at 2½ years; factor VIII activity was below 1%. In his youth, recurring joint hemorrhages caused him painful restriction while flexing his right knee and limited extension of his left elbow joint. Later he acquired hepatitis C infection from contaminated clotting factors; the hepatitis turned chronic, resulting in cirrhosis of the liver, from which he died in the late 1980s at age 38. HIV infection without clinical proof of an acquired immunodeficiency at the time was an incidental background finding. Two brothers of her father also died at a young age (between 21 and 40 years) of hemophilic complications; one brother died of AIDS acquired through contaminated clotting factors. Mrs. Landau reports several episodes of hemorrhage after a tonsillectomy at age 22 years. There were no other symptoms indicating a tendency for abnormal bleeding. Her menstruation is normal. Several readings of factor VIII activity were at 38% to 56%. The genetic counselor informs Mrs. Landau that she must be a carrier for hemophilia A and that future sons have a 50% risk of being affected. The counselor emphasizes that since the introduction of genetically engineered (recombinant) factor VIII, the risk of infection with viral diseases is very low. Occasionally the occurrence of antibodies for factor VIII may complicate therapy. Factor VIII does not cross the placenta; no major bleeding complications are to be expected in pregnancy, even if the child should be hemophilic. Severe bleeding after birth is rare, yet delivery in a tertiary medical center is recommended. Forceps and vacuum deliveries are to be avoided. Immediately after the birth of a son, factor VIII concentration should be measured in cord blood.

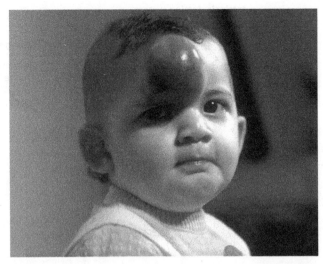

Figure 21.10. Hemophilia A. Forehead hematoma. (Courtesy of G. Tariverdian, Institut für Humangenetik Heidelberg.)

Epidemiology

Hemophilia A is the most frequent of the severe blood coagulation disorders. Prevalence among men is 1 in 10,000 for hemophilia A and 1 in 30,000 for hemophilia B.

Clinical Features

The severity of the disease varies considerably, from the most serious hemorrhages at birth (e.g., from the umbilical cord or after circumcision) to very mild forms (Fig. 21.10) that remain asymptomatic for several years. Severity correlates well with the basal activity of factor VIII or factor IX and can be predicted this way. See Table 21.6 for an overview.

Diagnosis

The typical finding of the initial coagulation studies is a **prolonged partial thromboplastin time (PTT**; a marker for the intrinsic clotting system) with **normal international normalized ratio (INR**; a marker for the extrinsic clotting system). In contrast to the more frequent VWD, the **bleeding time** is normal (Fig. 21.11).

A **detailed family history** (positive in two-thirds of cases) is of special diagnostic significance. Equally important is the exact history of hemorrhages. Spontaneous hemorrhages are frequent with hemophilia yet rare with VWD. **Determination of the activity levels of factors VIII and IX differentiates between hemophilia A and B.**

Table 21.6. Degrees of Severity of Hemophilia A and B

Classification	Activity of Factor VIII or Factor IX (%)	Clinical Symptoms
Severe hemophilia	<1	Spontaneous hemorrhage beginning in early childhood; obligatory presence of hemarthroses
Moderate hemophilia	1–5	Hemorrhages also with inadequate trauma; spontaneous hemorrhages rare
Mild hemophilia	6–35	Hematomas after severe trauma; secondary hemorrhages following surgery
Normal	>50	

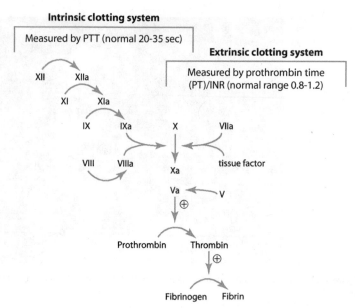

Figure 21.11. Intrinsic and Extrinsic Clotting System. Intrinsic Clotting System: measured by partial thromboplastin time (PTT; normal 20–35 sec). **Extrinsic Clotting System:** measured by thromboplastinogen time/ international normalized ratio (INR; normal 0.8–1.2).

Genetics

Hemophilia A. The *F8* gene for factor VIII is located close to the end of the long arm of the X chromosome (Xq28). Many different mutations have been described as causing hemophilia A. Especially frequent are larger **inversions** within the gene that are found in almost 50% of severe cases. Approximately 5% of patients have deletions in the *F8* gene that have also been associated with severe hemophilia.

Homozygous **hemophilia A in women** is extremely rare. If a girl or a woman proved to be hemophilic, Turner syndrome should be ruled out. Alternate explanations are skewed X inactivation, a translocation of the F8 gene, or antibodies against clotting factors (e.g., after pregnancy).

Hemophilia B. The *F9* gene for factor IX is located in the region Xq26-27.3. Point mutations are the most frequent cause for hemophilia B, followed by deletions. Inversions in the *F9* gene are rather rare.

Therapy

Therapy includes the **prophylaxis** of hemorrhages (e.g., no contact sports, wearing knee and elbow protection, no intramuscular injections), as well as careful local **hemostasis** (e.g., compression, sutures, fibrin patches) and **administration of clotting factors**. In cases of mild to moderate hemophilia, clotting factors are administered as needed. Severe hemophilia requires permanent treatment. High-quality recombinant or highly purified factor medications are available. Somatic gene therapy for hemophilia patients currently shows promise in clinical trials.

Von Willebrand Disease

Named after the Finnish physician Erik Adolf von Willebrand, **von Willebrand disease** is the most frequent congenital clotting disorder. It is caused by **quantitative or qualitative defects of VWF** that is coded by the large (52 exons) *VWF* gene on chromosome 12p13.3. Prevalence of the disorder is up to 1% of the population. This, however, also includes heterozygous mutation carriers who often only have very mild symptoms or no clinical symptoms at all. Prevalence of clinically relevant VWD is estimated at 1 in 10,000.

Clinical Features. Most patients have only discrete hemorrhaging or none at all. There are disturbances of primary and secondary hemostasis. VWD is usually suspected because of increased hemorrhaging during surgical procedures.

Pathogenesis/Genetics. VWF is a carrier molecule for factor VIII (and therefore part of the "factor VIII complex" and secondary hemostasis). In case of vascular damage it also mediates thrombocytic adhesion and thus is an important component of primary hemostasis (not affected by factor VIII deficiency). Of diagnostic significance is an increased bleeding time due to thrombocyte deficiency. In hemophilia, on the other hand, primary hemostasis and the bleeding time are normal.

> **Important**
>
> A deficit in VWF causes faulty thrombocytic adhesion as well as deficient coagulation. The clinical spectrum extends from asymptomatic disturbances to severe hemorrhaging.

21.7 Hereditary Thrombosis (Thrombophilia)

Hereditary causes for thrombophilia exist in up to 50% of all patients with deep venous thrombosis (DVT).

Indications for a possible genetic disposition are:
- First DVT before age 60 years
- Recurring DVTs
- Atypical localization of DVT
- Positive family history

Activated Protein C Resistance (Factor V Leiden)

About 30% of all patients with DVTs have a disturbed inactivation of factor Va through activated protein C (APC). This is called **APC resistance**. Prevalence of APC resistance is 5% of the general population. More than 90% of the cases are caused by a point mutation in the *FV* gene that codes for factor V. This is known by the name **factor V Leiden mutation** (named after the Dutch city) or R506Q (the correct nomenclature would be mutation p.R534Q at the protein level or c.1601G>A at the DNA level). The substitution of glutamine for arginine at this location removes the protein C cleavage site.

Heterozygosity for the factor V Leiden mutation increases the risk for thrombosis sevenfold as compared to the general population. Taking oral contraceptives results in a multiplication of the thrombosis risk (◻ Table 21.7).

Other Hereditary Causes for Thrombophilia

Prothrombin Mutation 2021G>A. This gain-of-function mutation in the 3' untranslated region of the *F2* gene for prothrombin results in an increased concentration of prothrombin. It is

◻ **Table 21.7.** Thrombosis Risk in Activated Protein C Resistance

Factor V Leiden Mutation	Oral Contraceptives	Thrombosis Risk
No	No	1-fold
No	Yes	4-fold
Heterozygous	No	7-fold
Heterozygous	Yes	30-fold
Homozygous	No	80-fold
Homozygous	Yes	>200-fold

heterozygous in 1% to 2% of Europeans and leads to a two- to sixfold increase in the incidence of DVTs. According to current knowledge, homozygosity for this mutation does not significantly increase that risk any further. Interestingly, the mutation affects the conserved transcription termination sequence in the *F2* gene, replacing a less efficient CG cleavage dinucleotide with a more efficient CA dinucleotide.

Protein C Deficiency. Protein C deficiency occurs if the level of activated protein C is less than 50% of normal. This results in a diminished inactivation of factor Va and factor VIIIa. A multitude of mutations of the *PROC* gene have been reported. Heterozygosity leads to an eightfold increase in thrombosis risk.

Antithrombin III Deficiency. This is also defined by an activity of less than 50% of normal. Type 1 has a quantitative reduction of the antithrombin III level in the blood, while type 2 has a normal level but the enzyme activity is diminished. Several studies have shown a 5- to 20-fold increase in thrombosis risk.

Protein S Deficiency. Mutations in the *PROS1* gene (if heterozygous) result in a fivefold increase in thrombosis risk.

If in one person several of the aforementioned defects occur simultaneously, the respective thrombosis risks are multiplied. Homozygosity for severe mutations of protein C, protein S, and antithrombin III results in severe clinical pictures, including prenatal onset of DVTs.

22 Respiratory System

LEARNING OBJECTIVES

1 In medieval times, infants with "salty" skin were considered "bewitched" because they usually died an early death. Which genetic disorder could be "diagnosed" by licking a child's forehead? Elaborate on how the genetic defect causes "salty" skin.

2 Explain how a patient's ethnicity might affect the predictive value of genetic testing. Use targeted mutation analysis in cystic fibrosis as an example, and calculate the likelihood of detecting two, one, or no mutation in an affected individual if the test has a mutation detection rate of 60%.

3 Evaluate the relationship of common disorders and rare genetic variants, using chronic obstructive pulmonary disorder (COPD) and α_1-antitrypsin deficiency as an example.

By far, the most significant genetic lung disease is cystic fibrosis. It is one of the most frequent autosomal recessive heritable disorders in the United States and Europe. Many other disorders of the respiratory system are multifactorial, with genetic factors playing a significant role. Genetic factors also have an influence on the susceptibility for respiratory infections.

22.1 Monogenic Lung Diseases

Cystic Fibrosis (CF, Mucoviscidosis)

Case History

Michael was diagnosed with cystic fibrosis when he was 3 months old. There were no complications throughout the pregnancy or at delivery, but Michael had postnatal failure to thrive. By the time he was 3 months old, he had developed severe anemia. During his hospitalization at 3 months, he had a positive sweat test, increased fecal fat, and decreased fecal elastase—all diagnostic for cystic fibrosis. Mutation analysis revealed homozygosity for the most frequent mutation, p.F508del. Michael is now being followed in the CF clinic at the local children's hospital. He receives enzyme capsules with his meals; in addition, he receives physical therapy for airway clearance, as well as nebulizer treatments for mucolysis on a regular basis. By now he is 14 months old. He has shown good growth and weight gain, and he has achieved his developmental milestones on time.

Epidemiology

Cystic fibrosis is the most frequent, life-limiting autosomal recessive disorder in the Caucasian population. The incidence is 1 in 2,000 to 1 in 3,500 among individuals of European descent. This corresponds to a heterozygote (carrier) frequency of 1:22 to 1:29.

■■■ **Why Is Cystic Fibrosis Occurrence so Frequent? A Hypothesis**

Cystic fibrosis is a serious disorder. Forty years ago, most patients died before 20 years of age. There was only a minimal chance that patients would have children of their own, and even the milder forms resulted in male infertility. Yet 3% to 5% of Caucasians are carriers for the disorder. How could such an unfavorable allele become so prevalent? As with other common recessive disorders, such as the hemoglobinopathies, it is assumed that heterozygous CF carriers may have had some kind of advantage in the past. The most widely accepted hypothesis is that carriers for *CFTR* mutations are better equipped to survive infectious intestinal diseases, such as cholera, than persons who, at the *CFTR* locus, are homozygous for the wild-type allele. Up until the 19th century, several cholera epidemics in Europe and North America caused hundreds of thousands of deaths, and even a small selective advantage may have had a substantial impact on the CF mutation allele frequency.

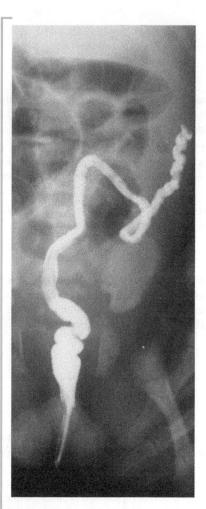

Figure 22.1. Meconium Ileus in a Newborn with Cystic Fibrosis. The obstruction usually occurs at the ileocecal junction before the ileocecal valve. Contrast agents show parts of the colon with a thin lumen (microcolon), while the ileum is massively distended and distally obstructed with viscous meconium. In most cases surgical intervention is necessary. (Courtesy of M. Mall, Universitäts-Kinderklinik Heidelberg.)

Clinical Features

Clinical symptoms for CF result from the obstruction of tubular structures by viscous secretions. In the classic type, these symptoms begin to occur in the first year of life. Of all newborns with CF, **20%** have **meconium ileus** (□ Fig. 22.1). The terminal ileum is blocked with thick, viscous meconium. Clinical symptoms in these children are progressive abdominal distension with deficient meconium clearance within the first 48 hours after birth. Meconium ileus is virtually pathognomonic for cystic fibrosis.

Respiratory symptoms are one of the most prominent features in patients with CF. It should be noted that the lungs are normal at birth but become damaged and diseased as a result of abnormal CFTR (i.e., the chloride channel, mutations of which cause CF) function. Respiratory problems—such as **chronic cough** and **recurrent pneumonia**—usually begin in the first few months of life. The cough is initially dry and later becomes productive with mucoid to purulent expectorant. The range of infectious agents that cause pneumonia in CF is different than in the general population. The most frequent pathogenic agent is *Staphylococcus aureus*. As the disease progresses and the chronic endobronchial damage worsens, infections with *Pseudomonas aeruginosa* occur more and more frequently. Other respiratory symptoms and complications include recurrent nasal polyps (in 10% to 15% of the cases), chronic sinusitis, chronic obstructive respiratory disease (COPD), bronchiectasis (□ Fig. 22.2), and pulmonary hypertension. Chronic hypoxia often leads to hypertrophic pulmonary osteoarthropathy with typical clubbing of the fingers (□ Fig. 22.3). Terminal respiratory insufficiency, often associated with secondary cardiac failure, is the most frequent cause of death in CF.

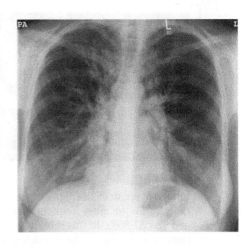

Figure 22.2. Chronic Pulmonary Disease with Cystic Fibrosis. The chest radiograph shows hyperinflation of the lungs, pronounced bronchiectasis, bronchial cuffing, and increased interstitial markings as a sign of chronic pulmonary inflammation. (Courtesy of J. Schenk, Pediatric Radiology, Universitäts-Klinikum Heidelberg.)

Complications from **exocrine pancreatic insufficiency** are the other major clinical component of classic CF. Beginning in their first months, affected children frequently show bulky, fatty, and malodorous stools; they develop significant **failure to thrive** (Fig. 22.4) and **hypoproteinemia**. Long-term symptoms can include a deficiency of the fat-soluble vitamins A, D, E, and K. The production of abnormal secretions results in an obstruction and dilatation of the pancreatic ducts. Since, initially, the production of pancreatic enzymes continues, the pancreas partially digests itself, resulting in **fibrosis** and the formation of cysts (hence the name "cystic fibrosis").

The **bile ducts** show a particularly high expression of CFTR. In the neonatal period, the involvement of the hepatobiliary system may be evident in prolonged hyperbilirubinemia. In the long term, the liver is affected by **focal** or **multilobular cirrhosis**, which occurs in more than three-fourths of all adult CF patients. This can lead to hypoproteinemia with edema. Hepatic failure is the second most frequent cause of death in CF patients.

Almost all men with CF are infertile with **azoospermia**, which results from congenital bilateral aplasia of the vas deferens **(CBAVD)**. Deficient secretions of the seminal vesicles result not only in chemical abnormalities but also in a diminished volume of the ejaculate. In mild forms of CF, CBAVD may be the only symptom or may be associated with chronic bronchitis/sinusitis. In these cases, there are usually hypomorphic mutations with residual function, including the so-called 5T intron variant on one copy of the *CFTR* gene (with a severe mutation on the other allele).

Genetics and Pathophysiology

CF is an **autosomal recessive** disorder that is caused by mutations in the *CFTR* gene on chromosome 7q31.2. The gene product, **cystic fibrosis transmembrane conductance regulator**, is an **adenosine triphosphate (ATP)-dependent chloride channel** located in the apical membrane of epithelial cells; it belongs to the so-called *ATP binding cassette* (ABC) transporter

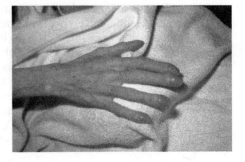

Figure 22.3. Digital Clubbing as a Clinical Sign of Chronic Hypoxia in Terminal Cystic Fibrosis. (Courtesy of M. Mall, Universitäts-Kinderklinik Heidelberg.)

III

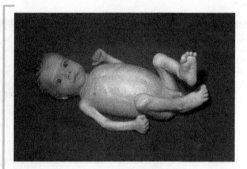

Figure 22.4. Infant with Cystic Fibrosis. Severe failure to thrive, as caused by exocrine pancreatic insufficiency and malabsorption, is one of the most frequent manifestations of cystic fibrosis during the first year of life. (Courtesy of M. Mall, Universitäts-Kinderklinik Heidelberg.)

family. More than 1,000 mutations in the *CFTR* gene have been reported, but most of them are rare. By far the most frequent mutation in Caucasians is **Delta-F508** (p.F508del, traditionally denoted ΔF508). In this mutation, the loss of the three nucleotides CTT in exon 10 causes the final gene product to have a deletion (Δ) of the amino acid phenylalanine (F) at position 508 in the nucleotide binding domain 1. The altered CFTR protein is processed intracellularly and disintegrates in the cell's proteasome complex, even before it reaches its destination in the apical cell membrane. The protein with p.F508del would have residual function if it were to reach the cell surface, and therefore, experimental therapy attempts to block the intracellular proteolysis of the mutated protein.

The majority (approximately 60%) of Caucasian patients with classic CF are **homozygous for the mutation p.F508del**. About 35% are compound heterozygous with involvement of the p.F508del mutation. Thus, it is rare that a Caucasian CF patient doesn't harbor at least one p.F508del mutation. The *5T intron* variant in the *CFTR* gene is also of clinical importance (see Section 3.5). **Compound heterozygosity** for p.F508del and the 5T/13TG variant typically results in a milder form of CF, such as CBAVD in men.

A core feature of CF pathogenesis is insufficient hydration of exocrine secretions caused by defective ion transport (CFTR participates in ion secretion as well as ion absorption). Viscous mucus in the small respiratory pathways disrupts mucociliary clearance; it also favors bacterial growth and results in recurring infections of the respiratory tract. The pancreas produces a secretion that is deficient in chloride, bicarbonate, and water, which not only blocks the pancreatic ducts but also significantly decreases the solubility of secretory proteins (enzymes). The abnormal composition of sweat is mainly caused by the disrupted reabsorption of sodium chloride. The fact that a CF patient's sweat is abnormally salty is of diagnostic significance (pilocarpine test); for hundreds of years this has been known as a symptom of CF.

"Woe to that child which, when kissed on the forehead, tastes salty. He is bewitched and soon must die." —Northern European folklore.

Diagnosis

The **sweat test** determines the salt concentration and is often used to diagnose CF. The parasympathomimetic agent pilocarpine, when applied to the skin, stimulates sweat production. Sweat with a chloride content of more than 60 mmol/L (in newborns, more than 90 mmol/L) is diagnostic for cystic fibrosis. An alternative test is the measurement of the **transepithelial nasal potential difference**. The level of **immunoreactive trypsin** (IRT) or the recently available **pancreatitis-associated protein** (PAP), as measured in a dried blood spot, can provide indications for cystic fibrosis. In some places, this is used for CF screening of newborns (sometimes in combination with DNA analysis).

Because the *CFTR* gene is so large and the types of mutations so vast, the initial genetic testing usually focuses on the most frequent mutations in the patient's population (**targeted mutation analysis/mutation panel**). A frequently used method has a mutation detection frequency of 88% in non-Hispanic Caucasians, which means that it will detect both mutations in 77% of CF patients (0.88^2), one mutation in approximately 21% ($0.88 \times 0.12 \times 2$) of patients,

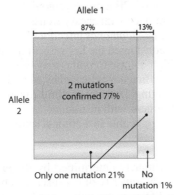

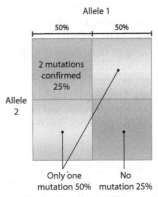

Figure 22.5. Sensitivity of the Standard Mutation Analysis for Cystic Fibrosis (CF). In non-Hispanic Caucasian patients, the standard method only recognizes 88% of CF alleles; this implies that, in approximately three-fourths of patients, both mutations are identified. If the mutation analysis only detected 50% of the mutated alleles in a given population, both mutations would only be confirmed in approximately one-fourth of the patients, while neither mutation would be found in another one-fourth of the patients.

and no mutation in approximately 1% (0.12^2) of patients of European descent. These numbers are considerably different with regard to other ethnicities (e.g., the mutation detection rate in African Americans is 69% and in Hispanics is 57%). Therefore, the ethnicity of the proband must be taken into account, especially when interpreting negative results (Fig. 22.5). The full sequencing of all exons, exon–intron boundaries, and promoter regions of *CFTR* has a sensitivity of greater than 98%, irrespective of the patient's ethnicity.

Figure 22.6. Young Adult with Cystic Fibrosis. While cystic fibrosis is the most common life-limiting autosomal recessive disorder in the Caucasian population, the life expectancy of affected individuals has increased dramatically over recent decades. Overall median survival is 36.5 years according to the Cystic Fibrosis Foundation report of 2006, and continues to improve. Early diagnosis, intensive surveillance, and prevention of primary and secondary complications allow for an active lifestyle, as seen in this young adult. (Photo courtesy of Rick Guidotti, www.positiveexposure.org.)

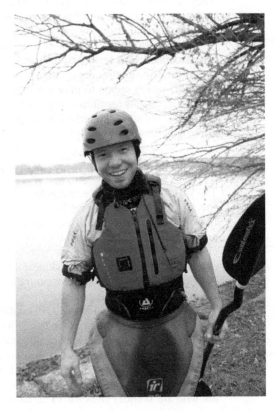

Therapy

The treatment of the pulmonary phenotype of CF aims at removing the viscous bronchial secretions (using mucolysis and postural drainage with chest percussions), as well as avoiding infections of the respiratory tract (especially *Pseudomonas* infections by inhalation of tobramycin). Lung or heart/lung transplantation is considered the last resort for patients with terminal disease. Nutritional therapy with special, high-calorie formulas may be used to increase weight gain and intestinal absorption. Pancreatic insufficiency is treated by administration of pancreatic enzymes. Ursodiol can help treat biliary sludging. Diabetes mellitus frequently develops during teenage or adult years and may require treatment with insulin.

Somatic gene therapy for CF is not yet applicable in a clinical setting.

Disease Progression and Prognosis

The natural course of cystic fibrosis is primarily determined by the extent of pulmonary involvement and by the nutritional status. The severity of the disease is highly dependent on the particular *CFTR* mutation. The average life expectancy has significantly improved over the past few decades, and currently the life expectancy is 37 years. With further improvements to treatments, CF patients born today are expected to have an average life expectancy of at least 40 to 50 years. (◻ Fig. 22.6)

22.2   Multifactorial Pulmonary Diseases

Asthma

Asthma is the most frequent chronic childhood disorder in the United States. Atopic disorders (e.g., bronchial asthma, allergic rhinitis, and atopic dermatitis) have a total incidence of 25%. They are etiologically related and characterized by an excessive production of immunoglobulin E (IgE; type I reaction). It has been known since the beginning of the 20th century that atopic disorders have a strong hereditary component. The heritability of asthma is approximately 50%, as determined by twin studies. Linkage analyses identified numerous genetic loci that are associated with bronchial asthma. In the majority of cases, these loci encompass **immunomodulatory genes**, among them those that code for CD14 (a component of the endotoxin receptor, which seems to play a role in the regulation of IgE), different **toll-like receptors** (whose mutations result in changes of the immune system's reaction to bacterial lipopolysaccharides), and several interleukins (especially IL-4 and IL-13) or their receptors (which in turn control the production of IgE).

Chronic Obstructive Pulmonary Disease

The WHO defines pulmonary emphysema as "a lung ailment that is characterized by a persistent blockage of airflow from the lung. It is an under-diagnosed, life-threatening lung disease that interferes with normal breathing and is not fully reversible." Among the risk factors for COPD are tobacco smoke (through tobacco use or passive smoking), air pollution, and recurring bronchopulmonary infections. Endogenous factors include antibody deficiencies (especially IgA deficiency), primary ciliary dyskinesia, and lack of protease inhibitors. The protease inhibitor α_1-antitrypsin has the highest concentration in plasma; it inhibits elastase, trypsin, chymotrypsin, thrombin, and bacterial proteases.

It is estimated that 1% of COPD patients actually have severe **α_1-antitrypsin deficiency**, which is caused by mutations in the *SERPINA1* gene on chromosome 14q32.1. More than 90 mutations are known; they were discovered by isoelectric focusing and given alphabetical names. Of special clinical significance is the deficiency allele **PI*Z** ("**Z allele**," allele frequency 0.5% to 2%) with an amino acid substitution E342K (glutamate to lysine). This results in abnormal folding of the gene product, causing defective hepatic secretion of α_1-antitrypsin. Individuals who are homozygous for PI*Z have a low plasma α_1-antitrypsin concentration (usually

12% to 24% of normal). As a result of protein aggregation and polymerization of the Z-type α_1-antitrypsin in the hepatocytes, affected individuals may develop liver disease. Prolonged hyperbilirubinemia and mild elevation of transaminases may be presenting features during the neonatal period. However, chronic liver disease with cirrhosis and fibrosis does not usually develop until adulthood (15% to 20% of patients with PI*ZZ genotype have hepatic cirrhosis at age 50). In adulthood, the progressive breakdown of the alveolar septae results in COPD with emphysema in the majority of cases.

> **Important**
>
> Severe α_1-antitrypsin deficiency can be detected by the absence of the α_1-globin fraction in serum electrophoresis.

23 Gastrointestinal and Digestive System

LEARNING OBJECTIVES

1 Describe how to differentiate between omphalocele and gastroschisis, and explain which of the two warrants a genetic evaluation.

2 Explain the phenomenon known as "Carter effect" using Hirschsprung disease as an example.

3 Name five clinical symptoms that could be presenting symptoms in a patient with hemochromatosis.

4 Develop a diagnostic algorithm for hyperbilirubinemia, and name at least three genetic disorders that should be considered in the differential diagnosis.

23.1 Malformations of the Gastrointestinal Tract

Malformations of the gastrointestinal tract include atresias, malrotation, abdominal wall defects, diaphragmatic defects, and anorectal malformations.

The gastrointestinal tract develops from a simple ectodermal tube between the 5th and 12th weeks (postmenstruation [p.m.]) of embryonic development. It extends from the buccopharyngeal membrane to the cloacal membrane and is divided into foregut, midgut, and hindgut. The **foregut** includes the esophagus, trachea, and respiratory diverticulum; the stomach; and the proximal duodenum with the liver, spleen, and pancreas. The **midgut** develops from the umbilical loop. As a physiological umbilical hernia beginning in the 6th week, the midgut is situated outside the body cavity inside the umbilical cord, where it rotates 90 degrees in a counterclockwise direction. Upon return into the abdominal cavity during the 10th week of development, the midgut rotates another 180 degrees in the counterclockwise direction. From the **hindgut** develops the distal third of the transverse colon, descending colon, sigmoid colon, and rectum. The embryological division into foregut, midgut, and hindgut is reflected in the arterial supply of the respective segments (by celiac artery, superior mesenteric artery, and inferior mesenteric artery).

Atresia

Esophageal Atresia. Esophageal atresia occurs in 1 in 3,000 to 1 in 4,000 live births. Type C esophageal atresia (classification by R. E. Gross), with distal tracheoesophageal fistula, is the most common type (85% of cases). Half of the children with esophageal atresia have additional malformations. An important differential diagnosis is **VACTERL** association (Section 13.3), which is characterized by malformations of the spine, heart, extremities, kidneys, and/or anorectal region.

Duodenal Atresia. Affected children present in the first days of life with bilious vomiting, scaphoid abdomen with epigastric fullness, hyperbilirubinemia, dehydration, and electrolyte imbalances. An important diagnostic clue is the "double-bubble sign" on anteroposterior (AP) abdominal radiographs. Between 20% and 30% of all children with duodenal atresia have **trisomy 21**.

Anal Atresia. Anorectal atresias result from an embryonic developmental disturbance of the urorectal septum. They occur in 1 in 5,000 live births. Up to two-thirds of the patients have additional malformations of other organs. Again, VACTERL association should be considered in the differential diagnosis (Section 13.3).

Abdominal Wall Defects

Gastroschisis. Typically, this is a right-sided paraumbilical abdominal wall defect. A hernial sac does not exist. The umbilical cord inserts normally and is not part of the defect. Because

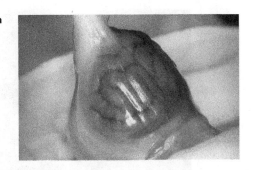

Figure 23.1. Omphalocele in a Newborn with Beckwith-Wiedemann Syndrome.

of the missing hernial sac, the protruding intestinal parts have contact with the amniotic fluid, which can cause edema and adhesion formation. Only 5% to 20% of patients have additional malformations. In most cases, gastroschisis does not seem to result from a genetic cause. Chromosomal aberrations are identified in only a very small proportion of cases (less than 2%).

Omphalocele. An omphalocele results when the intestinal loops fail to re-enter the abdominal cavity by the 12th week of gestation. Omphaloceles are covered by a hernial sac, which is the umbilical cord membrane (◼ Fig. 23.1). Up to 75% of the children have associated malformations. An important differential diagnosis is Beckwith-Wiedemann syndrome (Section 35.2). ◼ Table 23.1 shows the difference between omphalocele and gastroschisis.

Diaphragmatic Hernia

The prevalence of congenital diaphragmatic hernia is between 1 in 2,000 and 1 in 10,000 births. Most frequently, these are dorsolateral diaphragmatic defects (Bochdalek hernia). Additional malformations occur in 15% to 40% of the patients. Diaphragmatic hernias can be seen within the context of chromosome disorders, mainly in trisomy 21, 13, or 18. The prognosis is largely determined by secondary pulmonary hypoplasia and pulmonary hypertension.

Hirschsprung Disease

The phenomenon of "sluggish stools in newborns as a result of dilatation and hypertrophy of the colon" was first described in 1886 by the Danish pediatrician Harald Hirschsprung. The disorder is caused by the absence of intramural ganglion cells in the intestine, resulting in functional obstruction. In a large majority of cases, the **aganglionosis** is limited to the **rectum and sigmoid colon**. In only 8% of cases is the entire colon affected; the involvement of the entire intestine is even more rare.

Case History

Sarah was the firstborn child to her parents. The pregnancy was uncomplicated, and she was born vaginally at full term. Apgar scores were 8 and 9 at 1 and 5 minutes, respectively. While Sarah had normal muscular tone and was feeding well, she didn't pass meconium until 36 hours of life. She was discharged home with her mother 2 days after her birth, but returned to the emergency room after 2 weeks for chronic constipation and abdominal distension. Abdominal radiographs showed massive dilatation of the transverse and descending colon. A subsequent barium enema study demonstrated delayed emptying time and a funnel-like transition zone between proximal dilated and distal constricted bowel. A final confirmation of Hirschsprung disease was made histologically on examination of a suction biopsy specimen of rectal mucosa, which demonstrated

◼ Table 23.1. Comparing Omphalocele and Gastroschisis

	Omphalocele	Gastroschisis
Hernial sac present	Yes	No
Other malformations	Frequent	Rare

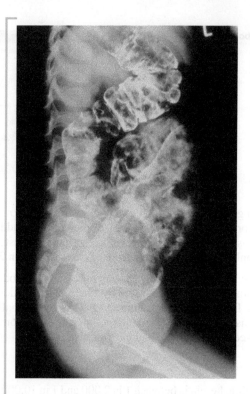

Figure 23.2. Hirschsprung Disease. Stenosis and massive proximal dilatation of the colon in a lateral abdominal radiograph. (Courtesy of Hj Müller, Department of Medical Genetics, University Children's Hospital Basel, Switzerland.)

the absence of enteric ganglion cells. The aganglionic segment was surgically resected and anastomosis of proximal bowel to the anus was achieved by a "pull-through" procedure. DNA array analysis and sequencing of the *RET* protooncogene were negative. The parents were counseled about the empiric recurrence risk for future children given the diagnosis of short-segment Hirschsprung disease in Sarah (i.e., 5% for males and 3% for females).

Epidemiology

With an incidence of **1 in 5,000**, Hirschsprung disease is the most frequent cause of intestinal obstruction in newborns. Boys are affected four times as often as girls.

Clinical Course

A first indication of Hirschsprung disease is the failure to pass meconium within the first 48 hours postnatally. Constipation, abdominal distension, emesis, and occasional intermittent explosive diarrhea typically manifest within days or weeks, but the diagnosis of Hirschsprung disease should also be considered in any child or adult with chronic constipation. The most important complication, even today, is a **toxic megacolon** where the intestinal bacteria penetrate the mucosal wall and can cause severe sepsis. The massive dilatation of the prestenotic intestinal sections (■ Fig. 23.2) can also result in bowel perforation. These life-threatening complications make it imperative that newborns suspected of having Hirschsprung disease rapidly undergo comprehensive diagnostic workup.

Approximately 70% of patients with Hirschsprung disease have no abnormalities in other organs. About 18% have additional malformations, among which genitourinary (6% to 7%), cardiac (2% to 5%), gastrointestinal (3% to 4%), and central nervous system (CNS) defects (3% to 4%) are most common.

Genetics and Pathophysiology

There are four times more boys than girls with Hirschsprung disease (male:female ratio **4:1**). The overall recurrence risk for siblings is about 4%, a 200-fold increase compared to the general population; it is higher for boys than for girls. It is interesting to note that the recurrence risk for subsequent siblings is higher if the index patient is a girl. For example, the recurrence risk for siblings of a girl with long-segment Hirschsprung disease is 33% in brothers and 9% in sisters. This so-called **Carter effect** (Section 5.6) characterizes a sex-specific threshold value and is typical for multifactorial inheritance.

The likelihood of a **familial type of Hirschsprung disease** is also higher if a long segment of the colon is affected. We now know several genes that are associated with Hirschsprung disease. In all cases the gene products take part in the migration and maturation of intestinal neural precursors. Most important in this group is the **receptor tyrosine kinase RET**. Mutations in the *RET* protooncogene account for 15% to 20% of sporadic cases of Hirschsprung disease, but the mutation makes up about 50% of familial cases. The inheritance pattern is autosomal dominant, with incomplete penetrance (50% to 70%). Other types of familial Hirschsprung disease are caused by mutations (e.g., in the genes for endothelin 3 or endothelin-B receptor) and can be inherited in autosomal dominant or autosomal recessive fashion. Nearly 12% of all patients with Hirschsprung disease have a chromosome disorder, most commonly trisomy 21.

> **Important**
>
> Mutations in the *RET* protooncogene cause two completely different types of disorders. Loss-of-function mutations cause the familial form of Hirschsprung disease, while certain activating mutations (gain of function) cause multiple endocrine neoplasia (MEN) type 2 (Section 32.5).

Diagnosis

A physical examination of children with Hirschsprung disease can be significant for a distended abdomen and an empty rectal ampulla. Diagnostic tests for Hirschsprung disease should include:

- **Barium enema:** Radiographs are taken immediately after hand-injection and again 24 hours later. A narrowed distal colon with proximal dilatation is the classic finding (Fig. 23.2). The retention of contrast for longer than 24 hours is also suggestive of Hirschsprung disease.
- **Suction biopsy of the rectal mucosa:** The absence of enteric ganglion cells on histopathological sections confirms the disease ("gold standard"). The biopsy should be obtained at least 1.5 cm above the dentate line on the dorsal side of the rectum.

Therapy and Management

The treatment of Hirschsprung disease is surgical, and it involves resection of the aganglionic segment and anastomosis of the proximal bowel to the anus ("pull-through"). Resection should involve a small segment of bowel proximal to the aganglionic zone, as the transitional zone might have altered motility.

Because of the frequency of associated malformations, all patients with Hirschsprung disease should undergo echocardiography and renal ultrasonography to evaluate for structural defects of the heart and kidneys.

23.2 Hepatic Dysfunction

Hemochromatosis

Hemochromatosis is an iron storage disorder, with **iron overload in the body** ("siderosis") resulting from excessive iron absorption.

The normal iron content of the body is approximately 3.5 g in men (about as much as in an iron nail) and approximately 2.2 g in women (due to the periodic blood loss of menstruation). A fivefold increase over normal iron content results in organ dysfunction. To be differentiated are **primary and secondary sideroses**. Classic hereditary hemochromatosis is the primary type. Among secondary sideroses are anemias in which excessive iron storage results from repeated blood transfusions (e.g., thalassemias and myelodysplastic syndromes) and sideroses associated with chronic liver diseases (including alcohol damage).

Case History

Mr. Moore, who is 42 years old, has suffered from undiagnosed chronic joint pain for the past 2 years. A few months prior to his evaluation in the genetics clinic, he started feeling tired. He was subsequently found to have elevated serum iron and plasma ferritin concentrations, which is suggestive of hemochromatosis. His family history is positive for a sister with hepatic cirrhosis, which is attributed to long-term alcohol abuse. The other siblings and the parents are healthy. Mutation analysis reveals homozygosity for the most frequent, disease-causing mutation in the *HFE* gene: p.C282Y. The geneticist tells Mr. Moore that arthropathy is a frequent complication of hemochromatosis. He suggests routine phlebotomy, even though the effect on arthropathy may be limited. Mr. Moore is referred to the hemochromatosis clinic of the department of gastroenterology. Since his siblings have a 25% chance of being affected, they are referred for genetic counseling.

Epidemiology

HFE hemochromatosis is, genetically, the most frequent autosomal recessive disorder among Caucasians, with a prevalence of risk genotypes (homozygosity or compound heterozygosity) of up to **1 in 200** and a carrier frequency of about 1 in 10 in various populations. Penetrance, however, is low, with published data in the range of 1% to 30%. Men are 10 times more likely than females to become symptomatic (male:female ratio 10:1). The onset of symptoms is usually after age 40 years.

Clinical Symptoms

In the 19th century, hemochromatosis was described as a triad of **hepatomegaly, diabetes, and bronze pigmentation of the skin**. These continue to be the most frequent symptoms. The following percentages apply to symptomatic patients, not to all homozygous carriers:
- Hepatic enlargement (90%), cirrhosis of the liver (75%)
- Diabetes mellitus (70%), also called "bronze diabetes" because of the skin pigmentation
- Dark skin pigmentation (75%), grayish to brown, especially in sun-exposed areas of the skin, due to an increase in melanocytes in the skin and an increasing thinning of the epidermis
- Painful arthropathy (30% to 50%), especially in metacarpophalangeal joints I through III and proximal interphalangeal joints. Joints of the hands and knees are involved later in the course of the disease
- Secondary cardiomyopathy (15% to 20%), due to iron deposits, and associated with congenital heart failure, and frequently with atrial fibrillation
- Additional symptoms including fatigue, abdominal pain, loss of libido in men, and amenorrhea in women

> **Important**
>
> **Symptoms of Hemochromatosis**
> Older patients often present with fatigue, abdominal pain, and arthritis, while younger patients more frequently complain of cardiac problems or possibly amenorrhea.

Genetics and Pathophysiology

The clinical picture of hemochromatosis can result from mutations in various genes. Mutations in four different genes (*HFE*, *TR2*, *hemojuvelin*, and *hepcidin*) have been described. Mutations in *ferroportin* result in a pathologically distinct disorder. The majority of patients with hemochromatosis have mutations in the *HFE* gene, the "classic type" of hemochromatosis. Thus, one speaks of **HFE hemochromatosis** and **non-HFE hemochromatosis**.

HFE hemochromatosis is caused by mutations of the ***HFE* gene** on chromosome 6p21.3. *HFE* codes for an atypical major histocompatibility class I (MHC I) protein that dimerizes on the cell surface with β_2-microglobulin, regulating iron absorption through transferrin. Among Caucasians, there are two frequent *HFE* mutations, p.C282Y and p.H63D. More than 90% of patients are **homozygous for mutation p.C282Y** (c.845A>G at the DNA level). Regardless of the body's actual need for iron, this results in a threefold increase of iron absorption in the epithelial cells of the duodenal mucosa. Five percent of patients are compound heterozygous for p.C282Y and p.H63D. Homozygosity for p.H63D does not result in clinically manifest hemochromatosis.

▪▪▪ Non-HFE Hemochromatosis

Some hemochromatosis patients with **juvenile hemochromatosis**, a severe type that occurs at a young age, are homozygous for mutations in the *HAMP* gene that codes for the protein **hepcidin**. Hepcidin is a central regulator of intestinal iron absorption and also inhibits the release of iron from macrophages. Some heterozygous mutation carriers develop clinical symptoms dependent on additional *HFE* mutations.

Other patients with autosomal recessive heritable juvenile hemochromatosis have mutations in the *HFE2* gene on chromosome 1q21.1. This gene codes for **hemojuvelin**, a modulator of the expression of hepcidin. This results in severe iron overload, with organ damage before age 30 years. Both sexes are equally affected. Iron overload occurs especially in the pituitary gland, the cortex of the adrenal glands, the thyroid gland, the parathyroid glands, and the gonads. Patients frequently die from heart failure. The therapy of choice for juvenile hemochromatosis also is periodic phlebotomy.

Some patients with hemochromatosis have nonsense or missense mutations in the *TFR2* gene that codes for the **transferrin receptor 2**. In contrast to transferrin receptor 1, which mediates cellular iron absorption via endocytosis, TFR2 regulates iron homeostasis through the hepcidin pathway. The exact pathophysiological mechanisms are not fully understood.

Mutations in the **ferroportin**-coding *SLC40A1* gene result in an **autosomal dominant** iron overload disorder. Affected individuals have relatively normal serum iron levels, but they show the accumulation of iron in macrophages. Ferroportin is necessary for intestinal iron absorption, as well as for the export of iron from macrophages and hepatocytes. Reduced ferroportin function, therefore, does not result in a primary increase of intestinal iron absorption (as seen in other types of HFE and non-HFE hemochromatosis). Complete absence of the protein results in embryonic lethality.

Iron Metabolism

▫ Figure 23.3 is a simplified version of our current understanding of iron metabolism in eukaryotic cells. While iron can enter a cell in a variety of ways (upper part of the illustration), there is only one known way for iron to exit the cell (i.e., via the protein **ferroportin**, whose

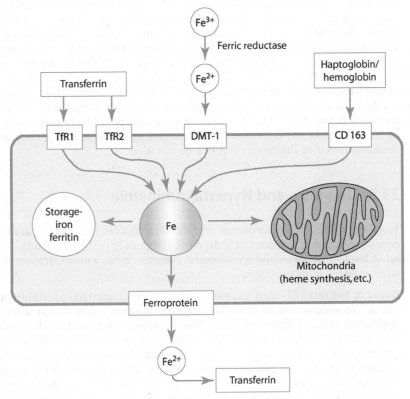

▫ **Figure 23.3. Iron Metabolism of the Cell**. (Simplified after Hentze et al. 2004.)

mutations result in an autosomal dominant iron overload syndrome). TfR stands for "transferrin receptor." DMT 1 signifies "divalent metal transporter type 1," which plays an important role in the reabsorption of iron from the intestine (after the trivalent iron of food is reduced by ferrireductase to Fe^{2+}). Monocytes and macrophages are capable of absorbing haptoglobin-bound iron via the CD163 receptor. Within the cell, a large part of the absorbed iron reaches the mitochondria, where heme biosynthesis takes place. Ferritin serves as an intracellular storage protein for Fe^{3+}; it can bind up to 4,500 mol Fe^{3+} per mol ferritin.

- **HFE:** HFE forms a complex with the transferrin receptor 1. *In vitro*, it inhibits the binding of transferrin to TfR, thus preventing the transferrin-mediated iron absorption of the cell.
- **Hepcidin:** Hepcidin is a peptide hormone that is synthesized by the liver. It is considered an inhibitor of intestinal iron reabsorption. It also regulates iron transport from macrophages and other cells. Recent studies show that hepcidin binds to ferroportin, permitting it to enter the cell and thereby inhibiting iron export from the cell.
- **Hemojuvelin:** It has been suggested that hemojuvelin interacts with bone morphogenetic protein (BMP), possibly as a coreceptor, and may signal via the SMAD pathway to regulate hepcidin expression. Individuals with mutations in the *HFE2* gene have lower hepcidin levels.

Diagnosis

- **Laboratory:** Plasma ferritin greater than 500 μg/L, transferrin saturation greater than 60%
- **Molecular genetic confirmation** of *HFE* mutation p.C282Y, or others
- **Liver biopsy**, with histology, to confirm hepatic iron overload, especially in individuals with presumed hemochromatosis who lack the common *HFE* mutations

Therapy and Prognosis

The therapy of choice is phlebotomy, especially in the presence of clinical endpoints. Phlebotomy is initiated twice weekly, until the serum ferritin concentration is 50 μg/L or lower. Then, weekly phlebotomies are continued until the hematocrit is 75% of the baseline hematocrit. At that time, the phlebotomies are performed less frequently. Serum ferritin concentrations are the most reliable way to monitor therapeutic phlebotomies. A **diet of low iron content** is advised, beginning with the choice of cooking utensils (e.g., a classic wok results in considerable iron concentration of the food). Drinking black tea with meals can reduce iron absorption.

The life expectancy of patients with classical HFE hemochromatosis is not affected if therapy is begun early. The risk of liver cirrhosis and, possibly, hepatocellular carcinoma (27% of untreated patients) mandates periodic screening examinations, including sonography and determination of α-fetoprotein (AFP) concentration.

23.3   Jaundice and Hyperbilirubinemia

Jaundice is a yellowish discoloration of the skin, mucous membranes, and sclerae, due to the deposit of bilirubin in tissues. It is the clinical sign of hyperbilirubinemia. While the total bilirubin level in serum should not exceed 1.1 mg/dL, it has a concentration of at least 2 mg/dL when scleral icterus is evident.

Direct or Indirect? The first question to answer with regard to hyperbilirubinemia is whether "direct" (conjugated, hydrophilic) bilirubin or "indirect" (unconjugated, lipophilic) bilirubin is elevated. While indirect hyperbilirubinemia reflects increased bilirubin release (e.g., due to hemolysis) or deficient conjugation with glucuronic acid in the liver, direct hyperbilirubinemia typically occurs in cases of liver cell damage (e.g., hepatitis) or cholestasis (arrest in the flow of bile). **Physiological neonatal jaundice** is an indirect hyperbilirubinemia. It is caused by increased hemoglobin breakdown after birth, in conjunction with the relatively low activity of immature hepatic glucuronosyl transferase. Excessive unconjugated (indirect) bilirubin cannot be glucuronidated sufficiently into excretable conjugated (direct) bilirubin.

Genetic or Not Genetic? There are multiple causes for hyperbilirubinemia and jaundice, most of them nongenetic (e.g., hepatitis, liver cirrhosis, cholangitis, and choledocholithiasis). Familial hyperbilirubinemia syndromes, however, should be considered as part of the differential diagnosis. Inherited, indirect hyperbilirubinemia is usually caused by a deficiency of the enzyme uridine diphosphate (UDP)-glucuronosyltransferase (asymptomatic Gilbert syndrome or symptomatic Crigler-Najjar syndrome). Genetic disorders associated with direct hyperbilirubinemia are Dubin-Johnson syndrome, Rotor syndrome, and Alagille syndrome.

Genetic Disorders of Bilirubin Glucuronidation

Based on the clinical consequences, two "syndromes" linked to a deficiency of the enzyme UDP-glucuronosyltransferase are distinguished. Both are caused by mutations/polymorphisms in the *UGT1A1* gene inherited in an autosomal recessive manner. **Gilbert syndrome**, also called **Meulengracht disease** or icterus intermittens juvenilis, is a benign metabolic variant caused by the reduction of UDP-glucuronosyltransferase activity to 25% to 40% of normal. It is found in up to 10% of Caucasians. Affected individuals are homozygous (or compound heterozygous) for common hypomorphic variants such as a dinucleotide (TA) repeat polymorphism in the promoter region of the *UGT1A1* gene. The diagnosis is often made in young adults based on the incidental observation of mild, largely indirect hyperbilirubinemia. Total bilirubin level is usually less than 6 mg/dL. Hyperbilirubinemia may occur intermittently in association with infection, stress, fasting, or menstrual cycles. Gilbert syndrome is observed more frequently in men than in women. Therapy is not necessary.

 Crigler-Najjar syndrome is the more severe form of UDP-glucuronosyltransferase deficiency and is caused by different loss-of-function mutations in the *UGT1A1* gene. Severity is variable, depending on the level of residual activity. The most severe type (type 1) is lethal, due to kernicterus after birth, unless rigorously treated with phototherapy and/or liver transplantation.

 Dubin-Johnson syndrome and **Rotor syndrome** are benign hyperbilirubinemia syndromes typically associated with direct hyperbilirubinemia, where the excretion of bilirubin glucuronides into the bile ducts is deficient. Affected individuals may present with jaundice but are otherwise asymptomatic.

Alagille Syndrome

Alagille syndrome is a multisystem disorder. Major clinical features include cholestasis, cardiac defects (peripheral pulmonic stenosis is typical), vertebral anomalies (e.g., butterfly vertebrae), ophthalmic findings (e.g., posterior embryotoxon), and characteristic facial features. As a result of bile duct paucity, Alagille syndrome manifests with direct hyperbilirubinemia. It is an autosomal dominant disorder most frequently caused by mutations in the *JAG1* gene (89%). A few cases (7%) result from a microdeletion in the short arm of chromosome 20, involving the *JAG1* gene. Less frequently, Alagille syndrome is caused by mutations in *NOTCH2*.

24 Metabolic Disorders

LEARNING OBJECTIVES

1 Describe the biochemical and functional differences between aminoacidopathies and organic acidurias.

2 Describe the three typical presentation patterns of fatty acid oxidation disorders.

3 Outline the treatment of phenylketonuria (PKU).

4 Name the single most important laboratory test for the diagnosis of urea cycle disorders.

5 Name two sphingolipidoses and their typical clinical features.

The term **inborn errors of metabolism** was coined in 1909 by Archibald Garrod. Congenital metabolic disorders affect approximately 1 in 500 newborns. Most follow an autosomal recessive inheritance pattern. Many cases represent a special challenge for the treating physician because of their severe, yet often nonspecific, symptoms. Because of the large number of individual enzyme deficiencies, metabolic disorders are frequently regarded as complicated. However, a pathway-based approach can help to engender a better understanding of metabolic disorders in terms of the major clinical and biochemical features.

24.1 Disorders of Intermediary Metabolism

Many classic metabolic diseases are enzyme defects in intermediary metabolism that affect the catabolism of "small molecules" of the three basic nutritional groups (i.e., carbohydrates, proteins, and fatty acids) or affect mitochondrial energy metabolism. The most important components of these metabolic pathways are summarized in ◘ Figure 24.1. The disease pictures resulting from these disorders are often dynamic; they fluctuate with the patient's metabolic status and therefore are often treatable. Most defects of intermediary metabolism can quickly be diagnosed through a few widely available metabolic assays. These include blood sugar analysis, acid-base status, urinary dipstick tests, and measurement of blood concentrations of lactate and ammonia, as well as more specialized selective screening tests such as plasma amino acids, urine organic acids, and plasma acylcarnitine profile (Chapter 16). Disorders of intermediary metabolism do not usually cause symptoms before birth, because metabolic changes can be corrected by the maternal–fetal circulation exchange.

> **Important**
>
> Disorders of intermediary metabolism are often treatable.

24.1.1 Disorders of Carbohydrate Metabolism

Patients with disorders of carbohydrate metabolism manifest a relatively broad spectrum of symptoms. Depending on the enzyme defect, clinical symptoms result from metabolite toxicity, energy deficiency, hypoglycemia, or glycogen storage. The most important diagnostic parameters, besides liver size and function, are the determination of blood sugar and lactate and occasionally galactose and its metabolites.

Disorders of Galactose or Fructose Metabolism

Patients with disorders of galactose or fructose metabolism develop clinical symptoms only after the ingestion of food containing lactose (glucose-galactose disaccharide, found in

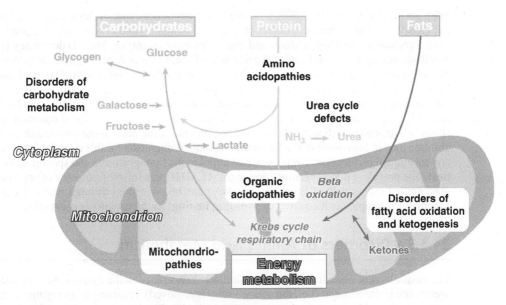

Figure 24.1. **Disorders of Intermediary Metabolism.**

milk and milk products) or fructose, (including saccharose table sugar is a glucose-fructose disaccharide). Galactose-1-phosphate and fructose-1-phosphate accumulate in classic galactosemia or hereditary fructose intolerance, respectively; they are toxic to the liver, kidneys, and brain. Clinical symptoms, diagnostics, and therapy of classic galactosemia are discussed in Section 16.4.

Glycogen Storage Diseases

The various glycogen storage diseases (GSDs) result from the diminished activity of the enzymes and transport proteins involved in glycogen and glucose metabolism. Clinical manifestations include pathological glycogen storage and associated organ dysfunction (e.g., hepatopathy, cardiomyopathy, and myopathy), as well as hypoglycemia (usually 4 to 8 hours after meals). The cumulative incidence is approximately 1 in 20,000. The most prevalent of these disorders are **von Gierke disease** (GSD type I; major symptoms include hypoglycemias and hepatomegalia) and **Pompe disease** (GSD type II; the major symptom is cardiomyopathy).

24.1.2 Disorders of Fatty Acid Oxidation and Ketogenesis

Fatty acids—when oxidized by the mitochondria—provide one of the most important energy sources for the organism. For example, during a prolonged fast, up to 80% of the total energy requirement is supplied by fatty acids. While the brain cannot utilize fatty acids, it can adapt to the catabolism of ketones synthesized in the liver, thus indirectly benefiting from this energy source. There are a large number of individual enzyme deficiencies affecting fatty acid oxidation and ketogenesis. These disorders often present clinically with severe **hypoketotic hypoglycemia** (i.e., low blood sugar and insufficient production of ketone bodies), causing seizures, coma, and sometimes death due to catabolic states (e.g., prolonged fasting for more than 8 to 12 hours, surgery, and infections); neonatal **lactic acidosis**, **cardiomyopathy**, and **hepatopathy**, resulting from the toxicity of long-chain fatty acid compounds and/or chronic **muscular symptoms** (e.g., muscle fatigue, pain, recurring rhabdomyolysis, or acute or chronic cardiomyopathy), which are typically seen in less attenuated variants of long-chain fatty acid oxidation.

Medium-Chain Acyl-Coenzyme A Dehydrogenase Deficiency

With an incidence of 1 in 6,000, medium-chain acyl-coenzyme A dehydrogenase (MCAD) deficiency is the most frequent defect of fatty acid oxidation and is now part of expanded newborn screening in the United States and many European countries. MCAD deficiency typically manifests during the second half of the first year of life, when children begin to sleep through the night and when their contact with other children exposes them to infections. The most dangerous symptom is acute **hypoglycemic coma** after prolonged fasting or other catabolic states that can, for example, occur in the course of an otherwise banal gastroenteritis with insufficient food intake and vomiting. Affected children become lethargic and deteriorate rapidly; if untreated they can suffer seizures and cardiac arrest within 1 to 2 hours. In the past, about one-fourth of affected children died in the course of the first manifestation. A diagnosis for this disorder is based on the typical clinical picture (i.e., the presence of hypoketotic hypoglycemia and specific **acylcarnitines**). The prevalent **p.K329E mutation** in the *ACADM* gene (allele frequency of approximately 70% among individuals of European ancestry) can be confirmed through molecular analysis. Treatment is simple, as it consists of **avoiding fasting**, so the prognosis is excellent.

24.1.3   Disorders of Amino Acid Metabolism

The catabolism of essential amino acids initially takes place in the cytosol. At some stage, the metabolite is deaminated (i.e., the amine group is removed), resulting in an organic acid that is then activated with coenzyme A and completely oxidized in the mitochondria. Disorders related to the metabolism of organic acids are called organic acidurias and are diagnosed by urinary organic acid analysis; they are described later in the chapter. Clinical symptoms in **aminoacidopathies** result primarily from the **toxicity of certain metabolites** that accumulate due to a specific enzyme defect (the same applies to defects of galactose and fructose metabolism). Some aminoacidopathies (e.g., histidinemia) remain asymptomatic, because the accumulating products are nontoxic. Mitochondrial energy metabolism usually is not affected. Therefore, only few diseases show acute metabolic crises. The concentrations of lactate, ammonia, and blood sugar, and the acid-base balance are usually normal. A diagnosis is made through the analysis of amino acids in plasma or by finding certain breakdown products in urinary organic acid analysis. Aminoacidopathies are often treatable through a **special diet** with low intake of the amino acid(s) whose catabolism is impaired and, sometimes, other measures. An unusual therapeutic approach is successful in tyrosinemia type I, a condition characterized by the accumulation of certain highly toxic metabolites. A substance called NTBC (nitisinone) is used to inhibit an enzymatic reaction two steps before the actual metabolic block, thus avoiding the development of toxic metabolites (Fig. 24.2). The most prevalent aminoacidopathy is phenylketonuria.

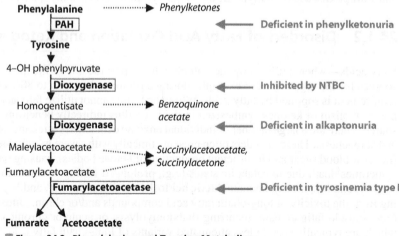

 Figure 24.2. Phenylalanine and Tyrosine Metabolism.

Phenylketonuria

Phenylketonuria (PKU) is caused by a genetic deficiency of the enzyme **phenylalanine hydroxylase** (PAH), which catalyzes the conversion of phenylalanine (Phe) to tyrosine (Fig. 24.2). This leads to a massive increase of Phe in the body and progressive brain damage. In genetics, PKU has been something of a "model disease," since it was the first identified neurogenetic disease (Følling, 1934), the first treatable genetic metabolic disorder (diet; Bickel, 1953), and the first disease that was recognized to be preventable by universal newborn screening (Guthrie test; 1963).

Case History

A few years ago, Mrs. Shabani moved to the United States from Albania. She now attends the genetics clinic because of intellectual disability and variable malformations in all of her seven children. One child died in infancy from tetralogy of Fallot. All other children (ages 2 to 17 years) have learning difficulties or intellectual disability associated with microcephaly; some have epilepsy or cardiac and vertebral defects. Mrs. Shabani admits to having had problems in school, and sometimes she finds it difficult to manage complicated household tasks. She has not had any formal neuropsychological evaluation. An analysis of her blood phenylalanine reveals elevated concentrations of approximately 1500 μmol/L (a normal level is less than 90 μmol/L); mutation analysis confirms the diagnosis of phenylketonuria (in her case compound heterozygosity for the severe mutation p.P281L and the mutation p.L48S, with residual activity). When she was born in Albania, no newborn screening for PKU existed; her own mental development was affected to a lesser degree than individuals with "classic" PKU because of residual PAH activity mediated by the mutation p.L48S and, possibly, favorable dietary factors (i.e., low-protein diet) during her childhood. Importantly, all of her children were exposed to the teratogenic effects of hyperphenylalaninemia during gestation, and thus are affected with maternal PKU (modified case history after Knerr et al., *BMC Pediatr* 2005, 5:5).

Epidemiology

The frequency of PKU varies greatly between different ethnic groups, ranging from 1 in 4,000 in Ireland and Turkey to just under 1 in 100,000 in Finland and Japan. In the United States the reported incidence ranges from 1 in 13,500 to 1 in 19,000 newborns, with higher incidences in European and Native Americans and lower incidences in African, Hispanic, and Asian Americans.

Clinical Symptoms and Course of the Disease

Newborns with PKU are completely asymptomatic, as the maternal–fetal circulation dispenses with excess phenylalanine. Blood Phe concentrations rapidly increase in the first few days of life until they reach a plateau of highly elevated Phe concentrations in the blood (**hyperphenylalaninemia**). If left untreated, this causes progressive psychomotor impairment that manifests itself roughly around the third month of life. If treatment does not ensue during early infancy, affected individuals will have severe intellectual disability (50% have an IQ lower than 35). Additional features include spasticity (◻ Fig. 24.3) and seizures, as well as aggressive, autistic, and psychotic behavior. The relative tyrosine deficiency also results in a reduced melanin synthesis, and untreated PKU patients have a lighter skin color than expected given their ethnicity. Untreated patients have a characteristic "musty" or "mouselike" odor due to the excretion of phenylacetic acid, a breakdown product of phenylalanine, in their sweat and urine.

Hyperphenylalaninemia Variants

- **Phenylketonuria** is the type of PAH deficiency that requires treatment (i.e., blood Phe concentrations exceed a certain threshold; this threshold is 600 μM in the United States, Germany, and other countries and 360 μM in the UK). Depending on Phe tolerance, severe, moderate, and mild forms of PKU are differentiated.
- **Mild hyperphenylalaninemia** (MHP) is the mild form of PAH deficiency in which plasma Phe levels are only slightly elevated (US guidelines: up to 600 μM), and treatment is not necessary.
- Hyperphenylalaninemia can also be caused by an inherited **deficiency in the biosynthesis or recycling of tetrahydrobiopterin (BH$_4$)**, the cofactor of PAH and other hydroxylases.

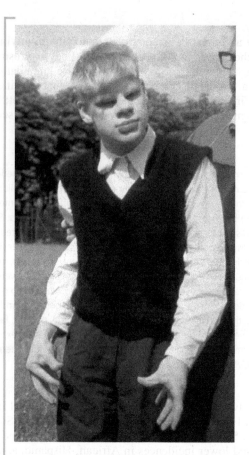

Figure 24.3. Untreated Phenylketonuria with Spasticity. (Courtesy of H. Bickel†, Universitäts-Kinderklinik Heidelberg.)

In addition to (and independent of) variably elevated Phe concentrations, affected patients have neurological symptoms of disturbed neurotransmitter metabolism; treatment is more difficult and less successful than in PKU.

Genetics and Pathophysiology

PKU is an **autosomal recessive** disorder. The ***PAH* gene** is located on chromosome 12q and contains 13 exons. Over 600 disease-causing mutations have been reported. Most of them are missense mutations that have variable effects on protein stability and function and are sometimes associated with residual enzyme activity. The range of mutations varies between different countries; in most populations there is a small number of specific, particularly frequent mutations, in addition to a large number of rare mutations. The population genetics of PKU is described in detail in Section 14.3.

Diagnosis

In most Western countries, PKU is recognized by **neonatal screening**; indeed, the concept of universal neonatal screening was first developed for PKU, as presymptomatic initiation of treatment is essential for a good prognosis. The **blood Phe concentrations** in individuals with PKU are usually normal at birth, but rise quickly during the first hours and days even without formula intake. Concentrations of Phe and tyrosine (typically low in PKU patients) are easily determined from a dried blood spot on a filter paper card. The classic **Guthrie test** used a bacterial inhibition test for this purpose (Section 16.2); the so-called expanded newborn screening is now done by way of **tandem mass spectrometry**, which can also detect numerous other treatable metabolic disorders. For newborn screening, blood samples should be taken between 24 and 48 hours of life.

Therapy

Internationally, there is no consensus about the blood Phe concentrations at which treatment should be started. In the United States and many other countries, treatment is started when Phe exceeds 600 µM (i.e., 10 mg/dL), while in the UK treatment is started when Phe exceeds 360 µM (although there is no evidence that blood Phe concentrations between 360 and 600 µM are harmful). Therapy for PKU consists primarily of a **phenylalanine-restricted diet**. Restricting natural protein intake ensures that blood Phe remains within a specific age-dependent limit. Individual **Phe tolerance** (the amount of Phe that can be ingested while blood concentrations remain in the therapeutic range) is mostly determined by the genotype; "mild" mutations with residual activity are associated with a higher Phe tolerance, since greater amounts of natural Phe can be metabolized. MHP does not require treatment, but women with PKU should be advised that in pregnancy, maternal Phe concentrations greater than 360 µM may be harmful to the fetus. The Phe content of various foods is available in tables.

This type of therapy, which is also being applied to numerous other metabolic disorders, is quite restrictive. Many children with classic severe PKU are only allowed 200 g of natural protein per day at age 5 years. Foods with high protein content, such as meat, fish, or eggs, are not allowed. Baked goods, fruit, and vegetables need to be weighed and their quantities limited. Low-phenylalanine foods such as special bread, pasta, and snacks are commercially available, yet are often three to five times as expensive as the traditional counterparts.

Without additional measures, this type of diet would result in serious protein deficiency. Therefore, the children need to receive the other amino acids (besides Phe) as well as **vitamins and trace elements as supplements**, usually as a prepared formula or powder mix.

For many patients with mild PKU, Phe tolerance is improved with the administration of the cofactor tetrahydrobiopterin (BH$_4$). Individuals with **BH$_4$-responsive PKU**, therefore, can eat more natural protein or may not need the special diet when prescribed the medication sapropterin dihydrochloride, which is currently approved by the U.S. Food and Drug Administration. Unfortunately, BH$_4$ therapy is not effective for individuals with classic PKU and thus does not benefit those patients who would need it most.

Care of PKU patients requires regular follow-up with frequent (initially weekly) monitoring of blood Phe concentrations. US recommendations stipulate that Phe is between 120 and 360 µM (2 to 6 mg/dL) up to age 12 years, and 120 and 900 [if possible: 600] µm (2 to 15 [10] mg/dL) thereafter. It is recommended that the diet be continued through adulthood. Because of the teratogenic effects of elevated Phe concentrations (i.e., greater than 360 µM), affected women must restart a very strict diet before they become pregnant (see Maternal Phenylketonuria).

■■■ Prognosis

If treatment is begun early and well managed, the prognosis is excellent. In such cases there are no cognitive sequelae. If therapy is delayed, irreversible brain damage is to be expected. It is estimated that in the first year of life, each week that classic PKU is left untreated causes loss of up to 1 IQ point. It should be noted that diet can be beneficial even in previously untreated adults. Although the intellectual deficit is irreversible, treatment may have positive effects on emotions and behavior.

■■■ Maternal Phenylketonuria

The level of Phe in the fetus is approximately 50% higher than in maternal blood. High maternal Phe concentrations during pregnancy are teratogenic and result in malformations and serious irreversible damage of the central nervous system in the fetus. Newborns with **maternal PKU** are typically microcephalic and at risk for congenital cardiovascular defects and other congenital malformations. Therefore, women with PKU should maintain a **strict diet and have appropriate medical monitoring prior to conception**. Maternal Phe levels must not exceed 360 µM during pregnancy. Of course, dietary treatment of a child affected by maternal PKU does not reverse or treat the congenital effects and is unnecessary unless the child him- or herself is affected with PKU (e.g., when the father also happened to be a carrier). Maternal PKU should also be considered as a differential diagnosis in cases of intellectual disability if the mother is from a country that did not have reliable newborn screening when she was born, if there are any questions as to the circumstances of her birth (e.g., home delivery), or if there are questions as to her access to medical care.

Organic Acidurias

Organic acidurias are **defects in the mitochondrial metabolism of coenzyme A–activated carboxylic acids**. They can be detected by analysis of organic acids in urine. Unlike amino acidopathies, organic acidurias also affect mitochondrial energy metabolism and, thus, are often associated with an elevated lactate. Other important laboratory findings include metabolic acidosis (out of proportion to that expected due to lactic acidemia), ketosis, hyperammonemia, and hypoglycemia. The majority of cases of classic organic acidurias (more than 70%) present in the neonatal period as **metabolic encephalopathy**, with lethargy, poor suck, vomiting, dehydration, and hypotonia. Acute management consists of reversing catabolism and withholding protein. Long-term therapy involves a protein-restricted diet with supplementation of nonaffected amino acids, vitamins, trace elements, and carnitine. The cumulative incidence of the organic acidurias is 1 in 6,000 newborns. The most frequent of these are **propionic aciduria**, **methylmalonic aciduria**, **isovaleric aciduria**, and **glutaric aciduria**.

Urea Cycle Defects

> **Important**
>
> Genetic disorders related to the detoxification of ammonia (NH_3), which is generated as a by-product of amino acid breakdown, are among the most frequent metabolic disorders (cumulative incidence is approximately 1 in 8,000). These conditions can become symptomatic at any age, are relatively easy to diagnose when the appropriate laboratory tests are performed, and are generally treatable. **An emergency ammonia level** should be performed in any patient with change in mental status or encephalopathy of unknown origin and in all newborns suspected of having "sepsis."

The urea cycle detoxifies ammonia to urea. There are five enzymes involved in the urea cycle, and each is associated with a genetic disorder (autosomal recessive or X linked; ◻ Fig. 24.4). An elevated ammonia level is seen in each condition.

Clinical Symptoms. Many urea cycle disorders manifest within the first few days of life with poor suck, lethargy, hyperventilation, seizures, loss of reflexes, and progressively severe encephalopathy that results in coma and death. Affected children also show thermal instability and, often, intracranial hemorrhages due to a progressive clotting disorder. Chronic (attenuated) disease types may present with intellectual disability, failure to thrive, and episodic neurological symptoms such as lethargy or ataxia. Recurring encephalopathy, with behavioral symptoms and confusion, are typically associated with high protein intake or catabolic state.

Diagnostics. The crucial laboratory finding is **hyperammonemia**. Ammonia (NH_3) values of greater than $150\,\mu M$ in newborns or greater than $100\,\mu M$ in older children call for immediate action, since irreversible organ damage usually occurs very rapidly in urea cycle defects. In addition, emergency analysis of amino acids in plasma and urine, as well as organic acids and orotic acid in urine, must be requested.

Therapy. As with organic acidurias, emergency treatment of hyperammonemia involves the immediate cessation of protein intake and reversal of a catabolic to an anabolic metabolic state by way of high-caloric infusion. The urea cycle is supported by the administration of arginine, which becomes an essential amino acid in those affected with urea cycle defects and which drives the urea cycle forward. Removal of ammonia is enhanced by the administration of sodium benzoate or sodium phenylbutyrate (Fig. 24.4). With very high ammonia levels, emergency extracorporeal detoxification by hemofiltration or dialysis must be initiated. Long-term therapy consists of a strict protein-restricted diet (with special attention to high-quality protein and essential amino acids), as well as the administration of detoxifying and supportive medications.

Ornithine Transcarbamylase Deficiency. X-linked ornithine transcarbamylase (OTC) deficiency is the most frequent urea cycle defect. Hemizygous males typically present with severe hyperammonemia that is fatal if not recognized and treated in the neonatal period. The clinical picture in females is variable; even within the same family, there is considerable variance between

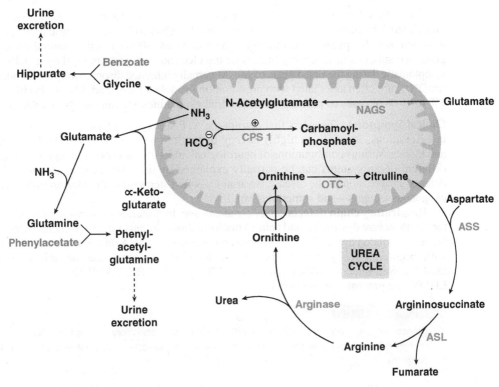

☐ **Figure 24.4. The Urea Cycle.** Index: Enzymes are depicted in yellow: N-acetylglutamate synthase (NAGS), carbamoylphosphate synthase I (CPS1, which requires activation (+) by N-acetylglutamate), ornithine transcarbamylase (OTC), argininosuccinate synthase (ASS), argininosuccinate lyase (ASL), arginase. In orange: mechanism of action of sodium phenylbutyrate and sodium benzoate as part of the emergency treatment of hyperammonemia in urea cycle disorders. (Modified from Zschocke J and Hoffmann GF, Vademecum Metabolicum, Stuttgart 2011.)

individuals, partly due to variable X inactivation in the liver. Often, heterozygous girls or adult women die from an acute metabolic crisis with irreversible brain edema during an apparently minor infection, without having had any previous decompensations. A detailed family history and molecular studies for *OTC* gene mutations are especially important.

24.1.4   Disorders of Energy Metabolism

Mitochondriopathies are genetic disorders of enzymes or enzyme systems that are directly involved in energy production through oxidative phosphorylation. They include, in particular, the **pyruvate dehydrogenase (PDH) complex**, **citrate cycle**, **respiratory chain**, and **adenosine triphosphate (ATP) synthase**. The various disorders overlap clinically, pathophysiologically, and genetically, since some proteins participate in several enzyme complexes, and the accumulation of some substances inhibits other enzymes. Many diseases of intermediary metabolism, especially organic acidurias and fatty acid oxidation defects localized in the mitochondria, also cause secondary impairment of oxidative phosphorylation. Conversely, inhibition of the respiratory chain (e.g., through hypoxia, genetic disorders, or inhibitors) causes a rise in the nicotinamide adenine dinucleotide plus hydrogen (NADH)/nicotinamide adenine dinucleotide (NAD$^+$) ratio; as a result, secondary inhibition of PDH and other enzymes occurs. The energy-producing function of the mitochondria, therefore, represents a complex network of interconnected metabolic processes that can be disrupted in multiple ways. Often it is difficult to identify the exact cause of disturbed energy metabolism.

These disorders are genetically heterogeneous (recessive, dominant, X chromosomal, or mitochondrial/maternal) and demonstrate variable expressivity and, in some individuals, lack of penetrance. Respiratory chain defects in children are often caused by mutations in nuclear genes for subunits or assembly factors of the electron transport chain; they usually become symptomatic during the first 5 years of life. Maternally inherited disorders of mitochondrial DNA (mtDNA) are often associated with presentation in adolescence or adulthood; in children, only 5% to 10 % of cases of primary mitochondrial cytopathies are caused by mtDNA mutations.

Clinical Symptoms. Disorders that disrupt the ATP supply of cells cause a variety of disease manifestations, especially in **highly energy-dependent organs** such as the brain, retina, heart, and kidney. Various combinations of neurological, muscular, and other symptoms arising from different organ systems can be partially explained by tissue-specific expression of genetic defects. Progression of the disease is variable—often stepwise with deterioration after certain exogenous triggers—and sometimes rapid.

Respiratory chain defects can occur at any age. Intrauterine presentation results in premature birth, severe dystrophy, and (brain) malformations. Infants may have encephalomyopathy; however, isolated myopathy is more frequent in adults. mtDNA mutations are often associated with specific, clinically defined syndromes, although the symptoms may be variable even within families. Well-known mtDNA syndromes (MELAS, MERRF, NARP, Kearns-Sayre, Pearson, LHON) are presented in Section 5.5.

Important

Elevated lactate (if not otherwise explained) is an important laboratory finding that points toward a primary mitochondrial disorder. However, consistently normal lactate does not exclude a mitochondriopathy.

Diagnostics. Clinical workup of a suspected mitochondrial cytopathy includes:
- A detailed examination of muscle status, including serum creatine kinase (CK); consider electromyography (EMG)
- A complete neurological examination, including electroencephalography (EEG)
- A precise assessment of other organ functions (e.g., liver, kidneys, heart, and eyes)

Mitochondrial cytopathies should always be considered if symptoms that indicate mitochondrial energy deficiency occur in **at least three organ systems**. Diagnostics should then focus on monitoring **lactate levels** in blood (repeated measurements throughout the day), urine, cerebrospinal fluid, and brain (determination of lactate peak on brain magnetic resonance spectroscopy). A modest elevation of alanine in the analysis of plasma amino acids can occasionally be a diagnostic clue. A cranial **magnetic resonance image (MRI)** might show characteristic abnormalities (e.g., T2 signal hyperintensities in the basal ganglia). **Surgical muscle biopsy** can be essential for the diagnosis, but due to its invasiveness should only be performed in a specialized center. Analysis of mitochondrial DNA is helpful if clinical symptoms are suggestive of a specific mtDNA syndrome.

■■■ mtDNA Depletion Syndrome

The close link between nuclear and mitochondrial genes is particularly evident in mtDNA depletion syndromes. A decrease in cellular mtDNA levels, as a significant diagnostic finding, was first reported in the 1990s. It has since proven to be an important pathogenetic principle. The mtDNA depletion can be caused by different primary defects; the underlying causes, however, are always **mutations in nuclear genes** that are necessary for the replication of mtDNA. Inheritance is usually autosomal recessive. Several clinical types can be differentiated. The first manifestation usually occurs within the first 2 years of life. The **hepatocerebral type** is characterized by acute liver dysfunction progressing to fulminant liver failure, "mitochondrial" central nervous system (CNS) symptoms (e.g., myoclonic seizures, ataxia, and encephalopathy) with episodic deterioration, and failure to thrive and dystrophy. It is frequently caused by mutations in the genes for mitochondrial deoxyguanosine kinase (purine recycling) or DNA polymerase γ (mtDNA replication). The **myopathic type** with nonepisodic, progressive myopathy and ragged red fibers in muscle histology typically is caused by mutations in mitochondrial thymidine kinase 2 (pyrimidine recycling). The main diagnostic test is the analysis of mtDNA levels in tissue, possibly together with specific molecular genetic analysis.

24.2 Disorders of Lysosomal Metabolism

While mitochondria are the power plants of the cell, lysosomes are the recycling centers that break down various small to very large molecules. For that purpose, they contain many different hydrolases in an acidic environment (pH 5). Genetic defects of lysosomal enzymes result in a defective catabolism of specific substrates, their intralysosomal accumulation, and a resulting functional loss of affected cellular systems and organs (Table 24.1).

Table 24.1. Overview of Disorders of Lysosomal Metabolism

Disorder	Deficient Enzyme	Type of Disorder	Coarse Facies	Cherry Red Spot	Corneal Clouding	Organomegaly	Dysostosis Multiplex	Intellectual Disability	Spasticity	Vacuolated Lymphocytes	ERT Available
MPS type I (Hurler-Scheie)	α-L-Iduronidase	M	X		X	X	X	X			P
MPS type II (Hunter)	Iduronate-2-sulphatase	M	X			X	S	X			P
MPS type III (Sanfilippo)	Four different enzymes of heparan sulphate metabolism	M	S			X	S	S	X	X	T
MPS type IV (Morquio)	Two different enzymes of keratan sulphate metabolism	M	X		S	X	X		S		T
MPS type VI (Maroteaux-Lamy)	Arylsulfatase B	M	S			X	X	X			P
Fucosidosis	α-Fucosidase	O	X			S	S	X	X	X	
α-Mannosidosis	α-Mannosidase	O	X		X	X	X	X	S	X	
Gaucher disease type I	Glucocerebrosidase	Sph				X					P
Gaucher disease type II	Glucocerebrosidase	Sph				X		X	X		P
Gaucher disease type III	Glucocerebrosidase	Sph				X		X	S		P
Niemann-Pick disease types A and B	Sphingomyelinase	Sph		S	S	X		X		X	
GM₁-Gangliosidosis	β-Galactosidase	Sph	X	X	X	X	X	X	S		
GM₂-Gangliosidosis (Tay-Sachs, Sandhoff)	β-Hexosaminidases A and B	Sph		X		S		X	X		
Krabbe disease	β-Galactocerebrosidase	Sph		S				X	X		
Metachromatic leukodystrophy	Arylsulphatase A	Sph		S				X	X		
Fabry disease	Ceramide trihexosidase = α-Galactosidase	Sph									P

M, mucopolysaccharidosis; O, oligosaccharidosis; Sph, sphingolipidosis.
X, symptom present; S, symptom sometimes present.
ERT, enzyme replacement therapy; P, clinical practice; T, clinical trials.
(Information as of June 2010.)

Mucopolysaccharidoses

Mucopolysaccharidoses (MPSs) are disorders related to the catabolism of glycosaminoglycans, which are modified (e.g., aminated, sulfated, or acetylated) polysaccharide chains derived from proteoglycans. These proteoglycans are glycosylated proteins that constitute a major component of the viscous extracellular matrix. Most show autosomal recessive inheritance. Children with MPS usually appear normal at birth but (in most MPSs) subsequently develop progressive skeletal deformities, including typical coarse facies, bone dysplasias (**dysostosis multiplex**), and contractures, as well as hepatomegaly. Depending on the MPS type, there may be progressive intellectual disability with loss of acquired skills, corneal clouding, and deafness. Hernias and recurrent upper and lower respiratory tract infections are common. All MPSs except type II (X-linked) are autosomal recessive. The diagnosis is typically made by analyzing glycosaminoglycans in the urine and is confirmed by enzyme analysis. Recombinant **enzyme replacement therapy (ERT)** has been approved for mucopolysaccharidosis type I (Hurler, Scheie; ◘ Fig. 24.5), type II (Hunter), and type VI (Maroteaux-Lamy); the intellectual disability, however, is not treatable with ERT. Bone marrow transplantation has proven to be beneficial in presymptomatic patients with MPS I. Otherwise, treatment of the mucopolysaccharidoses is symptomatic.

Sphingolipidoses

Sphingolipids are membrane lipids that contain ceramide (composed of sphingosine and a long-chain fatty acid) attached to a polar residue. They are found throughout the body but are of special importance in the nervous tissue, where they, for example, constitute important components of the myelin sheaths. Thus, sphingolipidoses usually present with primary disturbances in the central or peripheral nervous system. Typical, clinical features include progressive intellectual disability and neurological symptoms, including epilepsy, ataxia, and/or spasticity. Hepatosplenomegaly, caused by the accumulation of sphingolipids in reticuloendothelial cells, is not uncommon; dysmorphism or skeletal deformities are rare.

Diagnostic workup of suspected sphingolipidoses should include an ophthalmological examination; in most sphingolipidoses (except Gaucher and Fabry disease), the macula may

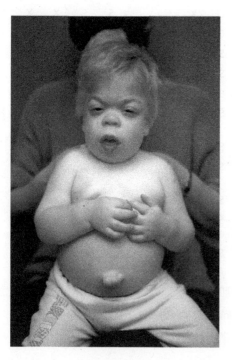

◘ **Figure 24.5. Hurler Disease.** Children affected by this mucopolysaccharidosis show progressive retardation, small stature with typical skeletal changes, coarse facial features, corneal clouding, and hepatosplenomegaly. Skin and hair are firm or thickened. Cardiac complications are the most frequent cause of death. (Courtesy of G. Tariverdian, Institut für Humangenetik, Heidelberg.)

appear as a typical **cherry-red spot** that is caused by lipid deposition in the periphery of the macula. Light microscopy may reveal foam cells in the bone marrow or vacuolated lymphocytes. The diagnosis is confirmed through enzyme analysis. With the exception of Fabry disease, sphingolipidoses show **autosomal recessive** inheritance.

Important sphingolipidoses with progressive neurodegeneration are **Tay-Sachs disease**, **Niemann-Pick disease**, and the severe form of **Gaucher disease (type II)**. More frequent is the nonneuronopathic form of Gaucher disease (type I), which is characterized by extreme (hepato-) splenomegaly and bone lesions. The chief symptoms of **Fabry disease** are intermittent, severe, burning pain and prickly paraesthesias in the fingers and toes, which often begin at elementary school age, as well as angiokeratomas of the skin. Recombinant enzyme replacement therapy is approved for Gaucher and Fabry disease.

24.3 Disorders of Lipid Metabolism

Disorders of lipid and lipoprotein metabolism are of special interest in adult medicine, because some are important risk factors for **cardiovascular disease**, which is the number one cause of death in the United States and many other countries. An elevated blood concentration of low-density lipoprotein (LDL) is a major predisposing factor for atherosclerosis and, consequently, myocardial infarction and stroke, while the concentration of high-density lipoprotein (HDL) has an inverse correlation with the risk for coronary artery disease. Most cases of atherosclerosis have a multifactorial etiology, but the less frequent monogenic disorders of lipid metabolism have contributed greatly to our understanding of the disease.

Familial Hypercholesterolemia (Low-Density Lipoprotein Receptor Deficiency)

Familial hypercholesterolemia (FH) is an important cause of recurrent myocardial infarction and other cardiovascular disorders within a family. It is an autosomal dominant disease caused by heterozygous mutations in the LDL receptor (*LDLR*) gene. The very rare homozygous form of LDLR deficiency causes childhood-onset cardiovascular disease.

Case History

Two-year-old identical twins of Turkish descent were referred for investigation of symmetrical skin lesions (xanthomas) on their elbows, knees, hands, and ankles (◻ Fig. 24.6A). Lipid analyses revealed severe hypercholesterolemia, with total cholesterol levels of 1.15 to 1.25 g/dL in both children. The consanguineous parents both had moderate hypercholesterolemia (250 to 350 mg/dL), which was previously unidentified. Family history was positive for cardiovascular disease. Conservative treatment of the twins had no therapeutic effect, while the xanthomas had significantly grown in size by the time they were 3 years old (Fig. 24.6B). Lipid apheresis, given every 2 weeks, was initiated and resulted in a softening and shrinking of the xanthomas; the affected twins have had no cardiovascular complications up to their present age of 11 years (case history from Zschocke and Schäfer, *Lancet* 2003, 361:1641).

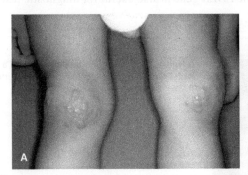
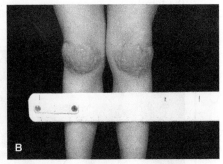

◻ **Figure 24.6. Homozygous Low-Density Lipoprotein Receptor (LDLR) Deficiency. A.** Bilateral xanthomas on the knees of a 2-year-old boy. **B.** Marked progression of xanthomas at 3 years of age.

Epidemiology

With an estimated **prevalence** of **1 in 500**, FH is one of the most frequent monogenic metabolic disorders. Nevertheless, less than 5% of the total number of hypercholesterolemias in the general population is attributable to LDL receptor deficiency. Homozygous LDLR deficiency has a predicted incidence of 1 in 1,000,000, but the deficiency is probably more frequent in consanguineous populations.

Pathophysiology

The LDL receptor plays a key role in the body's cholesterol metabolism. An organ's ability to eliminate LDL cholesterol from the blood depends on the density of the LDL receptors on the cell surface. About 70% of the body's LDL receptors are located on liver cells. Individuals with FH caused by a heterozygous *LDLR* gene mutation have a reduced number of LDL receptors in the liver; in homozygous individuals the receptors can be totally absent. As a result, cholesterol clearance from the blood is reduced, and circulating LDL (and LDL cholesterol) is removed independent of LDL receptors (e.g., by way of endocytosis in macrophages and monocytes). The migration of such cells into the vascular wall, their proliferation, and further endocytosis of LDL cholesterol constitute a first step toward atherosclerosis.

Clinical Symptoms

Individuals with FH and heterozygous *LDLR* gene mutations at birth have twice the normal levels of plasma LDL. Over a period of many years, the elevated LDL cholesterol (blood concentration usually 300 to 500 mg/dL) remains the only, silent indicator for a genetic disorder. Between age 30 and 40 years, many heterozygous persons have a myocardial infarction. Coronary artery disease in women occurs approximately 7 to 10 years later than in men. **Xanthomas** and **arcus cornealis** can be early warning signs (◻ Fig. 24.7).

　　Homozygous carriers of LDLR deficiency have a blood LDL cholesterol concentration of up to 1.2 g/dL (10-fold elevated) at birth. In early childhood, they develop xanthomas that may rapidly increase in size. Fatal myocardial infarctions, caused by progressive coronary artery disease, often occur in childhood or adolescence.

Genetics

More than 700 different mutations in the *LDLR* gene have been reported as causes for FH, among them point mutations as well as genomic rearrangements.

Diagnosis

FH should be suspected in every individual with LDL concentrations greater than 300 mg/dL in combination with elevated very low-density lipoprotein (VLDL), normal triglycerides, and low HDL. LDL concentrations greater than 600 mg/dL may indicate homozygous *LDLR* deficiency. A detailed family history and lipid studies in relatives are of particular importance. Mutation analysis of the *LDLR* gene is also useful for diagnostic testing within the family.

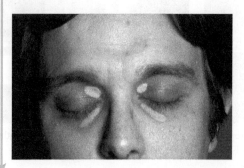

◻ **Figure 24.7. Palpebral Xanthelasma in a Patient with Familial Hypercholesterolemia.** (Courtesy of V. Voigtländer, Klinikum Ludwigshafen.)

Therapy

Therapy for **heterozygous patients** is aimed at normalizing LDL cholesterol concentrations using the following strategies:

- **Low-cholesterol diet:** Patients should reduce fat intake, substitute saturated animal fats with unsaturated vegetable fats, consume fish regularly (high content of omega-3 fatty acids), eat plenty of fruits and vegetables, follow a Mediterranean diet plan, restrict cholesterol intake, lose weight (if overweight), and exercise regularly.
- **Medication:** Statins (i.e., HMG-CoA reductase inhibitors) are the most effective LDL cholesterol–lowering drugs. They reduce the risk of myocardial infarction and overall mortality by primary and secondary prevention of cardiovascular disease. Additional medications include anion exchange resins (bile acid sequestrants), nicotinic acid, and fibrates.

In **homozygous LDL receptor deficiency**, even a strict diet and drug therapy do not achieve a sufficient reduction of serum cholesterol. LDL apheresis is the method of choice to remove excess LDL cholesterol; liver transplantation may be considered.

24.4   Other Metabolic Disorders

Peroxisomal Disorders

To protect cells from reactive oxygen species, **oxygen-dependent metabolic reactions** are carried out in special organelles called *peroxisomes*. Important reactions that occur in these organelles are α- and β-oxidation of different fatty acids (e.g., very long chain), as well as the biosynthesis (at least in several steps) of specific phospholipids, cholesterol, and bile acids. A considerable number of proteins, called **peroxins** (encoded by *PEX* genes), are necessary for the formation of peroxisomes and protein import. Thus, peroxisomal disorders include disorders in the formation of peroxisomes, disorders of membrane transport proteins, and deficiencies of individual peroxisomal proteins.

Clinical symptoms for peroxisomal disorders vary and include **neurological symptoms** (e.g., encephalopathy, hypotonia, epilepsy, and deafness), **skeletal anomalies** (especially short proximal extremities and epiphysial calcifications), **eye anomalies** (e.g., retinopathy, cataracts, and blindness), craniofacial **dysmorphisms** (e.g., macrocephaly and enlarged fontanelle), and **liver dysfunction** (e.g., neonatal hepatitis, hepatomegaly, cholestasis, and cirrhosis). Diagnostics include the determination of specific peroxisomal substances, such as very long-chain fatty acids (VLCFAs), phytanic acid, or plasmalogens.

Among the peroxisomal disorders are **Zellweger syndrome** (◻ Fig. 24.8); **X-chromosomal adrenoleukodystrophy,** which is characterized by progressive neurodegeneration (i.e., loss of myelin, resulting in dystrophy of the cerebral white matter) and Addison disease in boys; as well as **rhizomelic chondrodysplasia punctata**, discussed in Section 26.2.

Disorders of Sterol Synthesis

Cholesterol is synthesized endogenously from acetyl-CoA in a multistep process. Sterol synthesis disorders manifest themselves clinically with facial dysmorphisms and variable skeletal dysplasias;

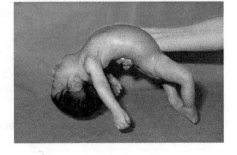

◻ **Figure 24.8. Zellweger Syndrome.** Neonates with the most severe form of peroxisome biogenesis disorders show extreme muscular hypotonia.

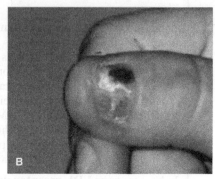

Figure 24.9. Lesch-Nyhan Syndrome. Severe self-mutilation of **(A)** mouth and tongue and **(B)** thumb in a young patient. (Courtesy of G. Tariverdian, Institut für Humangenetik Heidelberg.)

they should also be considered in unexplained miscarriages with specific fetal malformations. Among sterol synthesis disorders are chondrodysplasia punctata (Conradi-Hünermann syndrome), caused by an insufficiency of 3β-hydroxysteroid-Δ8,Δ7 isomerase (Section 26.2), as well as **Smith-Lemli-Opitz syndrome** (SLOS; see Chapter 19.3, Fig. 19.22). Inheritance is typically autosomal recessive.

Disorders of Purine and Pyrimidine Metabolism

Purines and pyrimidines are the precursors of nucleic acids; they are catabolized to uric acid (purines) or β-amino acids (pyrimidines). Numerous enzymatic defects have been described that present with disease-specific renal (e.g., kidney stones and renal failure), neurological (e.g., intellectual disability, epilepsy, and movement disorders), muscular (e.g., cramps and muscle wasting), hematological (e.g., anemia and immunodeficiency), or skeletal (e.g., gout and small stature) symptoms and signs. Children with **Lesch-Nyhan syndrome** (which is caused by a deficiency of the enzyme hypoxanthine-guanine phosphoribosyltransferase) have severe intellectual disability, neurological symptoms, and a characteristic tendency to self-mutilate (▪ Fig. 24.9).

Congenital Disorders of Glycosylation

Many proteins require posttranslational modification for normal function. Deficiencies of enzymes or other proteins that are involved in the generation and attachment of carbohydrate chains (mostly N-glycosylation) constitute the group of congenital disorders of glycosylation (CDGs). The spectrum of clinical symptoms caused by CDGs is as broad as the different functions of glycoproteins in the organism; all organ systems can be affected. Frequently, there are functional anomalies such as coagulation anomalies or endocrine or gastrointestinal symptoms. Most conditions cause neurological symptoms and intellectual disability. More than 20 different enzymatic defects affecting the N-glycosylation of proteins have been identified. The primary diagnosis is achieved by analysis of serum transferrin glycoforms (also called carbohydrate-deficient transferrin analysis); it is confirmed enzymatically or through mutation analysis. Treatment is symptomatic, except for phosphomannose isomerase deficiency (CDG Ib), which is treatable with oral administration of mannose.

> **Important**
>
> CDGs are among the few inborn errors of metabolism that can cause dysmorphic features in neonates. Analysis of serum transferrin glycoforms is a simple and cost-efficient screening test that should be done in all children with an unexplained multisystem disease and morphological anomalies.

Phosphomannomutase Deficiency (Congenital Disorder of Glycosylation Type Ia). Phosphomannomutase deficiency is by far the most frequent CDG, accounting for up to 80% of identified CDG patients. CDG type Ia typically presents in infancy as a **multisystem disorder** with severe failure to thrive, hypotonia, and developmental delay. Episodes of hypoglycemia, liver dysfunction, coagulopathy, and severe diarrhea might be present. Cerebellar atrophy is frequent and may provide an additional diagnostic clue. Older children usually have nonprogressive neurological symptoms and intellectual disability. Typical morphological features include an abnormal distribution of fatty tissue and inverted nipples. Diagnosis is confirmed enzymatically or through mutation analysis. Treatment is symptomatic and often requires G-tube placement and fundoplication.

Neurotransmitter Defects

The synthesis and catabolism of neurotransmitters are controlled by a number of enzymes, whose absence typically leads to severe, sometimes progressive, encephalopathies. Many of these disorders present in early childhood as epileptic encephalopathy; some can be effectively treated with specific vitamins or cofactors (e.g., pyridoxine-dependent seizures). Defects of dopamine biosynthesis cause progressive extrapyramidal symptoms, including intermittent focal dystonia, hereditary spastic diplegia or cerebral palsy, and severe (lethal) infantile encephalopathies. A diagnosis involves the measurement of neurotransmitters or their metabolites in cerebrospinal fluid. The indication for this test should be chosen with care; it is not indicated in cases of isolated intellectual disability or nonspecific behavioral disorders.

25 Endocrinology and Immune System

LEARNING OBJECTIVES

1 Identify monogenic causes of the typically multifactorial disorder diabetes mellitus.

2 Formulate a diagnostic algorithm on how to differentiate between pyloric stenosis and salt-wasting congenital adrenal hyperplasia (CAH) in a neonate with severe vomiting.

3 Identify at least four clinical presentations of nonclassic CAH, and discuss which molecular findings to expect upon sequencing of the *CYP21A2* gene.

25.1 Diabetes Mellitus

Both type 1 and type 2 diabetes are principally **multifactorial disorders** that are caused by a combination of genetic and nongenetic factors. Predictive analyses of known diabetes risk factors are of limited use, even though some genotypes are associated with a more than 20-fold increased probability of developing diabetes. Few forms of diabetes are inherited as monogenic traits; they constitute 1% to 5% of all cases.

Type 1 Diabetes

Type 1 diabetes (T1D) is caused by destruction of insulin-secreting β-cells in the islets of Langerhans of the pancreas via autoimmune insulitis. This results in an absolute insulin deficiency of the organism. Although T1D is **rarely familial**, genetic factors do play an important, predisposing role. Like many autoimmune disorders, T1D is strongly associated with certain variants of highly polymorphic human leukocyte antigen (HLA) genes. Since variants in adjacent *HLA* genes often show strong linkage disequilibrium, association studies are carried out with regard to specific haplotypes (combinations of variants). The HLA class II genes *DRB1*, *DQA1*, and *DQB1* are of particular importance for the development of T1D; more than 90% of patients carry the DR3 or DR4 haplotypes on at least one allele, whereas fewer than 40% of normal controls have these haplotypes. Individuals heterozygous for both DR3 and DR4 have a risk of approximately 1 in 15 of developing type 1 diabetes versus a risk of 1 in 300 in the general population. In contrast, there is also a protective DR2 haplotype that is found in 20% of the general Caucasian population but less than 1% of T1D patients. The HLA alleles are in close proximity to several immune-regulatory genes on chromosome 6. Within a family, the genetic risk for type 1 diabetes can be determined by identifying the HLA alleles of the index patient and his or her siblings. Monozygotic twins are at increased risk (30% to 35%), as are HLA-identical siblings (18% to 20% risk) and siblings sharing one HLA allele (5% risk). There is no increased risk for non–HLA-identical siblings.

In addition to HLA alleles on chromosome 6, there are other predisposition loci in the genome, such as *IDDM2*, which was mapped to a variable VNTR sequence upstream of the insulin gene on chromosome 11p15.

Type 2 Diabetes

Type 2 diabetes has become an epidemic in Western industrialized nations and is primarily caused by lifestyle factors and genetic predisposition(s). Pathophysiologically, two major factors that lead to type 2 diabetes are the derangement of insulin secretion and the development of insulin resistance.

A positive family history means a 2.4-fold increased risk for type 2 diabetes. Between 15% and 25% of first-degree relatives of an individual with type 2 diabetes develop impaired glucose tolerance or manifest with type 2 diabetes. Having one parent with type 2 diabetes increases one's risk for type 2 diabetes by 38%. The concordance rate for monozygotic twins is 35% to 60%; the rate for dizygotic twins is 17% to 20%.

Despite a strong genetic component and major research efforts, only a few risk-modifying genes have, thus far, been identified for type 2 diabetes.

Monogenic Forms of Diabetes

In the mid-1960s, the first cases of families with autosomal dominant heritable types of diabetes mellitus were identified. Despite having a young age of onset (at least one family member with age of onset younger than 25 years), their diabetes was not insulin dependent. The term *maturity-onset diabetes of the young* (**MODY**) was coined. However, this terminology has recently fallen out of favor, as it implies a resemblance to type 2 diabetes, even though all the subtypes of monogenic diabetes mellitus are very different from type 2 diabetes.

Monogenic forms of diabetes differ from type 1 in that they do not have circulating autoantibodies against pancreatic antigens, and there is measurable C-peptide in the presence of hyperglycemia. Yet, they are also distinct from type 2 diabetes in that they manifest in fairly young individuals in the absence of obesity, acanthosis nigricans, polycystic ovarian syndrome, or lipid profile abnormalities.

Diabetes diagnosed before 6 months of age is likely to be one of the monogenic forms of **neonatal diabetes** and not autoimmune type 1 diabetes. An underlying gene mutation can be identified in approximately 75% of cases. Transient and permanent forms of neonatal diabetes mellitus are known. The latter are frequently caused by mutation in the *KCNJ11* or the *ABCC8* genes, both of which encode subunits of an adenosine triphosphate (ATP)-sensitive potassium channel. It is important to identify patients with these mutations, as they will be best treated with oral sulfonylurea rather than insulin injections.

Patients who manifest familial, mild fasting hyperglycemia, with little deterioration with age, should be tested for heterozygous mutations of the **glucokinase** (*GCK*) gene. Glucokinase catalyzes the rate-limiting step of glucose phosphorylation, enabling pancreatic β-cells and hepatocytes to respond appropriately to hyperglycemia. Making this diagnosis provides important anticipatory guidance. Complications of this condition are rare, and medical treatment is typically not necessary. Pregnancy is the only exception, but insulin is required only in cases where there is excess fetal growth.

In contrast to patients with *GCK* mutations, individuals with familial young-onset diabetes caused by mutations in the **transcription factor genes** *HFN1A*, *HNF4A*, *HNFB4*, *PDX1*, or *NEUROD1* have progressive glucose intolerance with age and are at a high risk for developing diabetic complications. Mutations in the *HFN1A* gene represent the most common form of monogenic transcription factor diabetes. Low-dose sulfonylurea is the first-line pharmacological treatment for them.

Rare forms of monogenic diabetes manifest typical **extrapancreatic features**, including Wolfram syndrome (e.g., optic atrophy, deafness, and neurodegeneration), MIDD (i.e., maternally inherited diabetes with deafness), TRMA syndrome (i.e., thiamine-responsive megaloblastic anemia), and RCAD syndrome (e.g., renal cysts and diabetes).

25.2 Congenital Adrenal Hyperplasia

The term *congenital adrenal hyperplasia* (CAH) describes a group of autosomal recessive disorders that cause the impaired synthesis of cortisol and other steroid hormones from cholesterol by the adrenal cortex. In the most common form, insufficient **synthesis of cortisol and mineralocorticoids** is accompanied by **excessive synthesis of male sex hormones**. CAH represents the most frequent cause of adrenocortical (AC) insufficiency and of ambiguous genitalia in a chromosomally female (46,XX) infant. Several enzyme defects can cause CAH—all are inherited in an autosomal recessive manner:

- **21-Hydroxylase deficiency** (greater than 90% of cases) is discussed in greater detail in the following section.

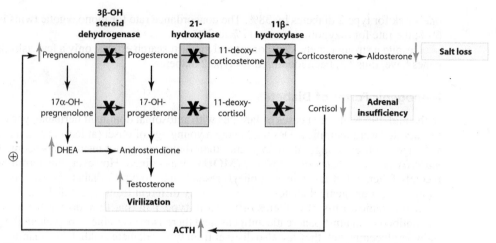

Figure 25.1. Deficiencies of Steroid Biosynthesis in Congenital Adrenal Hyperplasia (CAH). Enzymatic defects and resulting alterations are marked in blue; clinical symptoms are highlighted in yellow boxes.

- **11β-Hydroxylase deficiency** (5% to 8% of cases) causes virilization in females and hypertension but not usually salt-wasting crises, since the accumulating 11-deoxycorticosterone acts as a weak mineralocorticoid. Attenuated forms may present with menstrual irregularities and hirsutism in adolescent and adult women.
- **3β-Hydroxylase deficiency** (rare, 1% of cases) is characterized by impaired synthesis of all adrenal and gonadal steroids. It presents with adrenal insufficiency and salt wasting in both sexes. However, males show varying degrees of undervirilization, while females have normal genitalia or only mild virilization.
- **17α-Hydroxylase deficiency** (rare) is characterized by the reduced production of cortisol and sex steroids, as well as the accumulation of mineralocorticoid precursors. There are no adrenal crises; females have normal external genitalia and later sexual infantilism (primary amenorrhea), while male patients may present with 46,XY disorder of sex determination (DSD; Chapter 28) and show undervirilized, ambiguous or female-appearing genitalia (sex reversal).

See Figure 25.1 for an overview of the synthesis of adrenocortical steroids and the corresponding enzyme defects.

21-Hydroxylase Deficiency

Case History

Mr. and Mrs. Gonzalez present to your clinic for evaluation of infertility. They have been trying to conceive for 3 years. Mr. Gonzalez has had normal semen analysis. Mrs. Gonzalez has experienced oligomenorrhea. She also complains of excessive body hair. Recent endocrine studies revealed an elevated testosterone level for Mrs. Gonzalez (hyperandrogenism). Nonclassic 21-OH deficiency is identified in 2% to 10% of women with hyperandrogenism. Molecular genetic testing of the *CYP21A2* gene that codes for steroid 21-hydroxylase reveals compound heterozygosity for the mutations Q318X and V304M in Mrs. Gonzalez. While Q318X results in a total loss of enzyme activity, V304M has a high residual activity. The findings confirm the diagnosis of nonclassic 21-OH deficiency in Mrs. Gonzalez. Medical therapy with cortisol supplementation is initiated, which results in an improvement of hormone levels; Mrs. Gonzalez's menstrual periods become more regular. The chances of having a child with classic CAH are discussed with the family and molecular genetic testing is recommended for Mr. Gonzalez. In case Mr. Gonzalez was a carrier, the risk for this couple to have an affected pregnancy would be 50%. Prenatal treatment with dexamethasone prevents virilization of an affected female fetus.

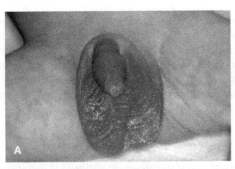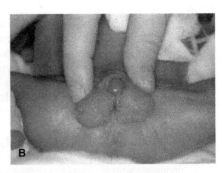

Figure 25.2. Congenital Adrenal Hyperplasia. A. Hyperpigmentation of the external genitalia in a boy. **B.** Ambiguous genitalia in a girl. (Courtesy of Universitäts-Kinderklinik Heidelberg.)

Epidemiology

The incidence of 21-OH deficiency worldwide is estimated to be 1 in 15,000. This translates into a heterozygous frequency of 1 in 60. CAH with salt loss is diagnosed three times more frequently than CAH without salt loss.

Variants

Clinically and genetically, we differentiate between three degrees of severity of 21-hydroxylase deficiency:
- **Salt-wasting CAH** (most frequent type): deficient biosynthesis of cortisol and aldosterone causes salt-wasting adrenal crisis typically at the age of 2 to 3 weeks.
- **Simple virilizing CAH:** there are no salt-wasting adrenal crises because of residual 21-hydroxylase activity.
- **Late-onset (nonclassic) CAH:** the typical biochemical changes are much milder. Often, clinical symptoms in girls are not noticed until puberty.

All variants of CAH manifest increased androgen synthesis.

Clinical Features

While the deficiency of cortisol and mineralocorticoids results in clinical problems in the peri- and postnatal period, the virilization due to CAH begins in the first trimester of gestation. At 6 weeks' gestational age, the fetal adrenal cortex produces increased amounts of androgens; therefore, **females** with classic CAH are typically recognized at birth because of their **ambiguous exterior genitalia**. Depending on the severity of virilization (classification after Prader), the affected female neonate might be mistaken for a boy with hypospadias (Fig. 25.2B). However, females affected with CAH would be expected to have normal ovaries and Müllerian structures. **Male** infants with CAH may have virilization (enlarged penis) or hyperpigmentation of the perineal region (Fig. 25.2A); yet, most often these **subtle physical features** are undetected. Thus, newborn screening for CAH is most helpful in males to prevent complications of the salt-wasting forms. Hyperplasia of the adrenal cortex can sometimes be visualized by sonography.

   Salt wasting with severe CAH begins to manifest clinically in the second week of life. Affected children (boys and girls) develop poor feeding, failure to thrive, and weight loss. **Severe vomiting** often causes dehydration. The analysis of serum electrolytes is important and can be the clue to the diagnosis: **hyperkalemic** metabolic acidosis with **hyponatremia**. If left untreated, hyperkalemia reaches life-threatening levels (up to 10 mmol/L) within 1 to 2 weeks, and the children die in their third or fourth week from electrolyte imbalance and cardiac arrest.

> **Important**
>
> An important differential diagnosis at this stage is pyloric stenosis. However, pyloric stenosis causes metabolic alkalosis, while salt-wasting CAH leads to metabolic acidosis. In addition, there always is hyperkalemia in salt-wasting CAH, which never occurs in pyloric stenosis.

Children **without salt wasting**, if untreated, develop the undesired virilization as they grow older. By the time they are 6 to 8 years old, boys and girls often begin to show signs of puberty (girls, however, without breast development). This is due to a **precocious pseudopuberty**, since the gonads are infantile to hypoplastic (androgens are formed ectopically in the adrenal cortex). Initially, affected children are much taller than their peers, while their bone age is many years advanced; epiphyses close prematurely, and the final body height is much shorter than normal.

■■■ Late-Onset Congenital Adrenal Hyperplasia or Nonclassic Congenital Adrenal Hyperplasia

Individuals with late-onset CAH typically have 25% to 50% residual activity of 21-hydroxylase. They produce normal amounts of cortisol and aldosterone with mild to moderately elevated levels of testosterone. Two-thirds of the cases of late-onset CAH are **compound heterozygous** with a "mild" mutation (i.e., with residual activity) on at least one allele. Prevalence is high; a New York study reports a prevalence of 1 in 100.

The most frequent symptom of women with late-onset CAH is **hirsutism** (60%), followed by oligomenorrhea (55%), acne (33%), and **infertility** (13%). At the same time, many women with late-onset CAH develop ovarian cysts. Late-onset CAH, therefore, is an important differential diagnosis for polycystic ovarian syndrome. Individuals with late-onset CAH do not always require glucocorticoid therapy. Many remain asymptomatic. Therapy is strongly indicated in cases of severe acne, hirsutism, menstrual irregularities, testicular tumors, and infertility. These require smaller doses of glucocorticoids than classic CAH.

Genetics

The gene for 21-hydroxylase is located on the short arm of chromosome 6 in close proximity to the HLA loci. Directly adjacent to the functional gene *CYP21A2* is another very similar pseudogene, *CYP21A1P*, that is inactive. Numerous mutations responsible for 21-hydroxylase deficiency stem from the exchange of genetic material between gene and pseudogene, resulting in a functional loss of the active gene.

Diagnosis

While the clinical presentation and typical electrolyte imbalances may suggest a diagnosis of CAH, the diagnosis of 21-OH deficiency is confirmed by biochemical findings such as an unequivocally elevated serum concentration of 17-OH progesterone. Plasma renin activity is markedly elevated in individuals with the salt-wasting form of 21-OH deficiency. Identification of the underlying mutations in the *CYP21A2* gene can help predict the severity of the disease, but it is especially important for directing prenatal therapy in subsequent pregnancies.

■■■ Prenatal Therapy

Treating the mother with dexamethasone during pregnancy suppresses the fetal pituitary-adrenocortical axis and thus prevents intrauterine virilization of the female fetus. This therapy, however, needs to start, at the latest, during the 6th week of gestation. This is only possible when both parents are known to be carriers of CAH-causing mutations. Treatment is initiated even though, statistically, it only benefits one in eight children. During the 11th week of gestation, chorionic villous sampling (CVS) will help determine whether therapy needs to be continued until birth. For a boy, therapy can be discontinued. A girl needs to have a DNA analysis. If the female fetus is affected, treatment is continued.

Therapy

Therapy consists of lifelong administration of glucocorticoids (cortisol). Patients should wear an ID bracelet, as stress doses of steroids are needed (e.g., during intercurrent illness, accident, or surgery). Additionally, mineralocorticoids (i.e., synthetic 9α-fluorcortisol) are administered in cases of aldosterone deficiency.

While feminizing genitoplasty for females with ambiguous genitalia and CAH has been the preferred treatment for decades, many patients treated in this manner have called into question the precedent dogma, which held that the ability to eventually bear a child should direct therapy in the infant and young child. Advocacy organizations, such as the Intersex Society of North

America (www.isna.org) and the Cares Foundation (www.caresfoundation.org), have called for increased awareness of the options for nonsurgical management and more systematic analysis of the psychological and physical outcomes of both the surgical and nonsurgical approach to CAH. Likewise, the American Academy of Pediatrics' (www.aap.org) revised "Consensus Statement on Management of Intersex Disorders" supports a more comprehensive approach to the infant and child with CAH and other DSDs.

25.3 Autoimmune Polyendocrinopathies

This group of disorders is also known as polyglandular autoimmune syndromes. They are characterized by two or more autoimmune endocrinopathies, such as Addison disease, hypoparathyroidism, and others. Often, it is possible to detect organ-specific autoantibodies even before the respective disorder becomes symptomatic, allowing anticipatory guidance about disease progression.

Various types are differentiated. **Polyglandular autoimmune syndrome type I** is an autosomal recessive disorder caused by mutations in the autoimmune regulator gene *AIRE*. Major characteristics are mucocutaneous candidiasis, hypoparathyroidism, and adrenal insufficiency (Addison disease). The more frequent **type II** is thought to be multifactorial in etiology, with several susceptibility loci. It manifests with immune thyroiditis (Schmidt syndrome) and/or diabetes mellitus type 1 (Carpenter syndrome) in addition to Addison disease. The less frequent **X-chromosomal polyendocrinopathy with immune deficiency and diarrhea**, also known as IPEX syndrome (**i**mmune dysregulation, **p**olyendocrinopathy, **e**nteropathy, **X** linked), typically manifests itself in newborns as a severe autoimmune disease picture with diabetes mellitus type 1; it is caused by mutations in the *FOXP3* gene.

For a detailed discussion of **immunodeficiencies**, a subject of great importance for differential diagnosis, see Chapter 37.

26 Skeletal System

LEARNING OBJECTIVES

1 Compose a clinical checklist for achondroplasia, and develop a management plan for a child affected with this condition.

2 Name four different types of craniosynostoses, and explain which sutures are fused prematurely in the respective conditions.

3 Elaborate on the concepts of gain-of-function and loss-of-function mutations, imprinting, and mosaicism using the *GNAS* gene and its associated disorders as an example.

26.1 Abnormal Bone Fragility

Osteogenesis Imperfecta

Also called "brittle bone disease," osteogenesis imperfecta (OI) is the most prevalent monogenic disorder associated with abnormal bone fragility. Before the molecular basis of OI was understood, OI was classified into four types based on clinical presentation, severity, and certain radiographic findings. Etiopathogenetically, all four types have mutations of the genes *COL1A1* or *COL1A2* that encode the chains of type I procollagen, the major protein in bone and most other connective tissues. See Section 4.2 for a detailed description of this disorder and its molecular genetic defects.

26.2 Skeletal Dysplasias

Skeletal dysplasias are a heterogeneous group of congenital disorders that, due to genetic defects in the formation of cartilage and bones, result in morphological abnormalities of the extremities, the torso, and/or the skull. In most cases, they also result in disproportionate short stature. Depending on where the growth defect occurs, we differentiate between rhizomelic, mesomelic, and acromelic types of disproportionate short stature. Pictorial representations of these types of short stature can be found in Section 35.1.

Based on the specific clinical and radiographic findings, there are more than 100 different skeletal dysplasias. Over the past few decades, the underlying genetic defects of many of these skeletal dysplasias have been uncovered.

Achondroplasia

Achondroplasia is the most common form of inherited disproportionate short stature. While a skeletal survey may be required to support the clinical suspicion of this diagnosis in the newborn, the physical features in a toddler, older child, or adult with achondroplasia are so characteristic that most physicians can make a diagnosis on initial presentation. Its depiction in ancient Egyptian art makes it one of the oldest recorded phenotypically evident genetic disorders.

Case History

Mrs. Border and her 3-year-old son, Phil, are seen at the pediatric genetics clinic. Shortly after birth, Phil was clinically diagnosed with achondroplasia; a targeted mutation analysis confirmed the diagnosis, showing that Phil is heterozygous for the common mutation p.G380R in the *FGFR3* gene. Since Mrs. Border wants to have additional children, she wishes to be informed of the chances of recurrence. Phil's physical examination reveals the typical findings of achondroplasia. Aside from frequent middle ear infections, Phil has been very healthy. He had mild muscular hypotonia at birth, which resolved with physical therapy by

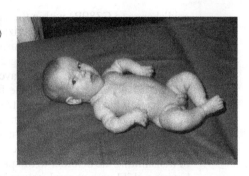

Figure 26.1. Achondroplasia in an 8-Month-Old Boy. (Courtesy of Universitäts-Kinderklinik Heidelberg.)

the age of 16 months. He was late to reach motor milestones (sat at 11 months and walked at 15 months), but his verbal and cognitive development have been completely normal. The family history is negative for achondroplasia or short stature. Mr. and Mrs. Border have no significant medical history, and they are both of normal height. Phil represents a de novo incidence of achondroplasia; the recurrence risk for additional children of his parents is small (less than 1%), owing to the possibility of either parent having germline mosaicism for the mutation.

Epidemiology

The prevalence of achondroplasia is approximately 1 in 20,000 individuals.

Clinical Symptoms

Disproportionate short stature is noticed **at birth**. Body size is mostly in the lower-normal range, while head circumference is in the upper normal range. Mild to moderate hypotonia is typically present during infancy, and the achievement of motor milestones is frequently delayed.

Craniofacial. All patients with achondroplasia have **relative macrocephaly**. The head appears large, with significant frontal bossing, and a relatively small cranial base (Fig. 26.1). Due to the growth defect of the cranial base, the foramen magnum and the venous outflow foramina are frequently too narrow, restricting cerebrospinal fluid circulation and occasionally causing **hydrocephalus**. **Midface hypoplasia** contributes to the typical facial features of achondroplasia and also predisposes the patient to recurrent otitis media.

Trunk/Extremities. The extremities are significantly shortened, especially the proximal parts (i.e., the upper arms and thighs), which is described as **rhizomelic short stature** (Section 35.1). The hands are broad, with short proximal and midphalanges and a **trident configuration**. There is ulnar deviation of the hands, incomplete extension of the elbows, and genu varum. Many children with achondroplasia have significant gibbus of the lower thoracic spine during infancy. Once they start walking, exaggerated lumbar lordosis develops. The most common complaint in adulthood is symptomatic spinal stenosis of L1–L4.

Development/Progression. Patients with achondroplasia have **normal intelligence**. Due to initial muscular hypotonia, most children are late in learning to sit and walk. The prognosis, however, is good since the hypotonia resolves over the course of the first 1 to 2 years. The disproportionate short stature, however, becomes more significant with time. This results in an average adult height of approximately 4 feet 3 inches (130 cm) in men and 4 feet 1 inch (125 cm) in women.

Genetics

Achondroplasia is an **autosomal dominant** disorder with 100% penetrance. It is caused by a defect of the **receptor for fibroblast growth factor 3** (**FGFR 3**), which controls the rate of cell division in the growth plates, particularly in the long bones. Achondroplasia is almost always caused by one of two different base changes (c.1138G>A or G>C) that cause the same amino acid change (p.G380R) within the transmembrane domain of the receptor. The mutation leads to a constitutional receptor dimerization, even without extracellular ligands (fibroblast growth factor [FGF]), consistent with a **gain-of-function** mutation. In 80% of the cases, this is caused by a new mutation; the remaining 20% are inherited from an affected parent. Parental germ cell mosaicism is rare. Studies have shown that de novo gene mutations for achondroplasia are exclusively inherited from the father. The chances of this occurring are associated with **advanced paternal age**, often defined as older than 35 years. After having one affected child, unaffected parents have a recurrence risk of 0.2%.

Patients with achondroplasia have no increased risk for infertility. Mothers with achondroplasia must deliver by C-section because of the small size of their pelvis. There is a 50% chance of transmitting the disorder to offspring. When both parents have achondroplasia, the chance of having a child with normal stature is 25%, of having a child with achondroplasia is 50%, and of having a child with homozygous achondroplasia (a typically lethal condition) is 25%.

▪▪▪ Hypochondroplasia

Hypochondroplasia is caused by heterozygous mutations of the *FGFR3* gene, different from the ones causing achondroplasia (mostly p.N540K). The clinical picture is similar, but the changes in hands and vertebral column are considerably milder, and the facial features do not vary much from unaffected family members. Adult height is between 4 feet 3 inches (130 cm) and 4 feet 11 inches (150 cm). Radiographs can help differentiate hypochondroplasia from achondroplasia.

▪▪▪ Thanatophoric Dysplasia

This severe clinical phenotype (Greek *thanatos*, "death") is also caused by certain dominant mutations of the *FGFR3* gene. Due to a massively narrowed bell-shaped thorax, most affected children die shortly after birth from respiratory insufficiency. With mechanical ventilation, it is possible to extend the life of an individual with thanatophoric dysplasia; however, the vast majority of physicians and ethicists agree that such treatment is futile and merely prolongs suffering and medical complications.

Diagnosis

Achondroplasia is diagnosed **clinically** and can be confirmed radiologically. Molecular genetic testing is usually not necessary to make the diagnosis, but it may be considered to confirm the diagnosis or to allow prenatal genetic testing for future pregnancies.

Therapy

- There is no causal therapy available. Growth hormone has been proposed as a treatment for short stature, and longitudinal studies to evaluate the usefulness of this approach are ongoing.
- Regular follow-up should occur with orthopedic surgery; otolaryngology and neurosurgery departments.
- A developing **hydrocephalus** needs to be monitored but rarely requires surgery, as it frequently resolves spontaneously. If symptomatic, a ventriculoperitoneal shunt is indicated.
- **Obstructive sleep apnea** may require adenotonsillectomy or continuous positive airway pressure (CPAP) by nasal mask.
- Due to adenoid growths, possibly in connection with midface hypoplasia, children with achondroplasia tend to have chronic or recurring otitis media. These should be treated consistently in order to prevent **conductive hearing loss**, which can lead to delayed speech development.
- **Suboccipital decompression** may be required if the narrow foramen magnum causes clinically significant compression of the medulla oblongata and spinal cord.
- **Spinal stenosis** is one of the most frequent complications in adulthood and may require decompression (most commonly at the L2-L3 level).

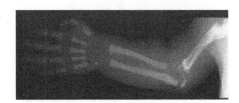

⬛ Figure 26.2. Rhizomelic Chondrodysplasia Punctata.
Shortening of the humerus with epiphyseal stippling.
(Courtesy of G.F. Hoffmann, Universitäts-Kinderklinik
Heidelberg.)

Chondrodysplasia Punctata

This term describes the radiologically visible small calcifications, especially in the cartilaginous epiphyses ("**epiphyseal stippling**") and in the vertebral column. This phenomenon, however, is unspecific and occurs in a great number of heritable and nonheritable disorders. The condition is associated with (mostly prenatal) disproportionate short stature.

The "classic" type of chondrodysplasia punctata is the X-linked **Conradi-Hünermann syndrome**. This disorder is caused by defects of the emopamil-binding protein (EBP) that, as 3β-hydroxysteroid-Δ8-Δ7-isomerase, catalyzes a reaction of sterol synthesis (Section 24.4). Conradi-Hünermann syndrome can be diagnosed by sterol analysis, which shows elevations of 8-dehydrocholesterol and 8(9)-cholestenol. The clinical picture includes shortening of the extremities, as well as scoliosis, cataracts, and various skin manifestations (e.g., linear and whorled atrophic and pigmentary lesions, striated hyperkeratosis, ichthyosis, and alopecia). The female-to-male ratio for Conradi-Hünermann syndrome is 5:1, and it has been suggested that mutations might be lethal when hemizygous; boys born with Conradi-Hünermann syndrome often are severely affected. The **rhizomelic type** (with shortening especially of the humeri and femora) of chondrodysplasia punctata is inherited in an autosomal recessive manner and is a peroxisomal disorder (⬛ Fig. 26.2; Section 24.8).

> **Important**
>
> **Warfarin Embryopathy**
> Warfarin use during pregnancy and a severe maternal vitamin K deficiency can induce a phenocopy of Conradi-Hünermann syndrome with identical skeletal changes, but without the manifestations in skin and hair.

26.3 Craniosynostoses

The term *craniosynostosis* signifies the premature closure of one or more cranial sutures. Diminished growth across the suture and increased growth along the suture can result in significant skull deformities. If, for example, the sagittal suture closes prematurely, cranial growth laterally is affected; the skull grows excessively long (frontally and occipitally). This results in dolichocephaly (long head). Craniosynostosis is recognized clinically from the characteristic skull deformity. Four important skull deformities and their underlying premature suture closures are represented in ⬛ Figure 26.3. Multiple synostoses can result in the clinically severe Kleeblattschädel (i.e., cloverleaf skull), with trilobed appearance of the skull. The prognosis is poor.

Craniosynostoses affect between 3 and 5 out of 10,000 neonates. Approximately 85% of cases are nonsyndromic, isolated cases, where the premature closure of the cranial suture is not associated with any additional morphological or functional symptoms. In 15% of cases, syndromic craniosynostoses with additional morphological and/or functional anomalies in the affected child occur. They are associated with primary genetic failure of the signaling system that governs the processes of growth and differentiation at the margins of the cranial sutures. Syndromic craniosynostoses are usually inherited as **autosomal dominant** traits.

If left untreated, skull deformity increases during the first years of life. Almost all types eventually result in **pansynostosis** (i.e., ossification of all cranial sutures). Aside from cosmetic (thus often social) problems, the insufficient cranial interior space (**craniostenosis**) can result in elevated intracranial pressure with the associated neurological complications. **Orbital stenosis**

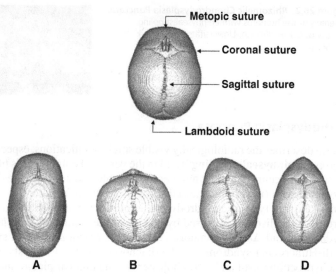

Metopic suture

Coronal suture

Sagittal suture

Lambdoid suture

A   B   C   D

▣ **Figure 26.3. Skull Deformities after Premature Closure of Cranial Sutures. A.** Dolichocephaly (long skull) after premature closure of the sagittal suture. **B.** Brachycephaly (short skull) after premature closure of the coronal suture. The skull can become relatively high (turricephaly). **C.** Plagiocephaly (oblique skull) after premature closure of the right coronal suture. **D.** Trigonocephaly (triangular skull) after premature closure of the frontal suture. (From Lentze et al. 2002.)

frequently results in exophthalmos, as well as optic nerve atrophy and blindness. Closure of the lambdoid suture can result in herniation of the brainstem and cerebellar tonsils into the foramen magnum and subsequent hydrocephalus.

Diagnostic evaluation involves cranial x-rays or computed tomography (CT) scans with three-dimensional reconstruction and an ophthalmological examination (funduscopic examination and evaluation for strabismus or field defects). A focused molecular genetic analysis based on the clinical picture may be indicated. **Treatment** is **neurosurgical** whenever craniosynostosis causes increased intracranial pressure. Consideration for cosmetic surgery depends on age of presentation and which sutures have fused prematurely. Molding helmets can be tried when surgery is not indicated. Surgery involves the opening of the calvaria by excision of the ossified suture. During the first year of life, the bone regenerates from the dura mater, while at later stages, the surgical defect may not be covered adequately by bone growth. Relapses are possible until 8 years of age.

■■■ **Fibroblast Growth Factors and Their Receptors**

FGFs are ubiquitously secreted signaling polypeptides that (assisted by FGF-binding proteins [FGFBPs]) activate cell surface tyrosine kinase receptors. FGF signaling has various biological functions, including mitogenesis and proliferation, angiogenesis, cellular differentiation, cell migration, and tissue-injury repair. The complex regulation of FGFs and FGFRs is reflected by the fact that, in humans, there are 22 FGF genes and 4 FGFR genes. Signaling is also mediated by alternative splicing of the immunoglobulinlike domain III of the FGFR protein; the "b" isoform of FGFR is expressed in epithelium and preferentially binds ligands secreted by adjacent mesenchyme, while the "c" isoform is expressed in mesenchyme and preferentially binds ligands secreted by adjacent epithelium. This mechanism avoids allowing FGFs to activate the cell that has secreted them (autocrine activation). Failure of this mechanism plays an important role in some of the FGFR-related disorders (i.e., Apert syndrome). The common mutations P253R and S252W in the *FGFR2* gene allow nonspecific binding of incorrect FGF molecules, which triggers inappropriate autocrine activation of the receptor.

Most craniosynostoses are caused by mutations in the **FGFRs 1 or 2** that trigger ligand-independent constitutional receptor activation. These mutations usually have a dominant gain-of-function effect; de novo mutations are frequent. Mutations of *FGFR3* typically result in defective growth of the long tubular bones (e.g., achondroplasia). The most important exception is mutation P250R in the *FGFR3* gene, which causes Muenke syndrome. Other important genes are *TWIST* (coding for a transcriptional regulator) and *EFNB1* (coding for the ligand of a receptor tyrosine kinase).

■■■ **Additional Fibroblast Growth Factor Receptor Mutations**

The proline-to-arginine mutations p.P252R in *FGFR1*, p.P253R in *FGFR2*, and p.P250R in *FGFR3* affect the exact same position in the linkage region between immunoglobulinlike domains II and III of the respective growth factor receptors. All three are frequent causes of craniosynostoses. Pfeiffer syndrome occurs in *FGFR1*, Apert syndrome in FGFR2, and Muenke syndrome in FGFR3 mutations. The clinical consequences of these mutations seem to be the result of similarly directed *gain-of-function* mutations that increase the binding affinity of specific ligands (fibroblast growth factors).

26.3.1 Craniosynostoses Due to Fibroblast Growth Factor Receptor Mutations

Crouzon Syndrome (Craniofacial Dysostosis)

With an incidence of 1 in 25,000, **Crouzon syndrome** is one of the more frequent craniosynostosis syndromes. It is usually caused by mutations in the immunoglobulinlike domain III of the **FGFR2 gene**. Clinical symptoms are limited to the head and neck. Premature closure of the coronal suture results in **brachycephaly** and **turricephaly**. Patients have a prominent forehead, hypertelorism with downslanting palpebral fissures, midface hypoplasia, and a beaked nasal bridge. Premature synostosis of the lambdoid suture results in **exophthalmus** and, in extreme cases, subluxations of the globe. **Pansynostosis** occurs relatively early (i.e., before the age of 4 years in three-fourths of cases). Patients with Crouzon syndrome have normal intelligence unless affected by complications from increased intracranial pressure.

Other Craniosynostoses

The craniofacial findings of **Pfeiffer syndrome** often resemble those of Crouzon syndrome, with additional broadening of the thumbs and great toes and variable cutaneous syndactylies of the fingers and toes. In most cases Pfeiffer syndrome is caused by mutations in the immunoglobulinlike domain III of the *FGFR2* gene (different from the ones causing Crouzon syndrome). Approximately 5% of the cases are caused by the mutation P252R in the *FGFR1* gene.

Apert syndrome is less frequent, but more severe, than other craniosynostoses (■ Fig. 26.4). In addition to the typical consequences of premature coronal suture synostosis (brachycephaly and turricephaly) and the typical facial features, affected children have severe syndactyly of the fingers and toes, and most patients manifest with intellectual disability even without elevated intracranial pressure. Apert syndrome is almost always caused by one of two mutations, S252W or P253R, in the *FGFR2* gene.

Muenke syndrome was first described in the late 1990s as a disorder caused by mutation P250R in the *FGFR3* gene. It is now considered the most frequent molecular genetically identifiable craniosynostosis (approximately 8% of all cases, including nonsyndromic craniosynostoses), yet it has a relatively mild clinical picture. Aside from the premature coronal suture synostosis, individuals may display discrete brachydactyly (short fingers) or (rarely) deafness.

26.4 Metabolic Bone Diseases

Familial Hypophosphatemic Rickets

Familial hypophosphatemic rickets, also called "vitamin D–resistant rickets," is the most frequent hereditary type of rickets. Incidence is 1 in 20,000 to 25,000 individuals. It is caused by mutations in the *PHEX* gene and inherited in an X-linked manner, with males typically

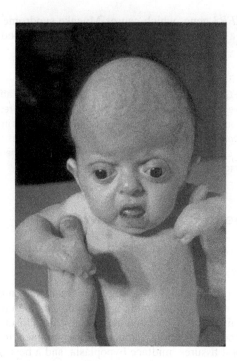

Figure 26.4. Apert Syndrome. (Courtesy of G.F. Hoffmann, Universitäts-Kinderklink Heidelberg.)

more severely affected than females. Impaired phosphate reabsorption in the proximal tubules of the kidney causes hypophosphatemia, and inadequate levels of inorganic phosphate impair the function of mature osteoblasts, resulting in **rickets and osteomalacia**. Affected children manifest with short stature, mostly between ages 2 and 3 years, with severe bowing of the weight-bearing bones. Important laboratory findings are low serum phosphate levels, in combination with normal calcium levels. Vitamin D metabolism is not affected. Therapy consists of 1,25-OH-vitamin D, phosphate replacement, growth hormone, and anticalciurics (such as thiazide diuretics). Differential diagnosis includes the rare autosomal recessive heritable form of **vitamin D–dependent rickets**, which is caused by a defective synthesis of active vitamin D or end-organ insensitivity.

Pseudohypoparathyroidism and Albright Hereditary Osteodystrophy

In contrast to hypoparathyroidism (HP), there is no parathyroid hormone deficiency in pseudo-hypoparathyroidism (PHP). Instead, there is **end-organ resistance** (of kidneys and skeleton) to parathyroid hormone. This results in **increased tubular phosphate reabsorption**, with hyperphosphatemia and simultaneous hypocalcemia due to decreased calcium mobilization from bones. PHP typically occurs in **Albright hereditary osteodystrophy** (AHO), a genetic syndrome with short stature, moderate obesity, short hands and feet (shortened metacarpals and metatarsals), and intellectual disability (average IQ 60). In addition to PHP, which is labeled **PHP type Ia**, endocrine disorders also include hypergonadotrophic hypogonadism and hypothyroidism. There are some patients with AHO **without** PHP, which is then labeled pseudopseudohypoparathyroidism (PPHP).

The complex links between AHO and PHP have only recently been elucidated. The key gene involved in the pathogenesis is *GNAS*, which utilizes multiple alternative promoters and splicing codes for several different proteins. The most important gene product is the α-subunit of a G protein (Gs alpha) that functions as a signal transduction protein for numerous hormonal and other receptors. The gene is **paternally imprinted** in the proximal renal tubules, as well as in the thyroid, pituitary, and ovaries; in those tissues, only the maternal gene copy is active.

Various mutations in *GNAS* result in distinct clinical manifestations:

- Heterozygous loss-of-function mutations on the **maternal** allele cause **PHP type Ia** (i.e., AHO plus resistance to parathyroid hormone, thyroid-stimulating hormone [TSH], and gonadotropin), since the paternal gene copy (e.g., in the kidneys) is inactive.
- Heterozygous loss-of-function mutations on the **paternal** allele cause AHO without PHP, labeled **PPHP**, or **progressive osseous heteroplasia**, which begins in early childhood with small ossifications of the skin and later involves other connective tissues.
- Paternal uniparental disomy of chromosome 20q13 causes **PHP type Ib**, which is characterized by parathyroid hormone resistance without AHO; familial types of this disorder are caused by mutations in the corresponding imprint center.
- Activating gain-of-function mutations of *GNAS* cause **McCune-Albright syndrome**, polyostotic fibrous dysplasia, and various endocrine tumors. These activating mutations are present in the mosaic state, resulting from a postzygotic somatic mutation in early embryonic development.
- The nonmosaic state of activating mutations of *GNAS* is presumably **prenatally lethal**.

■■■ G Proteins

G proteins (guanine nucleotide–binding proteins) are among the most important molecules of cellular signal transduction. As central second messengers, they transmit signals from receptors to subsequent effectors; their name refers to the fact that they utilize the switch between guanosine diphosphate (GDP) and guanosine triphosphate (GTP) as a signal mechanism. The large heterotrimeric proteins consist of three subunits: α, β, and γ. Each of these can be coded by different genes (13, 5, and 14 genes for α, β, and γ, respectively). For their research on G proteins, Gilman and Rodbell received the 1994 Nobel Prize for Medicine.

Inheritance of PHP type Ia depends greatly on the sex of the parent transmitting the mutation. If a father with PHP Ia or PPHP transmits his mutated allele, the affected offspring will develop PPHP. If, however, the same abnormal allele is transmitted by a mother with PHP Ia or PPHP, the offspring will develop PHP Ia.

Therapy for PHP Ia consists of the administration of active vitamin D, which normalizes serum calcium levels, and the oral application of enteric phosphate binders (e.g., calcium carbonate).

26.5 Congenital Multifactorial Skeletal Defects

Hip Dysplasia

See Section 5.6 for a discussion of this multifactorial heritable disease.

Clubfoot

Clubfoot (**talipes equinovarus, excavatus et adductus**) involves a defective positioning of the foot that cannot be passively corrected. The defect is complex and has four varieties: talipes equinus (downturned), varus (supinated), excavatus (high arched), and adductus (adducted). It is to be differentiated from positional clubfoot, which can be fully corrected either actively or passively.

Incidence is 2 to 3 per 1,000 newborns. **Males are affected twice as often as females**. Approximately 50% of the cases are bilateral. According to the degree of rigidity, the four types can be differentiated.

Clubfoot can be caused by exogenous, intrauterine factors (e.g., oligohydramnios) but also occurs with numerous (neuro-) genetic diseases. However, isolated clubfoot without known exogenous or genetic causes may be familial. Considering this a **multifactorial inheritance mechanism**, its recurrence risk is calculated on the basis of empirical data (i.e., a sporadic clubfoot has a recurrence risk of approximately 3% for subsequent siblings).

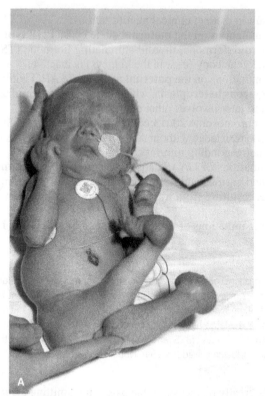
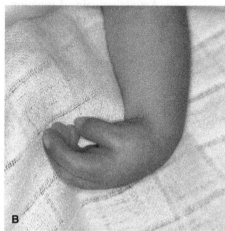

Figure 26.5. A, B. Arthrogryposis Multiplex Congenita. Note the absence of flexion creases in the hand **(B)**, indicating a defect in active movement that has been present since early embryonic development. (Courtesy of Universitäts-Kinderklink Heidelberg.)

Congenital Contractures/Arthrogryposes

The term *arthrogryposis multiplex congenita* describes multiple, nonprogressive contractures at the joints of extremities with or without spinal involvement (□ Fig. 26.5). The incidence in newborns is approximately 1 in 3,000. Arthrogryposis is caused by insufficient fetal movement (**fetal akinesia**), and it can be the only abnormality found or may be associated with an underlying disorder.

Classic arthrogryposis multiplex congenita (AMC, 30% of all cases), also called **amyoplasia**, is characterized by extensive lack of musculature; severe, nonprogressive contractures of all joints; typical posture of body and extremities; and a round face. The etiology of this condition seems to be mostly nongenetic; monozygotic twins are typically discordant. It is assumed that amyoplasia is caused by a generalized intrauterine circulatory defect during the development of the motor neurons of the anterior horns. The noninnervated muscle tissue is replaced by fibrous bands and fatty tissue. Intellectual development is normal; treatment is symptomatic (□ Fig. 26.6). The risk of recurrence is low (less than 1%).

The majority of cases of arthrogryposis multiplex, in which a diagnosis can be established, result from either **neurological disorders** (approximately 90%) or **genetic muscular diseases** (between 5% and 10%). Other causes may be severe **connective tissue disorders**, as well as **maternal disorders** (e.g., myasthenia gravis). The absence of flexion creases (e.g., at the fingers)

▣ **Figure 26.6. Arthrogryposis Multiplex Congenita.** Multiple joint contractures were evident at birth. Orthopedic therapy with splinting combined with vigorous physical therapy allows increased joint mobility and decreased muscle atrophy. (Photo courtesy of Rick Guidotti, www.positiveexposure.org.)

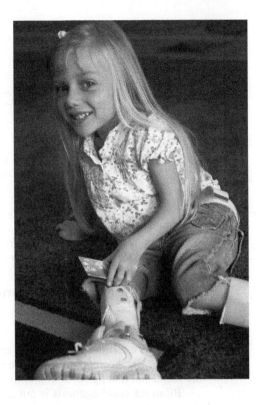

indicates that the respective joint has not been flexed since the first trimester. In the rarer cases of arthrogryposis, which result from **intrauterine space restriction** (oligohydramnios), the flexion creases are always present.

Numerous rare, monogenetic types of arthrogryposis have been identified. Among them are some that are autosomal dominant as well as several X-chromosomal heritable types. Sporadic cases that do not fit a specific disease picture have an empirical recurrence risk of 5%.

27 Urinary System

LEARNING OBJECTIVES

1 Describe the rationale for obtaining a renal ultrasound in females with Turner syndrome.

2 Identify five criteria that can help discriminate between autosomal dominant and autosomal recessive polycystic kidney disease.

3 Develop a five-point management plan for a 40-year-old patient with a new diagnosis of autosomal dominant polycystic kidney disease.

Malformations of the urinary system are frequent, accounting for **35% to 45% of all congenital anomalies**. In 72% of cases, there are other associated malformations. Renal defects have an incidence of 3 to 6 per 1,000 newborns.

27.1 Congenital Renal Anomalies

Renal Agenesis

Unilateral renal agenesis occurs in approximately 1 of every 1,000 newborns. It is caused by a developmental defect of the primitive ureter and the metanephrogenic blastema. Many cases are incidental findings of sonography.

   Bilateral renal agenesis is not compatible with extrauterine life. Incidence is about 1 of every 5,000 newborns. As the amniotic fluid consists mostly of fetal urine, the first manifesting symptom of fetuses with bilateral renal agenesis is typically severe oligohydramnios or anhydramnios, beginning at approximately 14 weeks of gestation. The oligohydramnios sequence results in multiple deformities of the fetus, also known as Potter sequence. It is to be noted that Potter sequence is not a specific result of bilateral renal agenesis but may have multiple etiologies (Section 13.3).

Horseshoe Kidney

Horseshoe kidney is the most frequent renal fusion anomaly (greater than 90% of cases). It is characterized by a parenchymal bridge at the inferior renal poles below the inferior mesenteric artery (□ Fig. 27.1). Horseshoe kidneys occur with a prevalence of approximately 1 in 500. Men are more frequently affected than women (male-to-female ratio, 2 to 3:1). In about 50% of cases, there are additional anomalies of the genitourinary tract (e.g., vesicoureteral reflux, ureteral duplication, urethral anomalies, and cryptorchidism).

> **Important**
>
> Congenital abnormalities of the urinary system and kidney occur in 30% to 40% of females with Turner syndrome. Horseshoe kidney is seen in approximately 10% to 15%.

27.2 Cystic Diseases of the Kidney

Autosomal Dominant Polycystic Kidney Disease

With an incidence of 1 in 1,000, autosomal dominant polycystic kidney disease (ADPKD) is considered to be one of the most frequent monogenic disorders. This is a **multisystem disorder**, as the cysts do not only occur in kidneys but also in the liver, seminal vesicles, pancreas, and arachnoid membranes. In addition, there are frequent vascular anomalies (intracranial aneurysms in approximately 10% of the cases, as well as aortic dilation and mitral valve prolapse).

Figure 27.1. Horseshoe Kidney in a Fetus with Trisomy 18.

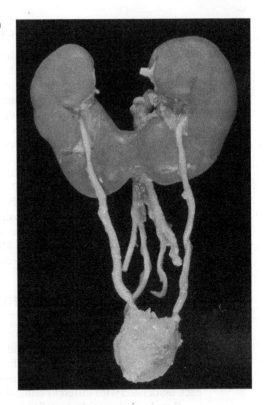

Clinical Symptoms. In most cases of ADPKD, renal cysts do not develop until adulthood. Typically, the **initial clinical manifestation** occurs **after 40 years of age**. Symptoms include abdominal and flank pain, macrohematuria, arterial hypertension, nephrolithiasis, and recurring urinary tract infections. In most cases, standard ultrasonography is diagnostic.

Frequent **complications** of ADPKD are cyst ruptures with macrohematuria, as well as bacterial infections of the renal cysts. Approximately 50% of all patients with ADPKD develop hypertension. Renal cell carcinoma does not occur more frequently in individuals with ADPKD than in the general population. Approximately half the patients with ADPDK have end-stage renal disease (ESRD) by the age of 60 years. Several mechanisms account for the decline in renal function. These mechanisms include compression of the normal renal parenchyma by expanding cysts, inflammation and fibrosis, and apoptosis of the tubular epithelial cells.

Genetics. Nearly 85% of cases of **autosomal dominant** polycystic kidney disease have a mutation in the *PKD1* **gene** on chromosome 16p, while the remaining 15% have a mutation in *PKD2* on chromosome 4q. The gene products are polycystin 1 and polycystin 2, respectively. A positive family history is found in 90% of all patients with ADPKD; the remaining 10% are *de novo* mutations. Patients with mutations in *PKD1* are usually more severely affected than patients with mutations in *PKD2* (younger age at diagnosis and earlier ESRD). The presence of a chromosomal deletion of 16p involving *PKD1* and *TSC2* explains the occurrence of both ADPKD and tuberous sclerosis in the same individual (Section 32.6) and is an example of a **contiguous gene syndrome**.

Therapy. Therapy for ADPKD is symptomatic or preventive with regard to complications. Good blood pressure control is considered critical, as this may delay development of ESRD. Hyperlipidemia is another correctable risk factor for ESRD. Screening for intracranial aneurysms by magnetic resonance angiography (MRA) or computed tomographic (CT) angiography is recommended for individuals with a positive family history of intracranial aneurysms.

Most individuals with polycystic liver disease have no symptoms and require no treatment.

Autosomal Recessive Polycystic Kidney Disease

Autosomal recessive polycystic kidney disease (ARPKD) is much rarer than ADPKD and has an estimated incidence of 1 in 20,000 to 1 in 40,000 newborns. The majority of patients manifest clinically either prenatally or in the perinatal period. Typically, affected individuals have bilateral flank masses at the time of birth, representing enlarged kidneys due to extreme dilatation of the collecting tubules (of note, macrocysts or cystic dysplasia are not features of this disorder, providing a diagnostic clue by ultrasonography). Approximately 30% of neonates with ARPKD die, typically due to respiratory insufficiency. Pulmonary hypoplasia is usually caused by severe oligohydramnios; however, pulmonary function is also affected by mechanical restriction of breath excursion due to the space-occupying cystic kidneys. More than 50% of children with ARPKD develop ESRD during the first decade of life. **Congenital hepatic fibrosis** is invariably present, yet it may not be clinically relevant in the neonatal period. Liver fibrosis frequently results in portal hypertension. Prognosis for patients with ARPKD depends on the severity of pulmonary complications during the neonatal period. Intensive medical care has increased the 1-year survival rate to 80% to 90%. ARPKD results from mutations in the gene *PKHD1* (*polycystic kidney and hepatic disease 1*).

27.3   Disorders of the Renal Tubular System

Bartter syndrome includes a group of autosomal recessive disorders that are characterized by hypokalemic metabolic alkalosis and hyperreninemic hyperaldosteronism. The cause of this disease is a defect in the tubular reabsorption of salt in the thick ascending part of the loop of Henle. Bartter syndrome can be caused by different transporter defects (six different genes), each associated with different clinical symptoms.

    Renal tubular acidosis (RTA) is a defect of acid-base metabolism that disrupts the kidney's ability to secrete H^+ ions (RTA type 1) into the distal tubule or to retain sufficient amounts of bicarbonate (RTA type 2) in the proximal tubule. This results in metabolic acidosis with hyperchloremia (**non-ion-gap acidosis**), bicarbonaturia, diminished excretion of titratable acids in urine, and elevated urinary pH. Metabolic acidosis results in calcium catabolism in the bones, nephrocalcinosis, and considerable growth retardation. Renal tubular acidosis can occur as an isolated disorder, as part of renal Fanconi syndrome, or within the context of numerous other diseases and disorders (e.g., in aldosterone deficiency or in chronic pyelonephritis). It is crucial that metabolic acidosis with RTA be treated with oral administration of bicarbonate. A timely correction of acidosis usually ensures that affected children grow to normal height.

28 Genital System and Sexual Development

LEARNING OBJECTIVES

1. Discuss how an individual's gender can be defined, and describe which different parameters are used in the process of gender assignment in a person.

2. Generate a list of physical and radiological examinations as well as laboratory tests that are indicated for the evaluation of a newborn with ambiguous genitalia.

There are three levels at which the sex of a person can be defined: chromosomal, gonadal, or anatomical. Based on the presence or absence of the Y chromosome, the chromosomal sex of the embryo is determined at the time of fertilization. Disorders that cause abnormal development of the gonads are sometimes called **sex determination disorders**, in contrast to **sex differentiation disorders**, where the gonads develop normally but the subsequent development of internal or external genitalia fails. Genital ambiguity occurs with an estimated frequency of up to 1%.

The key for determining the embryo's gonadal sex is the testis-determining factor (**TDF**) in the **SRY** region (sex-determining region of the Y) on the Y chromosome (Section 2.8). Sex-specific differentiation of the gonads starts between days 50 and 55 of embryonic development.

- With Y: In the presence of *SRY* and in concert with *SOX9*, which is downstream of *SRY*, Sertoli cells and Leydig cells develop, and the undifferentiated primordial gonads diverge toward testes organogenesis.

- Without Y: If the Y chromosome (or SRY) is absent or fails to act in time, the *SOX9* gene is silenced, and with the action of β-catenin, the gonadal balance is tipped toward ovarian development, proceeding with the action of ovarian determinants such as the *WNT4* and *FOXL2* genes.

The subsequent differentiation of the internal and external genitalia is normally determined by the action of **antimüllerian hormone** (AMH) produced by the testicular Sertoli cells, as well as **testosterone** and other androgens produced by the testicular Leydig cells.

- With testes: AMH triggers degeneration of all derivatives of the müllerian ducts (e.g., uterus, tubes, and upper vagina). Testosterone stabilizes the mesonephric ducts and promotes their differentiation to vasa deferentia, epididymis, and seminal vesicles. In the peripheral tissues, testosterone is metabolized by the enzyme 5α-reductase to **dihydrotestosterone**, which induces virilization of the external genitalia.

- Without testes: The absence of AMH allows the development of the Müllerian structures into Fallopian tubes, uterus, and upper vagina. Without testosterone, the Wolffian ducts regress, and the external genitalia remain female.

28.1 Disorders of Sex Development

Disorders of sex development (DSDs) are defined as congenital conditions in which the development of chromosomal, gonadal, or anatomical sex is atypical. While the traditional literature referred to individuals with abnormal sex development as "hermaphrodites," "pseudohermaphrodites," or "intersex patients," the current consensus is that the term *DSD* is more neutral, less pejorative, and a more accurate descriptor for these developmental disorders. Both the patient's karyotype and the radiological/physical/pathological examination of the patient's reproductive organs are used for the classification of DSD.

46,XX DSD: The chromosomal sex is female, but the external genitalia are ambiguous or male (abnormal virilization); testicles are absent. It is frequently caused by androgen excess.

46,XX testicular DSD: The chromosomal sex is female, but the external genitalia are male or ambiguous with palpable testicles. It is generally caused by the presence of the *SRY* gene on the X chromosome due to an Xp:Yp translocation.

46,XY DSD: The chromosomal sex is male, but the external genitalia are ambiguous (e.g., mild to severe penoscrotal hypospadias reflecting insufficient virilization); the gonads are underdeveloped (dysgenetic) with testicular elements. It is frequently caused by deficient androgen action.

46,XY gonadal dysgenesis: The chromosomal sex is male, but the anatomical sex is female with normal external genitalia, hypoplastic Müllerian structures, and fibrous streaks where ovaries would be expected. It is caused by mutations in *SRY* or other genes necessary for testes organogenesis.

Ovotesticular DSD: Both testes and ovarian tissues are present in the same individual (i.e., "true hermaphrodite" in the old nomenclature).

Gonadal Dysgenesis

An aberration in gonadal development can be caused by numerous genetic defects and does not necessarily cause abnormalities of the external genitalia. The most frequent causes of gonadal dysgenesis are sex chromosome aneuploidies, especially Turner syndrome (Section 19.1) and Klinefelter syndrome (Section 33.1). In the case of **Swyer syndrome**, the chromosomal sex is male, but gonadal differentiation to testes is abnormal (46,XY gonadal dysgenesis). This results in a female phenotype with nonfunctional streak gonads that have a high risk for malignancy. Between 15% and 20% of cases of pure XY gonadal dysgenesis are caused by mutations in the Y-chromosomal *SRY* gene. Mutations of other genes required for testes development have been identified; they are frequently associated with other syndromic features.

> **Important**
>
> **Malignant Transformation of Mixed Gonadal Tissue**
> Women with mixed gonadal tissue in Turner syndrome (with chromosomal mosaic 45,X/46,XY) or those with Swyer syndrome have a 15% to 35% risk for developing malignancy, especially gonadoblastoma, at a later stage. Gonadal tissue should therefore be removed before the age of 10 years.

XX Testicular Disorder of Sex Development

Development of testes in an individual with a female karyotype (46,XX testicular DSD) is most often caused by **translocations of *SRY* to an X chromosome**, which results from an uneven crossing-over between the pseudoautosomal regions of Yp and Xp in paternal meiosis. Inheritance is X linked; the clinical picture resembles Klinefelter syndrome. Affected men have small testes, sparse facial hair, and little body hair. Ambiguous genitalia may occur. One-third of affected individuals develop gynecomastia. Recently, there have been several case reports of males (infertile, but with otherwise normal virilization) who have a 46,XX and Y-negative chromosomal complement, indicating that genes other than *SRY* are important for sexual development in males.

Androgen Insensitivity Syndrome

The genetic deficiency of the nuclear **androgen receptor**, also called *testicular feminization*, is the most frequent cause of 46,XY DSD. Affected individuals have a male chromosomal sex (46,XY), normal testes with normal testosterone production, and normal peripheral production of dihydrotestosterone, but a female (or undervirilized male) physical appearance. Androgen insensitivity syndrome (AIS) is inherited as an X-chromosomal disorder and has an incidence of approximately 1 in 20.000. Nearly 70% of the mothers of affected girls are heterozygous mutation carriers, and in subsequent pregnancies these individuals have a 25% probability of having an affected daughter, a 25% probability of having a carrier daughter, a 25% probability of having an unaffected daughter, and a 25% probability of having an unaffected son.

The gender assignment for individuals with complete androgen insensitivity is **female**. No abnormalities are noted in the newborn or child; rather, medical attention is sought in early adolescence because of amenorrhea or suspected inguinal hernia (that turns out to be an inguinal testis). Women with complete AIS have sparse axillary and pubic hair; a shortened, blind-ending vagina; absence of the uterus; and bilateral intra-abdominal or inguinal testes. Gender identity is typically female. More than 300 mutations in the *AR* gene that cause variable functional effects have been reported. Depending on the activity of the androgen receptor, the phenotype and presentation can vary from infertility in an adult male (mild AIS) (Section 33.1), to undervirilized or ambiguous genitalia in a newborn (partial AIS), to primary amenorrhea in a young woman (complete AIS).

■■■ Gender Identity

Gender identity refers to a person's self-representation as male or female (with the caveat that some individuals may not identify exclusively with either). Perceived gender identity and behavioral differences between the sexes are transmitted to the brain through the direct effects of sex hormones. Animal studies (e.g., with animals of complete androgen resistance) indicate that normally functioning androgen receptors are necessary for "masculinization" of the brain.

Treatment. Therapy depends on the predominant external appearance and on the perceived gender identity of the affected individual. In cases of incomplete androgen resistance, virilization may be avoided if the testes are removed before puberty. Otherwise, the testes are left in situ until the end of puberty to allow normal development and progression of puberty. The risk of malignancy indicates subsequent gonadectomy, to be followed by cyclic estrogen administration.

Defects of Androgen Biosynthesis

A female phenotype with a male chromosome complement (46,XY DSD) also occurs in androgen synthesis defects. The most frequent is the autosomal recessive **5α-reductase deficiency**, where the endocrine function of the testes is normal and the androgen receptor is intact, yet the **peripheral cells** fail to convert testosterone to the many times more potent dihydrotestosterone. Most individuals with 5α-reductase deficiency are born with external genitalia that appear female but with a short, blind-ending vagina due to the regression of Müllerian structures. Ambiguous genitalia or undervirilized male genitalia (micropenis and hypospadias) are also seen in a portion of patients. During puberty, individuals with 5α-reductase deficiency develop increased muscle mass; undergo a deepening of the voice; develop pubic, facial, and body hair; show enlargement of the phallus; and have a growth spurt; however, secondary sexual characteristic development is markedly less than that expected for an unaffected male. Children with 5α-reductase deficiency are often raised as girls. About half of these individuals adopt a male gender role in adolescence or early adulthood. The diagnosis is typically made by the characteristic elevation of the testosterone/dihydrotestosterone ratio. Cultured fibroblasts from the perineal region can be studied for enzyme activity. Mutation analysis is also available.

Congenital Adrenal Hyperplasia

Congenital adrenal hyperplasia (CAH) is a genetic disorder of insufficient synthesis of cortisol and mineralocorticoids, as well as excessive synthesis of male sex hormones. It is the most frequent cause of 46,XX DSD. Actually, the vast majority of virilized 46,XX infants will have CAH. For a detailed discussion, see Section 25.2.

■■■ Differential Diagnosis for Ambiguous Genitalia
▬ Ambiguous genitalia, together with **additional anomalies** (e.g., congenital malformations), occur with heritable steroid biosynthesis defects (especially Smith-Lemli-Opitz syndrome) and other genetic syndromes (e.g., campomelic dysplasia).
▬ In the absence of additional morphological anomalies, the probable diagnosis depends on the karyotype:
  ▬ 46,XX: Congenital adrenal hyperplasia or exogenous androgen administration
  ▬ 46,XY: Androgen insensitivity syndrome, defects of androgen biosynthesis

28.2   Genital Malformations

Hypospadias

Hypospadias refers to a defective opening of the urethra on the ventral aspect of the penis (❑ Fig. 28.1). Its frequency is estimated at 0.5% of all male newborns. According to where the opening occurs, glandular, penile, penoscrotal, scrotal, and perineal types of hypospadias can be differentiated. Etiology is usually considered multifactorial. Hypospadias can be considered the very minimal form of ambiguous genitalia. Therefore, one should always look for associated malformations.

Epispadias

In this very rare defect (1 in 30,000) the urethra opens on the dorsal aspect of the penis. Usually, epispadias occurs with a split urethra and bladder exstrophy. In bladder exstrophy, the anterior wall of the bladder extends through an abdominal wall defect, exposing the posterior wall of the bladder.

Undescended Testicle

This is a developmental defect where (unilaterally or bilaterally) the testicle does not completely descend into the scrotum. The following types can be differentiated:
▬ **Cryptorchidism:** Nonpalpable testes reside in the abdominal cavity.
▬ **Testicular ectopia:** Normal descent occurs, but to an abnormal location (e.g., femoral or suprapubic locations).
▬ **Canalicular testis:** The testicle is located above its natural position in the scrotum but still outside the abdominal cavity.
▬ **Retractile testis:** The testis moves between the scrotum and lower inguinal canal. This is considered normal in prepubertal boys.

Undescended testicles are seen in 4% to 5% of all male newborns. In most cases, there is a spontaneous descent during the first year of life. If this does not happen, treatment should be initiated, which can be hormonal (human chorionic gonadotropin [hCG] injections, sometimes

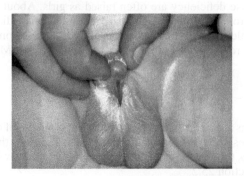

❑ **Figure 28.1. Third-Degree Hypospadias.**

in combination with gonadotropin-releasing hormone [GnRH]) or surgical (orchidolysis and orchidopexy).

It is assumed that undescended testicles result from insufficient prenatal androgen secretion. This is typically idiopathic, but also seen in defects of androgen synthesis and androgen receptors.

Malformations of Female Genitalia

Septations and duplications of female genitalia are frequent (estimated incidence is 1% to 3%) and result from the insufficient fusion of the caudal segments of the Müllerian ducts. One of the most frequent anomalies is bicornate uterus; in extreme cases, there is a duplex uterus with a common vagina. Another group of defects results from complete or partial atresia of one or both Müllerian ducts. Morphological malformations of female genitalia are always to be considered in the differential diagnosis of female sterility.

29 Visual System

LEARNING OBJECTIVES

1 Explain how nonallelic homologous recombination (NAHR) can cause defects of red–green color perception, and describe why men are more frequently affected than women.

2 Discuss the differential diagnosis of bilateral cataracts in a 2-week-old neonate.

3 Summarize the clinical and ophthalmoscopic findings of retinitis pigmentosa, and name at least three genetic causes of this clinical appearance.

29.1   Congenital Defects of Color Vision

Congenital defects of color vision are grouped into three major categories:
- Defects of red or green perception (◻ Fig. 29.1)
- Defects of blue–yellow perception
- Total color deficiency (achromatopsia)

Also to be differentiated are color vision weaknesses (e.g., prot**anomaly** indicates red weakness) from color blindness (e.g., prot**anopia** indicates red blindness). By far, the most frequent color vision disorders involve X-chromosomal heritable defects of the genes that code for the red-perceiving pigment and the green-perceiving pigment. Their cumulative prevalence is 3% to 9% in men and 0.4% in women (depending on ethnic origin). The most frequent defect in this group is deuteranomaly (green weakness), with an incidence of 4% to 5% among men.

Defects of Red and Green Perception. Located on the distal long arm of the X chromosome (Xq28) is a sequence of several homologous genes that code for the visual pigments of red and green cones. The genes are 98% identical, while their structures differ only by a 1.3-kb insertion in intron 1 of the gene for the red cone pigment. The first gene in the sequence codes for red cone pigment (*OPN1LW [opsin 1 long wave sensitive]*) and always occurs once, while the number of the subsequent *OPN1MW* genes for green cone pigment (*opsin 1 medium wave sensitive*) is variable; approximately 50% of X chromosomes have three, while 5% have five or more *OPN1MW* genes. Only the first two genes of this sequence are expressed, as controlled by a locus control region (LCR). Due to functional polymorphisms, the spectral sensitivity of the range of normal color perception varies between different normal individuals. Severe deficiencies of red or green perception occur due to deletions resulting from an **unequal crossing over** (nonallelic homologous recombination [NAHR]) between the different cone pigment genes. Due to the complex sequence variability, the phenotype in the deficiencies of either the red- or the green-perceiving systems is also highly variable. In the case of the very rare **blue cone monochromacy** (e.g., through an LCR deletion), both red and green cone function are absent, resulting in a severe defect in both color perception and central acuity. If only the red cone pigment or only the green cone pigment is altered or defective, color perception is altered, but visual acuity is normal. All of these deficiencies follow **X-chromosomal inheritance**. Approximately 15% of all women are carriers for deficiencies of either red or green color defects. If an unfavorable X inactivation occured, a heterozygous female would have defects in red or green perception.

Other Color Vision Defects. Deficiencies of **blue vision** are much rarer than deficiencies of red or green perception. The gene that codes for the blue cone is located on chromosome 7 (*opsin 1 short wave sensitive*). The prevalence of tritanopia (blue color deficiency) is estimated at 1 in 500 individuals. All reported cases have had missense mutations in the *OPN1SW* gene. The inheritance of this disorder is autosomal dominant with variable expressivity. The rare **complete achromatopsia** (autosomal recessive inheritance) is due to deficiencies of the intracellular signaling pathways of cone phototransduction.

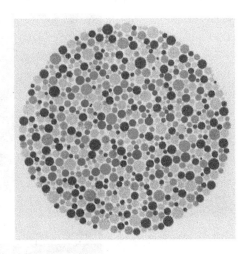

Figure 29.1. Ishihara Color Test for Red–Green Color Deficiencies. Persons with normal color vision see the number 26. (From Grehn, 2006.)

> **Important**
>
> Deficiencies of red or green cone pigments are inherited in X-chromosomal fashion. The deficiency of blue cone pigment is inherited in autosomal dominant fashion.

29.2 Cataracts

With a prevalence of 90% in older individuals, **senile cataract** is the most frequent type of cataract. Numerous causes for this disorder exist; twin studies have shown that genetic factors are important. Human genetics differentiates between the four major types of lens clouding:
- Isolated hereditary congenital cataract (i.e., unassociated with any extraocular defects)
- Cataract as part of a congenital ocular disorder
- Cataract as part of a more generalized genetic syndrome
- Cataract as part of a metabolic disorder

Congenital cataracts account for approximately 10% of the cases of childhood visual impairment. One in 250 newborns has a congenital cataract, which is not always clinically significant.
- Numerous genes whose mutations cause **isolated hereditary congenital cataracts** have been identified. Many autosomal dominant heritable types of congenital cataract are due to **gene defects of crystallin proteins**.
- Cataracts as part of **congenital ocular disorders** occur in (or in association with) aniridia, microcornea, microphthalmia, and other disorders.
- Cataracts are signs of some **monogenic disorders**: **myotonic dystrophy**, neurofibromatosis type 2, all progeria syndromes, pseudohypoparathyroidism, and many others. Congenital cataracts also occur with **chromosomal aberrations**, among them trisomy 13 and trisomy 18. Between 10% and 15% of children with trisomy 21 develop cataract, some of them as early as 6 months of age.
- Important differential diagnoses for cataracts occurring at an early age are the following **metabolic disorders**: **galactosemia** (Fig. 29.2), diabetes mellitus ("snowflake cataract"), peroxisomal disorders (e.g., chondrodysplasia punctata, Zellweger syndrome, and Refsum disease), Smith-Lemli-Opitz syndrome, Wilson disease ("sunflower cataract"), Fabry disease, and glucose-6-phosphate dehydrogenase deficiencies.

> **Important**
>
> Galactosemia should be considered in the differential diagnosis if a cataract, especially a central nuclear cataract, develops in the first week of life.

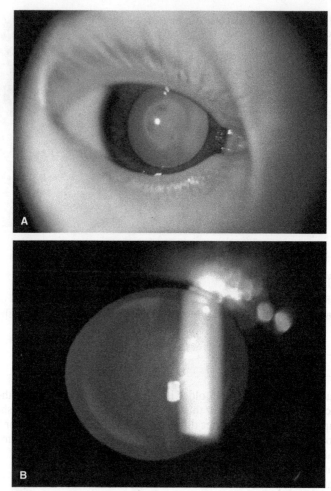

□ Figure 29.2. Cataract in an Infant with Galactosemia. A. In an infant with galactosemia, the early change in the lens is a condensation of the nucleus, creating an "oil-droplet" distortion centrally, which is more easily visualized when the pupil is dilated. **B.** Later, if the disorder is not treated, the nucleus becomes opaque, as the cells in its margins die and create spokelike changes. Eventually, the entire lens turns white. (Courtesy of Richard A. Lewis, Baylor College of Medicine, Houston, TX.)

29.3   Blindness

The estimated prevalence for childhood blindness is 30 to 100 per 100,000 individuals. The majority of cases are congenital (approximately 90%); blindness at a later stage of childhood or in adulthood occurs much less frequently. The following paragraphs list several human, genetically relevant causes of congenital or acquired blindness.

Retinitis Pigmentosa

The term *retinitis pigmentosa* refers to an ophthalmological finding and is not a specific diagnosis. More than 75 different ocular and constitutional disorders may have retinitis pigmentosa associated with them. These include, but are not limited to, deficiencies of the mitochondrial or peroxisomal energy metabolism and an entire group of isolated heritable disorders of either the retinal pigment epithelium or photoreceptors whose common characteristics are progressive degeneration of retinal pigment epithelium, pigment migration in macrophages into the neuroepithelium, night blindness, reduction of the peripheral visual field, and ultimately loss of central visual acuity. The cumulative frequency in most studied populations is 1 in 3,500 individuals.

Clinical Relevance. Most affected individuals notice difficulties seeing in relatively low light (night blindness is referred to as nyctalopia). Later, the visual field progressively narrows until only a small, central field of vision remains (e.g., tunnel vision). At this point, spatial orientation is extremely difficult. Different types of retinitis pigmentosa progress at different speeds. The benefit of **dietary treatment** (e.g., with vitamin A, vitamin E, or docosahexanoic acid [DHA]) remains controversial.

Retinal Findings. Retinal examination reveals characteristic mottling of retinal pigment epithelium with migration of pigment into the retina within macrophages. Due to the shape of some of those deposits, these are described as "bone spicules". Other ophthalmoscopic features include pigmented cells in the vitreous, attenuation (i.e., narrowing) of the retinal vessels, waxy pallor of the optic nerve, and occasionally cystoid macular edema (◻ Fig. 29.3).

Genetics. Retinitis pigmentosa manifests a considerable **genetic heterogeneity** (i.e., defects in many different genes cause the same clinical appearance). Approximately 50% of patients with retinitis pigmentosa have a positive family history. Between 30% and 50% of these are autosomal dominant, 10% to 40% are autosomal recessive, and 10% to 30% are of X-chromosomal inheritance. A substantial fraction of the autosomal dominant cases are caused by mutations in the *RHO* gene that codes for the visual pigment **rhodopsin**.

Syndromic Types. Between 20% and 30% of cases of retinitis pigmentosa occur as part of an underlying syndrome. The most frequent syndromic types (10% to 20% of all cases) are the **Usher syndromes**, which additionally manifest moderate to severe bilateral hearing loss and vestibular dysfunction; the hearing impairment invariably precedes the onset of the retinal disease. Thirteen different genes have been associated with Usher syndromes. They all follow autosomal recessive inheritance. The **Bardet-Biedl syndromes** (BBSs, approximately 5% of all cases of retinitis pigmentosa) additionally manifest obesity, polydactyly, hypogenitalism, structural and functional renal disorders, and intellectual disability. Mutations have been identified in at least 14 different genes that cause the same phenotype, each of which is transmitted in an autosomal recessive manner. In about 15% of individuals, mutations in two different genes at different BBS loci may result in the clinical phenotype, called digenic triallelic inheritance. Among the rare yet potentially **treatable** variants of retinitis pigmentosa are abetalipoproteinemia, Refsum disease, and familial vitamin E deficiency.

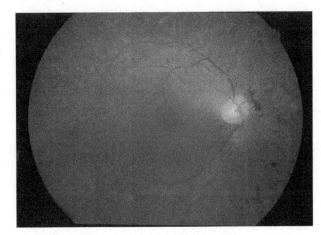

◻ **Figure 29.3. Retinitis Pigmentosa.** Note mottling of the retinal pigment epithelium, dark pigment deposits, and attenuated vessels. (Courtesy of Richard A. Lewis, Baylor College of Medicine, Houston, TX.)

Retinoblastoma

Retinoblastoma is a genetically caused malignant tumor of the retina. After choroidal melanoma, it is the second most frequent primary tumor of the eye and the most common ocular malignancy in children. The clinical presentation and genetic mechanisms leading to retinoblastoma are discussed in more detail in Section 32.2.

Leber Hereditary Optic Neuropathy

Leber hereditary optic neuropathy (LHON), first described by Theodor Leber in 1871, is inherited maternally through mutations in the mitochondrial DNA. It typically affects young men between the ages of 15 and 35 years and results in an acute to subacute progressive neuropathy of the optic nerve with a large irreversible central scotoma. A discussion of this disorder, in the context of mitochondrially heritable diseases, is found in Section 5.5.

X-Linked Juvenile Retinoschisis

Mutations of the retinoschisin-coding gene *RS1* on the distal tip of chromosome Xp cause X-linked juvenile retinoschisis, one of the more frequent causes of juvenile macular degeneration. The disorder is characterized by bilateral schisis (i.e., splitting of the nerve fiber layer of the retina), which causes deterioration of visual acuity during the first decade of life. The retinal examination shows radial striations (spoke-wheel pattern) and cystic lesions. The estimated prevalence of X-chromosomal juvenile retinoschisis depends on the ethnic background; in some countries (e.g., Finland) it is up to 1 in 15,000 individuals. About half of cases have peripheral retinoschisis that can become so extensive that inner and outer retinal holes lead to retinal detachment.

30 Auditory System

LEARNING OBJECTIVES

1 Distinguish various classifications of hearing loss, and elaborate on how those can help narrow down the differential diagnosis.

2 Name at least four genetic syndromes that can present with hearing loss, and identify associated clinical findings for each syndrome.

In the general population, the prevalence of hearing loss increases with age, from 1 in 1,000 at the time of birth to between 1 in 4 and 1 in 3 at the age of 65 years, reflecting the impact of genetics and the environment, as well as the interaction between an individual's genetic predisposition and environmental triggers. Hearing loss is described by type (e.g., conductive, sensorineural, or combined), associated symptoms (e.g., syndromic or nonsyndromic), and time of onset (e.g., prelingual or postlingual). If deafness occurs before the age of 7 years, the previously acquired speech is mostly lost. This is defined as **prelingual hearing loss**. Beginning at the age of 7 years, however, the acoustic memory for speech remains. This is called **postlingual hearing loss**. Hereditary hearing loss can be of an autosomal recessive, autosomal dominant, X-linked, or maternal (mitochondrial) inheritance.

30.1 Hereditary Hearing Loss

Of all cases of congenital hearing loss, approximately 50% are considered genetic, whereas the other 50% are considered environmental or idiopathic. As for the genetic causes of congenital hearing loss, mutations in several hundred genes have been identified. It is helpful to differentiate between the syndromic types (30%) and nonsyndromic types (70%) of congenital hearing loss. Most genetic causes of nonsyndromic hearing loss follow **autosomal recessive** inheritance, and the most frequent identifiable genetic cause is a homozygous mutation of the **connexin 26** – coding *GJB2* gene. The carrier rate for hearing loss–associated *GJB2* mutations in the general population is approximately 3%. Another recessive, heritable type of deafness is caused by mutations of the *GJB6* gene, which codes for connexin 30.

> **Important**
>
> **Genetic Heterogeneity of Hereditary Hearing Loss**
> Hereditary hearing loss is characterized by considerable **heterogeneity**. Therefore, it is possible—if not more likely—that parents who both have an autosomal recessive type of hearing loss have children with normal hearing. If, for example, the father is homozygous for a mutation of the *GJB2* gene and the mother is homozygous for a mutation of the *GJB6* gene, all the children from this relationship will be heterozygous for the mutation of *GJB2* and heterozygous for the mutation of *GJB6*. In theory, none of these children will have congenital deafness.

Less frequent are cases of autosomal dominant, nonsyndromic hearing loss or cases of syndromal hearing loss. ◻ Figure 30.1 offers an overview of the causes of prelingual hearing loss.

Examples of Syndromic Hearing Loss

— **Waardenburg syndrome:** Congenital sensorineural hearing loss with various degrees of severity; pigmentary anomalies of hair, iris, and skin (most typical involves a white forelock and heterochromia of the iris); and dystopia canthorum (lateral displacement of the inner canthi of the eyes). It is of autosomal dominant inheritance.

— **Neurofibromatosis type 2:** Bilateral tumors of the eighth cranial nerve (vestibular schwannomas) with hearing loss. The average age of onset is between 18 and 24 years, with autosomal dominant inheritance (Section 32.6).

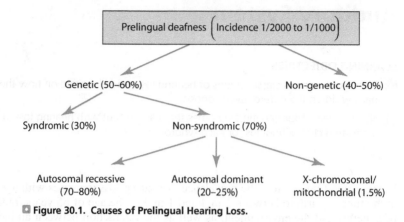

Figure 30.1. Causes of Prelingual Hearing Loss.

- **Crouzon syndrome:** Craniosynostosis syndrome (Section 26.3). Conductive hearing loss occurs in more than 50% of the cases. This is partially due to complete atresia of the external acoustic meatus; it involves autosomal dominant inheritance.
- **Usher syndrome:** Autosomal recessive congenital sensorineural hearing loss **plus** development of retinitis pigmentosa beginning in the second decade of life (Section 29.3).
- **Pendred syndrome:** Congenital hearing loss **plus** euthyroid goiter (mostly in adolescence and later), resulting from defective iodine binding in the thyroid gland.
- **Alport syndrome:** Variable sensorineural hearing loss **plus** progressive renal failure due to glomerulonephropathy. Most cases involve X-chromosomal inheritance.

30.2   Environmental Factors of Deafness

Important differential diagnoses of congenital deafness are prenatal infections with pathogens of the TORCH spectrum (**to**xoplasmosis, **r**ubella, **c**ytomegalovirus, and **h**erpes). Bacterial meningitides are etiologically significant in hearing loss of postnatal onset. The acquired hearing loss in adults is largely attributed to environmental influences (especially long-lasting noise exposure to more than 90 dB [A]), but susceptibility to such hearing loss, again, is a combination of genetic predisposition and environmental factors. As an example, a variant in the mitochondrial 12S ribosomal RNA (A→G at position 1555 of mitochondrial DNA) increases the risk for acquired hearing loss when exposed to aminoglycoside therapy.

31 Neurological and Neuromuscular Disorders

LEARNING OBJECTIVES

1 Formulate a plan on how to counsel and test a presymptomatic individual at risk for Huntington disease.

2 Compose a table indicating how deletions and copy numbers of *SMN1* and *SMN2* influence the clinical phenotype of spinal muscular atrophy.

3 Name at least six characteristics necessary to make the clinical diagnosis of Rett syndrome.

4 Sketch a pedigree of a family with CAG repeat expansion in the 5′ untranslated region (UTR) of the *FMR1* gene, discuss the various clinical phenotypes that might be present, and explain the phenomenon of maternal anticipation based on your pedigree.

5 Discuss three different treatment options for individuals with Duchenne muscular dystrophy.

31.1 Neurodegenerative Disorders of the Central Nervous System

Neurodegenerative disorders are characterized by a progressive loss of structure and function of neurons. Among this large group of disorders are several that were already mentioned in Chapter 24 (neurometabolic disorders). In lysosomal storage diseases, for example, the accumulation of certain metabolites causes degeneration and premature loss of neurons and/or white matter in the central and peripheral nervous system. A particular characteristic of neurodegenerative disorders in childhood is **developmental regression**: after a period of seemingly normal age-appropriate psychomotor development, the child ceases to develop further, and previously learned abilities are eventually lost.

Many neurodegenerative disorders affect primarily the gray matter of the brain, resulting in neuronal loss with behavioral changes, seizures, and dementia as early symptoms. The **leukodystrophies** are clinically, pathophysiologically, and neuroradiologically distinct, as they primarily affect the white matter (Greek *leukos*, "white") and are distinguished by an early involvement of the motor system (with its long nerve fibers). Spasticity, paresis, and ataxia occur early on, whereas seizures and dementia occur as later symptoms of leukodystrophies.

31.1.1 Basal Ganglia Diseases

Parkinson Disease

Clinically, Parkinson disease is characterized by the cardinal symptoms of resting tremor, bradykinesia, rigidity, and increasing dysfunction of postural reflexes. Pathophysiologically, it is considered the result of functional loss of the dopaminergic systems of the brain. The etiology of Parkinson disease is complex, multifactorial, and not completely understood. In most cases, the disease occurs sporadically, yet 10% to 30% of all parkinsonism patients have a positive family history for Parkinson disease. Families with autosomal dominant heritable types of Parkinson disease have been described.

Several Parkinson disease–associated genes have been identified, among them *SNCA*, which codes for the protein **α-synuclein** and is associated with autosomal dominant parkinsonism. α-Synuclein is a competitive inhibitor of the enzyme tyrosine hydroxylase, which catalyzes the synthesis of L-DOPA from tyrosine. Several different types of *SNCA* mutations have been described, including missense mutations, duplications, and triplications of the gene. Median age of onset of Parkinson disease, secondary to *SNCA* mutations, is approximately 45 years.

Mutations in *PINK1*, *DJ1*, and *PARK2* each are responsible for autosomal recessive Parkinson disease. In many cases, these occur in early to midadulthood (typically between the ages of 20 and 40 years). Mutations (mostly point mutations) in *PARK2* are responsible for up to 50% of all juvenile familial cases of Parkinson disease, as well as 18% of all sporadic cases that occur before the age of 50 years. *PARK2* codes for **parkin**, an important component of the intracellular ubiquitin–proteasome complex.

Identifying familial cases of Parkinson disease and clarifying the underlying molecular defects have significantly contributed to an improved pathophysiological understanding of the disease while also making it possible to develop new therapeutic strategies.

Huntington Disease (Huntington Chorea)

Huntington chorea is the first disease whereby genetic analysis was used for asymptomatic individuals who were at risk in order to predict their neurological fate. It continues to be one of the most prominent examples of **predictive** testing in the absence of curative therapeutic options.

Case History

A 40-year-old mother seeks genetic counseling with her 13-year-old son Kevin. She is extremely concerned that her son may one day show signs of Huntington disease, because the boy's father has the disease. She requests molecular genetic testing for Kevin so she will know for certain. She separated from her husband when, at the age of 45 years, he became increasingly aggressive and erratic. After the separation, the husband was hospitalized with severe psychosis. Later he developed choreiform movements and dementia and is now completely dependent, living in a chronic health care facility.

After Kevin's grandfather was diagnosed with Huntington disease, Kevin's father opted for molecular genetic testing, which confirmed the diagnosis for him as well (45 repeats). Kevin has developed appropriately for his age and has a normal neurological examination. In the counseling session, the mother and son are informed of the clinical presentation and natural course of the disorder. The genetics of the disease and the ethical challenges of presymptomatic testing are discussed. They are told that consensus holds that asymptomatic individuals younger than 18 years should not have testing. Testing before age 18 years not only raises the possibility of stigmatization but also can have serious educational and career implications. It is recommended that Kevin has another counseling session after he reaches the age of 18 years.

Epidemiology

The incidence in Western Europe is approximately 1 in 20,000 individuals. It appears less frequent in Japan, China, and Finland and among African blacks. Men and women are equally affected.

Clinical Symptoms and Progression

Carriers for Huntington disease are almost always asymptomatic in childhood and adolescence. The **age of onset for the disease** is typically between 30 and 50 years, with a **peak around 45 years**. Only in 5% to 10% of the cases does the disease manifest before age 20 years.

The **classic triad** of symptoms for Huntington diseases includes:
— Movement disturbances (especially extrapyramidal motor symptoms)
— Cognitive disturbances (including dementia)
— Psychiatric abnormalities

Often the disease begins with increasing clumsiness, agitation, and irritability. Family members report personality changes with morose and depressive moods. In most cases, close examination of the patient reveals early signs of movement disorders, which the patient typically tries to hide or integrate into motion sequences. This is especially true for the **involuntary grimacing** of facial muscles.

> **Important**
>
> There is significant danger of suicide, especially during the early stages of the disease, due to depressive moods.

Motor Disturbances. The name *Huntington chorea* refers to the most conspicuous characteristic of this disease (i.e., the typical choreiform movements). These are jerky, typically brief and abrupt **involuntary movements,** initially in the face and upper extremities, that cannot be controlled. In the extremities, these movements include sweeping, swinging, and sometimes writhing movements. Sometimes hyperkinesis begins unilaterally and later extends to the other side. As the disease progresses, there are increasing abnormalities of voluntary movements and abnormal eye movements. Rapidly alternating movements are often limited (**dysdiadochokinesis**). Speech becomes dysarthric (i.e., increasingly incomprehensible and choppy). Over time, patients develop **dysphagia**, because chewing muscles and the tongue are in constant dysfunctional motion. At the later stages, there is considerable weight loss, incontinence, and the inability to speak.

Psychiatric Disturbances. Among the early psychiatric changes is depression, often with suicidal ideations. The type and extent of personality change, however, depend largely on the primary personality prior to disease onset. Introverted patients tend toward depression, whereas extroverted individuals tend to be more aggressive and uninhibited (e.g., hypersexual behaviors). These patients can be very irritable, difficult to live with, and, in some cases, so uninhibited that they commit violent crimes. Additional symptoms include delusions (e.g., paranoia and manic jealousy) and hallucinations, as well as paranoid psychoses, taken together as **choreophrenia**.

Cognitive Disturbances. Learning, attention, and memory are increasingly affected as the disease progresses. **Slowing down of thought processes** and comprehension defects are frequent. Over time, there is manifest **dementia**. In contrast to many Alzheimer patients, those suffering from Huntington disease are mostly aware of their cognitive losses.

Genetics and Etiology

Huntington disease is one of the very few **autosomal dominant** heritable diseases for which the manifestation of the disease does not significantly differ for homozygous and heterozygous carriers (**complete phenotypic dominance**). The time of onset of the disease is the same; the only difference is that homozygous patients progress somewhat faster. New mutations are extremely rare; a lack of family history of the disease is usually due to missing clinical data or the early death of family members.

The disease results from the **expansion of a polyglutamine sequence (CAG)$_n$** in the coding sequence (5′ gene region) of the *HTT* **gene** on chromosome 4p16.3, which codes for the protein **huntingtin**. Individuals with 10 to 35 CAG repeats have no disease risk. In the case of 27 to 35 repeats, however, a repeat expansion can occur in the germ line, so that children may be affected by the disease (premutation). Individuals with 36 to 39 repeats may or may not develop symptoms of Huntington disease (incomplete penetrance). Beginning with 40 CAG repeats, all affected individuals will develop Huntington disease. There is an inverse correlation between the number of repeats and the age of onset of the disease; the higher the number of repeats, the earlier the onset. It is impossible, however, to predict the age of onset in individual cases.

The extended (CAG) repeat, not the normal allele, is unstable during meiosis, especially during spermatogenesis. Anticipation, the phenomenon in which increasing disease severity or decreasing age of onset is observed in successive generations, is known to occur in Huntington disease, and it takes place more commonly in paternal transmission of the mutated allele (paternal anticipation). Patients who inherit the diseased allele from the father should anticipate an earlier onset of the disease. *De novo* mutations have not been described.

Neuropathology

Neuropathological features include the selective degeneration of neurons in the **corpus striatum** (caudate nucleus, putamen) and subthalamic nucleus. Most affected neurons are medium sized and produce specific neurotransmitters (γ-aminobutyric acid [GABA] and enkephalin or "substance P"). Atrophy of the **corpus striatum** can be seen postmortem and may manifest on magnetic resonance imaging (MRI) as enlarged lateral ventricles. In advanced stages, the entire brain is often **atrophic**. This results in hydrocephalus ex vacuo, with expansion of the lateral ventricles, widened sulci, and considerably atrophic gyri. The entire cerebral mass is reduced.

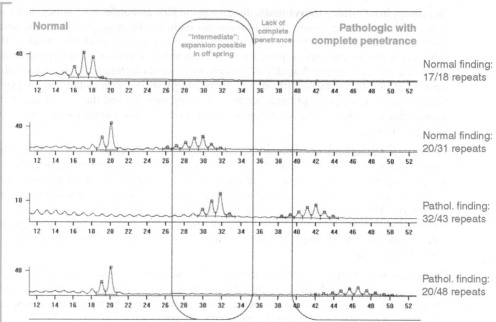

Figure 31.1. Molecular Genetic Diagnostics in Huntington Disease. The generally fast and reliable process of fragment length analysis on the sequencing apparatus shows repeat sizes on both alleles. (Courtesy of B. Janssen, Institut für Humangenetik Heidelberg.)

Diagnosis

In symptomatic patients, the diagnosis of Huntington disease is made **clinically**, based on the disease picture, the progression, and positive family history. Molecular diagnostics with detection of the typical CAG repeat expansion in the *HTT* gene (polymerase chain reaction [PCR] amplification) has a 100% sensitivity and specificity, and the method is technically simple and fast (Fig. 31.1).

> **Important**
>
> Molecular genetic analysis can easily prove carrier status for Huntington disease in presymptomatic, at-risk individuals. **Predictive genetic testing** usually involves pretest interviews and physical examination in which the proband's family history, current neurological status, and motives for testing are assessed. The interviews also include extensive counseling about Huntington disease, the testing process, and the possible impact of positive and negative test results. Potential implications with regard to health, life, and disability insurance; employment; and educational discrimination should be discussed. Blood samples are typically not drawn on the same day, but as part of a second encounter. The test results should not be provided over the phone, and long-term follow-up needs to be arranged for individuals with a mutant allele.

■■■ **Genetic Information Nondiscrimination Act**

The Genetic Information Nondiscrimination Act (GINA) protects against the improper use of genetic information in health insurance and employment. It is a federal law that prohibits health insurers from denying coverage or charging higher premiums based on a genetic predisposition of developing a disease in the future.

Therapy

Causal therapy is not available. Hyperkinesis can at least be alleviated, temporarily, by administration of dopamine antagonists. Psychiatric disturbances can be treated with antidepressants or neuroleptics; however, these are only effective in early stages of the disease. More important than any pharmacological therapy is the emotional and psychological support for the patient and his or her family. A high-calorie diet helps to delay significant weight loss and cachexia.

■■■ **Juvenile Progression (So-Called Westphal Variant)**

Up to 10% of individuals with Huntington disease experience onset before age 20 years. The vast majority of these patients (greater than 80%) have long (CAG) expansions, which are paternally derived; occasionally, the children manifest clinically even before their fathers. The clinical presentation differs from classic Huntington disease and is characterized by seizures, muscular rigidity, and bradykinesia/akinesia. The disease picture progresses rapidly.

31.1.2 Ataxias

Chronic progressive ataxia with **increasingly unsteady gait, disturbances of fine motor skills, slurred speech, and disturbances of eye movement** can be seen in multiple neurodegenerative disorders. More than 50 different genetically defined types of hereditary ataxias are known, and inheritance patterns include autosomal dominant, autosomal recessive, X-linked, and matrilineal (mitochondrial) types.

Spinocerebellar Ataxias

The spinocerebellar ataxias are a group of inherited neurological disorders that are both clinically and genetically heterogeneous. Most of these display **autosomal dominant** inheritance, but recessive and X-linked types have also been recognized. The autosomal dominant types are numbered in the order of which their genetic loci are described—spinocerebellar ataxia types 1 to 31 (**SCA1 to SCA31**).

Clinical Symptoms. The onset of spinocerebellar ataxias occurs in most cases after 25 years of age. Symptoms of cerebellar ataxia include gait disturbance, difficulty with balance, slurred speech, and fine motor impairment. Speech disturbances include dysarthria, tremulous voice quality, and slow speech rate, as well as hoarseness and an inability to control the breath while speaking (so-called *wasting air* phenomenon). Additionally, there are accompanying symptoms such as spasticity, ophthalmoplegia, maculopathy, dementia, epilepsy, tremor, dystonia, and polyneuropathy, all of which are observed in specific subtypes and help prioritize molecular genetic testing.

Genetics. The most frequent SCAs are due to disturbances in nucleotide expansion. As in Huntington disease, most of these are trinucleotide disorders with **polyglutamine expansion** caused by an increased number of CAG repeats in the respective gene. These disorders result from altered protein function when the repeat number is 40 or greater. Another essential factor in genetic counseling of affected families is **anticipation** (i.e., the fact that the severity of the disease increases in subsequent generations in a family). In one type, SCA7, anticipation can be extreme, and it is possible that severely affected children die from complications of SCA before the affected parent or grandparent becomes symptomatic (Section 3.6).

Friedreich Ataxia

Friedreich ataxia (hereditary spinal ataxia) is the most notable **autosomal recessive** heritable ataxia. In contrast to most SCAs, the clinical onset of symptoms in Friedreich ataxia is before the age of 25 years, usually between 10 and 15 years. With a prevalence of 1 in 25,000 to 1 in 50,000, it is the most frequent heritable ataxia in Europe and the Middle East.

Clinical Symptoms. The disorder begins very gradually, usually with poor balance when walking, followed by slurred speech and upper limb ataxia. Deep tendon reflexes in the lower extremities are typically absent, and plantar responses are upgoing (Babinski positive). Lower extremity spasticity can be significant, and impairment of sensory function and proprioception is commonly seen. As the disease progresses there are secondary skeletal changes (e.g., ankle inversion, pes cavus, "Friedreich hand," and scoliosis); however, the skeletal changes may also present as an early symptom, even before significant neuropathy develops. **Hypertrophic cardiomyopathy** is present in two-thirds of individuals with Friedreich ataxia and represents the most common cause of death (50% of cases). Other complications include optic atrophy with nystagmus, diabetes mellitus, dysautonomic symptoms (e.g., constipation, urinary frequency/urgency, bradycardia, and cold and cyanosed feet), and dysphagia. Cognitive function and memory are spared. Approximately 10 years after onset, the majority of patients are wheelchair bound, while the average interval from symptom onset to death is 36 years. Approximately one-fourth of the patients show an atypical disease course with later manifestation and slower progression.

Genetics. Friedreich ataxia is caused by a relative deficiency or functional loss of the mitochondrial protein **frataxin**, which plays a major role in the biogenesis of enzymes of the respiratory chain. The vast majority of patients with Friedreich ataxia are homozygous for an unstable expansion of a **GAA trinucleotide repeat in intron 1** of the *FRDA* **gene**. While normal alleles have 5 to 33 GAA repeats, that number increases to between 66 and 1,700 in patients with Friedreich ataxia. The increase of repeat lengths disrupts the transcription and normal splicing at the *FRDA* locus, resulting in a diminished function of the cell's frataxin. Frataxin deficiency causes intramitochondrial accumulation of iron, decreased activity of mitochondrial enzymes, increased sensitivity for oxidative stress, and ultimately apoptotic cell death.

Ataxia Telangiectasia (Louis-Bar Syndrome)

Ataxia telangiectasia (AT) is an autosomal recessive **DNA repair defect** (Section 32.7). The disorder is caused by mutations of the *ATM* gene (*mutated in ataxia telangiectasia*). Patients are particularly sensitive to ionizing radiation, a fact that can also be confirmed cytogenetically as increased chromosome fragility.

Clinical Symptoms. Cerebellar ataxia has an early onset, usually between ages 1 and 2 years. Additional findings include oculomotor apraxia (disturbances of rapid eye movements), muscular hypotonia, choreoathetosis, and an increased risk of infections. Typical oculocutaneous telangiectasias are usually evident by age 6 years. The majority of patients with AT have a humoral and/or cellular immune defect. The resulting **vulnerability to infections** is the most important reason for the considerably decreased life expectancy (still below 40 years) of affected individuals. The second most frequent cause of death in AT is malignancy, especially **leukemias** and **lymphomas**. The lifetime risk for malignancy is 35% to 40%.

Genetics. The *ATM* gene on chromosome 11q is the only gene known to cause ataxia telangiectasia. Most frequent are null mutations that result in a complete loss of protein function.

31.1.3   Disorders of the Pyramidal Tract

Amyotrophic Lateral Sclerosis (Lou Gehrig Disease)

Amyotrophic lateral sclerosis (ALS) is a progressive **neurodegenerative disorder of the upper and lower motor neurons**. It rarely manifests before the age of 50 years. The complete disease picture is a combination of atrophic and spastic paralyses. Among the initial symptoms are pareses, fasciculation and atrophy of the small muscles of the hand, atrophic or spastic pareses of the calves and feet, and bulbar paralyses. In most cases, the disease progresses rapidly. In two-thirds of the cases, it is fatal within 5 years of onset. Swallowing disturbances, with aspiration pneumonia and paralysis of the respiratory muscles, lead to respiratory insufficiency and are among the most frequent causes of death.

Incidence of ALS is 1 to 3 per 100,000 individuals. Approximately 1 in 10 patients with ALS has a positive family history. **Autosomal dominant**, **autosomal recessive**, **and X-linked types** of ALS are known, and various disease-associated genes and chromosomal susceptibility loci have been identified.

Spinal Muscular Atrophy

Spinal muscular atrophies (SMAs) are **disorders of the lower motor neurons**. A progressive degeneration of anterior horn cells in the spinal cord results in increasing muscular hypotonia and atrophy. According to the age at onset and the progression, four types of SMA are differentiated. The most serious neonatal type with prenatal onset, severe contractures, and respiratory failure is occasionally designated as type 0. Spinal muscular atrophy is inherited in an **autosomal recessive** manner. Carrier frequency is 1 in 50, while the incidence of the disorder is approximately 1 in 10,000 newborns.

Type I (Werdnig-Hoffmann). This type manifests within the first 6 months of life. At birth, many infants already have **generalized muscular hypotonia,** with lower extremities more affected than upper, and proximal muscles affected more than distal. Affected infants may also present with poor feeding, swallowing problems, or abdominal breathing. Deep tendon reflexes are usually absent. Fasciculations of the tongue are seen in most, but not all, individuals. Children with SMA type I have normal and lively facial expressions, as the facial musculature is not affected. Paresis of intercostal musculature predisposes patients to the development of atelectases. Without intervention, 80% of children die within the first year from respiratory failure or complications of aspiration pneumonias.

Type II (Intermediate Type). Onset occurs between the 6th and 12th months of life. Affected children may learn to sit without support; however, they do not ambulate independently.

Type III (Kugelberg-Welander). Patients with SMA type III learn to walk on time or with a slight delay. The first clinical symptoms develop mostly between ages 2 and 8 years with a "swaying" gait or a positive Gowers sign as they get up from the floor (similar to Duchenne muscular dystrophy). Their ability to walk continues for a considerable time but worsens during the growth spurt in puberty. Life expectancy is the same as that of the general population. **Type IV (Adult SMA).** The clinical findings of **adult SMA type IV** are similar to those of type III, but onset is later (second or third decade of life).

Diagnosis and Genetics. There are two genes associated with spinal muscular atrophy: *SMN1* and *SMN2*. The two genes are adjacent to each other and almost identical; they differ in only five base pairs. While *SMN1* is the primary functional gene whose mutations cause SMA, the number of copies of *SMN2* modifies disease severity. The gene product participates in RNA processing in the neurons. *SMN1* produces full-length transcripts, while *SMN2* typically produces transcripts lacking exon 7 caused by a C-to-T transition in *SMN2*'s exon 7, which disrupts splicing of this exon. Only 10% of *SMN2* transcripts produce a full-length SMN protein; the gene product of the remaining 90% is nonfunctional. The number of *SMN2* copies varies greatly. While 50% of individuals in the general population have two copies, others may have zero, one, three, or four. SMA is caused by the homozygous **loss of the *SMN1* gene**. In 95% of cases, there is a typical **deletion of exon 7 and exon 8** of the gene; point mutations are rare. Due to the splicing variant, *SMN2* cannot compensate for the loss of *SMN1*. The number of copies of the gene, however, modifies the severity of the disease. While patients with SMA type I almost always have one or two copies of *SMN2*, individuals with type III typically have three or four copies of *SMN2*.

31.1.4 Leukodystrophies

Pelizaeus-Merzbacher Disease

This X-chromosomal disorder is caused by a disturbed function of proteolipoprotein 1 (PLP1), the main component of myelin sheaths in the brain. Typically the disorder manifests itself during the time of myelination, which is during the first years of life. The major radiographic characteristic is **primary hypomyelination** and patchy demyelination of the brain. The peripheral nervous system is not affected. Classic first symptoms of the disorder are nystagmus and muscular hypotonia; cerebellar and pyramidal symptoms develop later and lead to dystonic movement disorders. Affected individuals have intellectual disability. The disease progresses slowly; in the classic type, survival into the sixth or seventh decade of life has been reported.

■■■ Genetics of Pelizaeus-Merzbacher Disease

The molecular basis for Pelizaeus-Merzbacher disease is complex. Although only one gene is affected, **different pathomechanisms** are involved. The most frequent identifiable cause of PMD is a duplication of the entire *PLP1* gene, which results in overexpression that probably affects myelination through an imbalance of normal myelin components. It is interesting to note that null mutations in the *PLP1* gene, which cause an absence of the functional gene product, result in a relatively mild disease, with mild myelin defects, but more severe axonal degeneration. Some missense mutations result in the formation of abnormally folded PLP. This results in a major disturbance of protein processing in the endoplasmic reticulum, premature apoptotic death of myelin-forming oligodendrocytes, and an especially severe neonatal presentation of the disease. Neonatal Pelizaeus-Merzbacher disease also occurs if three or more copies of the *PLP1* gene are present. Finally, there are *missense* mutations in the *PLP1* gene that cause a clinically distinct disorder, **spastic paraplegia type 2**. The latter is characterized by weakness and spasticity of the legs, while central nervous system (CNS) symptoms are largely absent. **Heterozygous women** can also manifest neurological anomalies. Paradoxically, this is observed more frequently in families wherein the hemizygous boys have a mild phenotype.

31.1.5   Other Neurodevelopmental Disorders

Rett Syndrome

With a prevalence of **1 in 8,500 girls**, Rett syndrome is one of the most frequent heritable causes of intellectual disability in females. Affected children are **clinically normal at birth** and develop normally during the first 6 to 18 months (■ Fig. 31.2A). Most developmental milestones (e.g., social smile, sitting, crawling, and walking) are reached on time. The first symptom is typically postnatal **deceleration of head growth** that eventually leads to microcephaly. After a short period of developmental stagnation, previously acquired developmental milestones are lost (**regression**).

One of the cardinal symptoms of Rett syndrome is the loss of purposeful hand movements, which occurs between age 6 months and 2½ years. Those are replaced by the typical **stereotypical hand movements**, which have been described as washing and kneading (Fig. 31.2B). Diagnostic criteria for Rett syndrome have been defined.

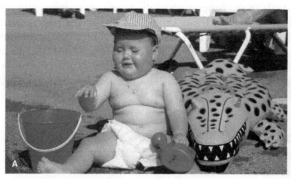
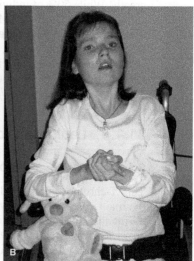

■ **Figure 31.2. Rett Syndrome.** The same girl **(A)** at age 1 year after normal development during infancy and **(B)** at age 12 years with typical hand stereotypies.

Diagnostic criteria for Rett syndrome include the presence of eight disease characteristics that are considered necessary for the diagnosis:

1. Normal prenatal and perinatal period
2. Normal psychomotor development in the first 6 months of life
3. Normal head circumference at birth
4. Postnatal deceleration of head growth
5. Loss of purposeful hand movements between 6 months and 2½ years
6. Stereotypical hand movements
7. Regression of cognitive, motor, behavioral, and social skills
8. Impairment or deterioration of locomotion

Supportive clinical findings include breathing disturbances, impairment of sleeping pattern, and progressive **scoliosis** (◻ Fig. 31.3). Other findings would be considered as exclusion criteria: organomegaly, cataract, retinopathy, optic atrophy, and a history of perinatal or postnatal brain damage.

The treatment of Rett syndrome is mostly symptomatic. Life expectancy is not necessarily lower than normal. However, cases of sudden death are reported as a result of cardiac arrhythmias or nocturnal apneas.

Genetics

Rett syndrome is an X-linked disorder caused by mutations in the *MECP2* **gene** on chromosome Xq28. The normal gene product, MeCP2 (methyl-CpG-binding protein 2), binds to methylated DNA in the human genome and functions as a master regulator of gene transcription. Thus, when MeCP2 function is lost, the transcription of thousands of genes is altered.

Mutations in *MECP2* are much more deleterious in hemizygous males. Affected male fetuses often die in utero. Boys with *MECP2* mutations are typically affected with severe encephalopathy, microcephaly, seizure disorder, and profound psychomotor impairment. Most of these boys die before the age of 2 years.

Most cases of Rett syndrome are caused by missense or nonsense mutations in *MECP2* (approximately 80%), while exon deletions or whole gene deletions are less frequently observed. The vast majority (99.5%) of the cases of Rett syndrome are caused by de novo mutations; however, germline mosaicism has been documented in this disorder.

◻ **Figure 31.3. Rett Syndrome.** Severe scoliosis in a 14-year-old girl with Rett syndrome.

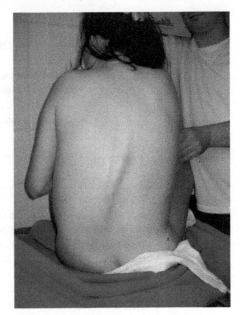

▪▪▪ *MECP2* Duplication Syndrome

Duplications in Xq28, ranging from 0.3 to 2.3 Mb but always involving the *MECP2* gene, cause a mental retardation syndrome in hemizygous males that is characterized by infantile hypotonia, severe intellectual disability, absent speech, progressive spasticity, recurrent **severe respiratory infections** (75% of patients), and epilepsy (50%). About half of the affected patients die before age 25 years, most of them secondary to complications of severe infections. Mothers who are carriers of the duplication show skewed X inactivation (favoring the normal allele) but may still display subtle neuropsychiatric phenotypes, including anxiety disorder, compulsivity, and rigid personality.

31.2   Other Disorders of the Central Nervous System

31.2.1   Structural Malformations of the Central Nervous System

Prenatal development of the CNS clearly takes longer than that of other organ systems and spans the entire fetal period. Even after birth, the development of the nervous system is not complete. Subsequently, the CNS is vulnerable not only to disturbances of morphogenesis during the first 3 months of pregnancy but also to ischemic and toxic events in late pregnancy.

The two cerebral hemispheres can be detected at approximately **5 weeks after conception** (postconception [p.c.]). At that time, the telencephalon (cerebrum), diencephalon (interbrain), mesencephalon (midbrain), metencephalon (hindbrain with cerebellum and pons), and myelencephalon (medulla) are recognizable as distinct structures. Disturbances of **neuronal proliferation** during early embryonic development cause microcephaly and simplification of the gyration pattern.

This initial period is followed by the **migration phase**, during which time neurons travel into the cortex, and by the **organization of cortical layers**. This phase lasts until the mid–second trimester. Neuronal **migration defects** include distinct entities such as **lissencephalies**, polymicrogyria, subependymal (periventricular) heterotopias, and others. Several monogenic causes of abnormal neuronal migration have been identified.

CNS developmental disturbances **in the third trimester** are less frequently caused by genetic alterations. Instead, they are more likely attributable to infectious or ischemic causes. Periventricular lesions or defects of the cortical or deep gray matter are the result of disturbances during this phase of fetal development.

> **Important**
>
> **Developmental Disturbances of the Central Nervous System**
> ▬ First and second trimester: The causes tend to be genetic:
>   ▬ Disturbances of proliferation (e.g., primary microcephaly)
>   ▬ Disturbances of migration (e.g., lissencephaly)
>   ▬ Disturbances of organization and late migration (e.g., bilateral polymicrogyria)
> ▬ Third trimester: The cause tends to be infectious/ischemic.

Neural Tube Defects

Normally, the neural tube closes at the end of the fourth week of embryonic development. Failure to close completely results in **neural tube defects** (NTDs), which range in severity from anencephaly to spina bifida occulta. Neural tube defects are among the **most frequent** congenital defects, with an incidence at birth of 0.2% to 1.0%. Etiology is multifactorial and is influenced by both genetic and environmental factors (e.g., maternal folate deficiency).

Anencephaly (▫ Fig. 31.4A) is the most severe type of neural tube defect. It is caused by a failure of the neural tube to close at its rostral (upper) end, resulting in the absence of a major portion of the skull and cerebral hemispheres. In most cases, the cerebellum is absent and the brainstem often is hypoplastic. Infants with anencephaly either are stillborn or die within several hours.

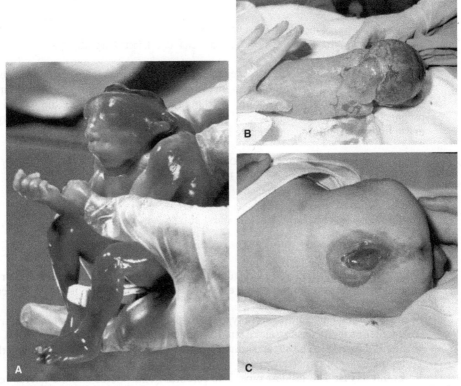

🔲 **Figure 31.4. Neural Tube Defects. A.** Anencephaly. **B.** Encephalocele. **C.** Meningomyelocele. (Courtesy of Universitäts-Kinderklinik Heidelberg.)

Encephalocele (Fig. 31.4B) is a herniation of brain tissue caused by a defect in the skull (mostly occipital). The protruding tissue is covered by skin or a thin membrane. **Meningocele and myelomeningocele** (Fig. 31.4C) are caused by incomplete closure of the caudal part of the neural tube. In a meningocele, the meninges protrude through the vertebral cleft, while in a myelomeningocele, the spinal cord also protrudes. Clinically important is the fact that patients with a skin-covered meningocele frequently have **no** neurological deficits. Exposure of neural tissue to amniotic fluid typically results in neurological defects, ranging from clubfoot to paraplegia. Frequently, hydrocephalus will also develop.

Spina bifida occulta represents the mildest form of spina bifida. It refers to a defect of the vertebral arch that does not involve protrusion of the cord or membrane. Often, there is abnormal hair growth, pigmentation, or formation of pits in the affected area. A clinically relevant consequence is **tethered cord syndrome**, an abnormal attachment of the distal spinal cord (i.e., conus medullaris) in the vertebral canal that, during growth, can result in neurological complications in the lower extremities (e.g., initially pulling pain, then motor and sensory dysfunction of the lower extremity and sphincter weakness with incontinence); it needs to be surgically corrected.

Etiology. Isolated neural tube defects are considered to be of **multifactorial etiology**. Mothers with diabetes mellitus (risk of up to 1%) and/or on valproate medication (risk of up to 5%) have an increased probability of having children with neural tube defects. **Administration of folic acid** reduces the incidence of neural tube defects, especially in women who already have one child with such a defect. However, it is crucial that folic acid be administered in the very first days and weeks of pregnancy (**periconceptionally**). Therefore, it is recommended that women planning a pregnancy take folic acid preconceptionally, which results in a 70% decrease in the incidence of neural tube defects.

■■■ **Preconceptual/Periconceptional Administration of Folic Acid**
— For all women: 0.4 mg daily
— For women who already have a child with a neural tube defect: 4 mg daily

Today, most neural tube defects are identified by ultrasonography; they can also be recognized by **elevated titers of AFP** (α-fetoprotein) in the maternal blood. AFP is one of the four biomarkers tested as part of the maternal serum screening ("quad screen") during the second trimester of pregnancy (typically 16 to 18 weeks' gestation). Elevated titers of **AFP and acetylcholinesterase in amniotic fluid** can indicate a neural tube defect.

■■■ **Recurrence Risk of Neural Tube Defects**
— Incidence in the total population: 1 in 300 to 1 in 1,000
— Total population with administration of folic acid: 1 in 2,000 or less
— One sibling with an NTD: 1 in 25
— One sibling and administration of folic acid: 1 in 100

Holoprosencephaly

Holoprosencephaly (HPE) is a structural malformation of the brain with failed or incomplete separation of the forebrain during gestation. Holoprosencephaly is differentiated into three classic subtypes (after DeMyer):

— **Alobar HPE:** The most severe type. It involves no separation of cerebral hemispheres, no interhemispheric fissure, and a single "monoventricle" (instead of two lateral ventricles).
— **Semilobar HPE:** The left and right frontal and parietal lobes are fused. The interhemispheric fissure exists only posteriorly.
— **Lobar HPE:** The mildest type. The cerebral hemispheres and the lateral ventricles are mostly separated. There is a lack of separation of only the most anterior regions of the frontal lobes.

Case History

Mr. and Mrs. Roberts seek genetic counseling, as their first child was born 1 year ago with holoprosencephaly and died after 5 days of life. The couple wants to be informed about the recurrence risk. The pregnancy was uncomplicated, and prenatal maternal screening tests and chromosome analysis at birth were normal. Neither partner has significant health problems. Mr. Roberts, a 35-year-old investment banker, was adopted at 4 months and lacks any information about his biological parents. Mrs. Roberts, a 32-year-old attorney, has a family history that is noncontributory. Clinical examination of Mr. Roberts reveals a slight hypotelorism with a narrow (i.e., "pinched") nasal bridge, a single upper incisor, no upper frenulum, and a bifid uvula. These are considered microforms of holoprosencephaly, which can be caused by mutations in the sonic hedgehog (*SHH*) gene that has autosomal dominant inheritance and variable intrafamilial expressivity. Molecular genetic testing identifies a disease-associated mutation in the *SHH* gene. The couple is counseled about a 50% chance for future offspring of inheriting the abnormal *SHH* gene copy, and variable expressivity is discussed. After lengthy discussions about the consequences of the finding, this couple decides against molecular genetic testing in a subsequent pregnancy but opt for close prenatal observation with frequent ultrasonography.

Epidemiology

Holoprosencephaly represents the most frequent malformation of the human brain, with an incidence of 1 in 250 in embryos and 1 in 10,000 in newborns.

Etiology

Causes of holoprosencephaly are outlined in ▢ Figure 31.5.

Clinical Symptoms

Clinical symptoms largely depend on the severity of the HPE. Patients with **alobar HPE** have microcephaly and mostly severe to profound intellectual disability, frequently with seizure disorder. Additional symptoms and associated malformations may depend on the exact cause

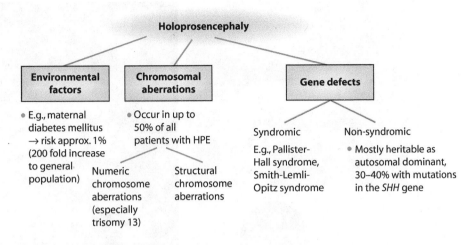

Figure 31.5. Etiology of Holoprosencephaly.

of holoprosencephaly, especially in syndromic cases. Typical **craniofacial symptoms** do not always correlate with the severity of the brain malformation (Fig. 31.6). The range extends from **cyclopia** (with or without proboscis) in alobar HPE over microphthalmia and/or absent nasal septum to (almost) **normal facies**, possibly with microsymptoms in autosomal dominant heritable HPE. Frequently, there are orofacial malformations (e.g., bilateral cleft lip and midline cleft lip and palate).

Important

Microsymptoms in Holoprosencephaly

Nonsyndromic, nonchromosomal, autosomal dominant heritable HPE is characterized by incomplete penetrance and extremely variable expressivity, even within the same family. Individuals with normal intelligence and normal physical examination can be identified as harboring a disease-causing mutation when tested following the birth of a severely affected child. Possible microsymptoms and minimal findings include:

- Hypotelorism
- A single upper incisor
- Anosmia/hyposmia with missing olfactory bulb
- Missing superior labial frenulum
- Narrow ("pinched") nasal bridge
- Bifid uvula

Diagnosis

The diagnosis is made by brain imaging, preferably **MRI**. This allows for classification of the subtype. **DNA array analysis** should be requested for all individuals with HPE. This will detect aneuploidies (e.g., trisomy 13), as well as microdeletions and microduplications. Between 30% and 50% of patients with a positive family history of HPE and 2% to 5% of those with no family history have an identifiable mutation in a gene associated with non-syndromic HPE. Among the genes most commonly involved are *SHH*, *SIX3*, *TGIF*, *ZIC2* (often severe HPE with less pronounced facial anomalies), and *GLI2* (often typical facies without brain malformation). **Molecular genetic analysis** by gene sequencing should be considered. Often there is compound heterozygosity with mutations in two different genes, blurring the line between monogenic and polygenic or multifactorial inheritance. In 18% to 25% of the patients, HPE occurs as one symptom of an underlying syndrome (e.g., Pallister-Hall syndrome or Smith-Lemli-Opitz syndrome). Diagnostic testing is performed according to the presumptive diagnosis.

III

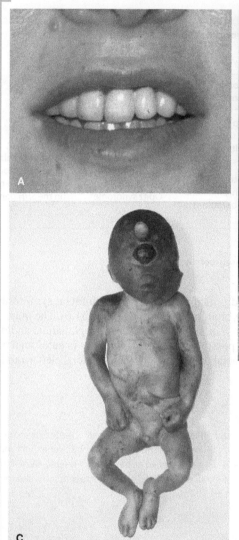

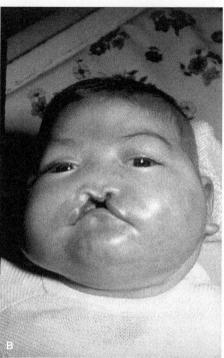

Figure 31.6. Holoprosencephaly. A. Single upper incisor. B. Cleft lip/cleft palate. C. Cyclopia with proboscis.

Clinical Management

Careful clinical examination and focused diagnostic evaluation within the first days of life are extremely important. Treatment is symptomatic and supportive. Etiopathological clarification of HPE is essential for counseling regarding inheritance, recurrence risk, and anticipatory guidance.

Prognosis

Patients with cyclopia typically die within a few hours or days postnatally. Roughly 50% of patients with alobar HPE die within the first 4 to 5 months of life, 80% in the first year. About 50% of patients with semilobar HPE survive the first year of life. Due to nonpenetrance or variable expressivity, patients with autosomal dominant nonsyndromic HPE may have a normal life expectancy and normal intellectual development.

31.2.2 Intellectual Disability

Definitions of intellectual disability (ID) vary greatly and often are controversial. According to the American Association of Intellectual and Developmental Disabilities, "Intellectual disability is a disability characterized by significant limitations both in intellectual functioning and in adaptive behavior, which covers many everyday social and practical skills. This disability originates before the age of 18." The ICD-10 defines intellectual disability (formerly termed *mental retardation*) as "a condition of arrested or incomplete development of the mind, which is especially characterized by impairment of skills that contribute to the overall level of intelligence, i.e., cognitive, language, motor, and social abilities. ID can occur with or without any other mental or physical condition. Degrees of ID are conventionally estimated by standardized intelligence tests. These can be supplemented by scales assessing social adaptation in a given environment."

Using standardized intelligence tests, intellectual disability is defined as an **IQ of under 70**. The IQ value of 70 is not randomly chosen: since the average IQ is set at 100, with a standard deviation of 15, an IQ of 70 is two standard deviations below the mean. In common clinical practice, the term *developmental delay* is used for children younger than the age of 5 years, while *intellectual disability* is used to describe children 5 years and older.

To be differentiated are patients with mild ID (IQ 50 to 69) and those with more severe forms of ID (IQ less than 50; ▢ Table 31.1). Mild ID accounts for 80% to 85% of all cases of ID. Individuals with lower socioeconomic statuses are overrepresented in this group (i.e., mild ID), while persons with more severe forms of ID are of normal socioeconomic distribution.

The total prevalence of ID in the population is 1% to 3%, while IQs of less than 50 are detected in 0.3% to 0.5%. Several studies have shown that an underlying etiology can be identified in up to 90% of cases of severe and profound ID, while 50% to 80% of cases of mild ID remain unclassified. Parents with borderline intellectual functioning (IQ 70 to 84) are overrepresented among those who have children with mild ID.

Causes of intellectual disability are extremely varied. A detailed evaluation by developmental specialists and clinical geneticists can identify the cause of ID in up to 50% of cases. In up to 25% of cases, ID is caused by a monogenic disorder (the Online Mendelian Inheritance in Man [OMIM] database has more than 1,700 entries under "mental retardation"). Chromosomal abnormalities and copy number variants are identified in up to 20% of individuals with ID. Teratogenic factors during pregnancy appear to be an infrequent cause of ID (less than 5% of the cases), as are complications during delivery (less than 5%). The most frequent cause for severe ID, with an incidence of 1 in 650, is trisomy 21.

While mild ID affects both sexes with equal frequency, the more severe forms of ID manifest a clear **imbalance in gender distribution**. Boys are disproportionately more frequently affected (1.3 to 1.5 times more affected than girls). This is attributed mostly to the X-chromosomal forms of intellectual disability. X-linked intellectual disability (XLID) accounts for 16% of males with ID. This is in part related to hemizygosity of all X-chromosomal genes (except those of the pseudoautosomal regions) in males. It is estimated that more than 200 genes on the X chromosome may be associated with XLID. Almost half of these have been identified, and molecular genetic testing is offered on a clinical basis. Another 20% have been regionally mapped to specific loci. The most frequent cause for XLID is fragile X syndrome.

▢ **Table 31.1.** Intellectual Disability: Levels of Severity

Severity	IQ
Profound	<20
Severe	20–34
Moderate	35–49
Mild	50–69

Diagnosis

The diagnostic evaluation of all children with ID should include a **complete neurological and dysmorphological examination**, as well as formal developmental testing (IQ testing). High-resolution **DNA array analysis** should be performed on all cases, regardless of the degree of severity and additional accompanying symptoms. **Cranial MRI** should be done on all children with neurological abnormalities, including microcephaly and macrocephaly. Molecular genetic **analysis for fragile X syndrome** is important for all boys with mental retardation and should be considered in the female patient with ID, especially if family history is supportive or is not attainable. In individual cases, **additional studies** are to be considered (including metabolic analyses) depending on the clinical presentation and differential diagnoses.

Fragile X Syndrome

The most frequent cause of X-chromosomal ID is fragile X syndrome, also called Martin-Bell syndrome. The disorder was named for a particularity that occurs during chromosome analysis of affected individuals: culturing their lymphocytes in folate-deficient medium (or after adding the folic acid antagonist methotrexate) causes an increased incidence of chromosome break-age at the terminal end of the long arm of the X chromosome, such that the terminal region of Xq appears "fragile." Since 1991, it has been known that the disorder is caused by a marked increase in the number of CGG repeats, resulting in hypermethylation of the *FMR1* promoter that blocks the expression of the *FMR1* gene.

Case History

Sabrina Jennings, 15 years old, was recently diagnosed with fragile X syndrome. Her parents wish to be informed about the implications of the diagnosis for Sabrina and other family members. Sabrina was born at term after an uncomplicated pregnancy; her size and weight at birth were within the normal range. Her development was delayed; she walked at 16 months and spoke her first words at 3 years of age. Sabrina was enrolled in speech and occupational therapy. She now receives special education. Mr. and Mrs. Jennings have another 11-year-old daughter and a 9-year-old son; both are healthy and attend regular schools. Mr. Jennings is an engineer. A brother of his father was intellectually disabled, but a diagnosis is not known. Mrs. Jennings graduated from high school and works in sales at a local department store. Her 68-year-old father was recently diagnosed with dementia and some unexplained neurological symptoms (shakiness and unsteady gait). The family receives counseling about fragile X syndrome, including the etiology, the genet-ics, and the natural course of the disorder. Given the unexplained neurological symptoms in Mrs. Jennings' father, the possibility of him having fragile X-associated tremor/ataxia syndrome is discussed in some detail. It is recommended to test Mrs. Jennings' DNA for CGG trinucleotide repeat expansion in the 5' untranslated region of the *FMR1* gene.

Epidemiology

Fragile X syndrome is the most frequent known monogenic cause of intellectual disability. According to estimates, at least 6% of all cases of intellectual disability in males result from this disorder. Prevalence in men is about 1 in 4,000. Prevalence in women is approximately 1 in 8,000.

Clinical Symptoms

At birth, infants frequently weigh more and have a larger head circumference than normal (around the 97th percentile). Additionally, there is poor sucking and feeding, as well as frequent gastroesophageal reflux. Milestones of development are delayed; walking occurs after 18 months, and speech often occurs after age 3 years.

   In childhood, patients with fragile X syndrome are rather shy and have little social inter-action. Often they manifest autistic behavior, with aversion to touch, little eye contact, and verbal perseverations. They are increasingly hyperactive, with stereotypical movements, hand flapping, and hand biting. Intellectual development is impaired; there are marked deficits in speech. Measured IQ is typically between 30 and 50 (98% with IQ less than 70).

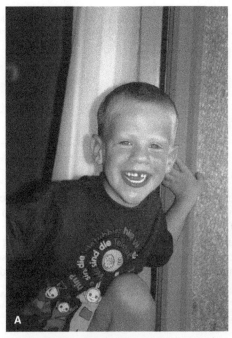
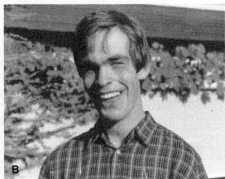

Figure 31.7. Fragile X Syndrome. A. Fragile X syndrome at school age: rather mild facial symptoms with large ears and prognathism. **B.** Fragile X syndrome in a 28-year-old man: broad nose, prognathism, and large ears.

Craniofacial symptoms become more prominent as children grow older (◻ Fig. 31.7). Patients are said to "grow into" the typical phenotype, which includes a long face with prominent forehead, prognathism (large jaw), and large ears.

There is a congenital **weakness in connective tissues** that manifests itself in soft velvety skin. Additionally, there are fleshy hands and feet with marked creases (◻ Fig. 31.8), hyperextensible joints, and not infrequently myopia, scoliosis, flat feet, and mitral valve prolapse.

Figure 31.8. Fragile X Syndrome. Deep plantar creases. (Courtesy of G. Tariverdian, Institut für Humangenetik Heidelberg.)

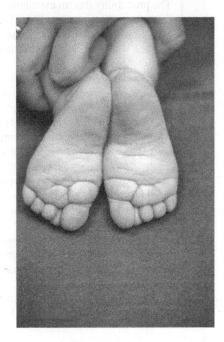

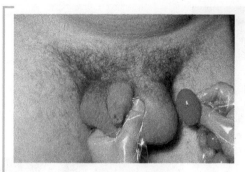

Figure 31.9. Fragile X Syndrome. Macroorchidism. (Courtesy of G. Tariverdian, Institut für Humangenetik Heidelberg.)

In puberty, affected males manifest another cardinal symptom: **macroorchidism** (□ Fig. 31.9). The testicles grow beginning at age 9 years and throughout puberty, to a total average volume of 50 mL (normal 15 to 20 mL) in adulthood.

Heterozygous women with full mutation have an overall milder phenotype, usually with discreet facial dysmorphisms (e.g., prominent chin). In 50% to 60% of the cases, there is also intellectual disability. Neuropsychiatric abnormalities are commonly observed.

> **Important**
>
> Microcephaly makes the diagnosis of fragile X syndrome very unlikely.

Genetics and Etiology

Fragile X syndrome is caused by a CGG **trinucleotide expansion** in the 5′ untranslated region of the **FMR1** (*fragile X mental retardation 1*) gene. This gene is located on the long arm of the X chromosome and codes for a protein named FMRP (fragile X mental retardation protein). Normally, this gene has 6 to 54 CGG repeats. A **full mutation** of more than 200 repeats results in hypermethylation of the *FMR1* promoter, causing inhibition of *FMR1*, resulting in decreased FMRP production. Cases of 55 to 200 repeats are considered to be in the "**premutation**" range. These mutations are not associated with intellectual disability; however, the repeat is unstable, and especially in females, meiotic amplification to a full mutation of more than 200 repeats can occur. The probability that an expansion will occur depends on the size of the premutation. Numbers of more than 100 repeats are likely to expand to a full mutation in the next generation. As a rule, there is no amplification in male meiosis. This is consistent with the concept of **maternal anticipation**. Women who are premutation carriers are at increased risk for premature ovarian failure (POF).

■■■ Fragile X-Associated Tremor/Ataxia Syndrome

Premutations of fragile X syndrome result in a neurological disease picture, especially in older men. The term *fragile X–associated tremor/ataxia syndrome* (FXTAS) has been coined for this recently described condition. It is characterized by progressive cerebellar ataxia with intention tremor. Additionally, there are other neurological symptoms, such as deficits in short-term memory, Parkinson disease, peripheral neuropathy, neuromuscular weakness of the lower extremities, and increasing autonomic dysfunction. The penetrance of these symptoms is age related. The symptoms are seen in 20% of men between 50 and 60 years of age with premutation, in 40% of men between 60 and 70 years with premutation, in 50% of men between 70 and 80 years with premutation, and in more than 75% of men older than 80 years with premutation. Fewer women with premutation develop FXTAS, but a considerable proportion (25%) show early menopause due to premature ovarian failure. Interestingly, neurodegeneration underlying FXTAS is not related to loss of function of the *FMR1* gene but is caused by overproduction of expanded *FMR1* messenger RNA (mRNA) strands and depletion of CGG-binding proteins. Thus, pathogenesis involves RNA gain of function, like some other conditions with trinucleotide repeat expansion, such as myotonic dystrophy. This also explains why individuals with a fragile X full mutation do not develop FXTAS.

An overview of the relationships between trinucleotide expansion, gender, and clinical presentation is provided in □ Table 31.2.

Table 31.2. Repeat Expansions of *FMR1* and Corresponding Clinical Symptoms

Type	Number of (CGG)$_n$ Trinucleotide Repeats	Methylation at *FMR1* Promoter Locus	Clinical Manifestation in Men	Clinical Manifestation in Women
Normal	<55	Nonmethylated	Healthy	Healthy
Premutation	55–200	Nonmethylated	Initially asymptomatic, with increasing age frequently FXTAS	Mostly asymptomatic, possibly FXTAS; Approximately 25% with premature ovarian failure
Full mutation	>200	Hypermethylated	100% Affected, full clinical picture after puberty	50% Variably affected; 50% Clinically initially asymptomatic

Mosaics. Mosaics of cell lines with full mutation and premutation, or cell lines with or without hypermethylation at the promoter, occur in 15% to 20% of boys with fragile X syndrome. These children have an overall milder clinical picture. On a cellular level, these findings correspond to X-chromosomal heterozygosity in women.

Inheritance. Expansion of a premutation in the female (not the male) germ line is possible; the reverse (i.e., regression from a full mutation to a premutation) has not been observed. Full mutations are not transmitted by affected men. Accordingly, the following rules of inheritance apply:
- Each patient with full mutation has a mother with premutation or full mutation.
- The offspring of women with premutation, as a rule, have a 50% risk of premutation or full mutation. Whether a premutation during maternal meiosis expands to a full mutation strongly depends on the size of the premutation: the probability of expansion is under 20% for less than 70 repeats, about 80% for more than 90 repeats, and nearly 100% for more than 100 repeats.
- Approximately 50% of the offspring of women with full mutation have a full mutation but never a premutation.
- Daughters of men with a premutation or full mutation (mosaic) always have a premutation.

Diagnosis

The molecular diagnosis of fragile X syndrome is made by PCR amplification and Southern blot analysis. PCR amplification is used to determine the repeat numbers in the normal and premutation loci. Southern blot analysis is added for larger repeat expansion. Southern blot analysis should also be used to determine the methylation state (by utilizing methylation-sensitive restriction enzymes) in order to functionally differentiate premutations from full mutations (see Chapter 15, Fig. 15.5D).

Clinical Management

There is no causal therapy. Children with fragile X syndrome should be enrolled in early childhood intervention programs with speech, occupational, and physical therapy; later they should receive special education. Diagnostic testing for autism should be considered. Pharmacological treatment for attention-deficit/hyperactivity disorder (ADHD), which can be quite disruptive in children with fragile X syndrome, should be considered. Early detection of ophthalmological problems (especially strabismus and myopia), which occur in up to 50% of the patients, requires regular ophthalmological examinations.

31.2.3 Epilepsy

Seizure disorders are among the most common neurological disorders. Annual incidence is approximately 1 in 2,000, and prevalence is 0.5% to 1%. Etiology usually is multifactorial; it is estimated that a **genetic disposition** exists in roughly **40% to 50%** of all cases of epilepsy. However, only an estimated 2% of all epilepsies follow monogenic inheritance. Seizures during the neonatal period, for which no infectious cause has been determined, are very unusual; thus, all children with **neonatal seizures** should have a detailed genetic and metabolic evaluation.

The **recurrence risk** in families can only be estimated for the most frequent, generalized, idiopathic epilepsies whose cause is unknown or multifactorial. The disease risk for first-degree relatives is approximately 4% to 10% in sporadic cases. The concordance rate for monozygotic twins is considerably higher than for dizygotic twins (76% versus 33%, respectively).

Monogenic Epilepsies. During the last few years, mutations in many different genes have been identified as causes of specific epilepsy syndromes. In most cases, formal genetic inheritance is autosomal dominant; the gene products typically are proteins of ion channels. Individual epilepsy syndromes (e.g., juvenile myoclonic epilepsy) manifest themselves as etiologically **polygenic**, which means that they can be caused by mutations in different genes. Conversely, different mutations of the same gene can result in different types of epilepsy (**pleiotropy**). Mutations of the *SCN1A* gene, which codes for the α-subunit of a neuronal sodium channel, are seen in both the severe type of myoclonic epilepsy of childhood and the much more benign "generalized epilepsy with febrile seizures."

Neonatal Seizures. All newborns who manifest with seizures within the first days of life should undergo a detailed infectious workup, including a lumbar puncture. However, spinal fluid should also be sent for cerebrospinal fluid (CSF) neurotransmitter, CSF lactate, CSF glucose, and CSF amino acid analysis. A plasma amino acid analysis, sent at the same time, allows calculation of the CSF/plasma glycine ratio, which can be used to evaluate for nonketotic hyperglycinemia (a rare cause of severe epilepsy and profound intellectual disability). Other tests that should be considered include urine organic acid analysis, acylcarnitine profile, blood glucose, lactate and ammonia (to evaluate for inborn errors of metabolism), plasma total homocysteine, testing for carbohydrate-deficient transferrin (to evaluate for congenital disorders of glycosylation), urine polyols and urine purines, and DNA array analysis (to evaluate for chromosomal aberrations and copy number variants), depending on the exact clinical presentation. All children with neonatal seizures should receive a trial of intravenous (IV) pyridoxine for pyridoxine-dependent seizures, which is a treatable metabolic defect; if not successful, IV pyridoxal phosphate and IV folinic acid should be considered.

31.2.4   Autism

Autism spectrum disorders (ASDs) affect 1 in 110 children born in the United States and are highly heritable, with a concordance of 88% among monozygotic twins (as compared to 30% in dizygotic twins); boys are more likely to be affected than girls (male-to-female ratio, 3:1). There is a high comorbidity with other mental disorders and physical illnesses, especially with intellectual disability (approximately 30% of cases) and epilepsy (approximately 20% of cases).

Idiopathic autism (90% of cases) and syndromic autism (approximately 10% of cases) can be differentiated. Syndromic autism is a symptom of an underlying syndrome. Important differential diagnoses of **syndromic autism** are fragile X syndrome, Rett syndrome, tuberous sclerosis, and Smith-Magenis syndrome. The recurrence risk after having one autistic child is estimated to be 2% to 7% (i.e., three to eight times higher than in the general population).

Several susceptibility genes for idiopathic autism have been identified (e.g., *NRXN1*, which codes for neurexin 1, and *SHANK3*). DNA array analysis should be performed on every patient presenting with autism, as copy number variants are identified in 10% to 20% of all individuals referred for an evaluation of ASDs. Common copy number variants in individuals with autism include deletions and duplications of 15q13.3, 16p11.2, and 22q13.3. However, each single susceptibility locus accounts for a very small fraction of cases (typically less than 1% of all cases). The total number of autism susceptibility genes has been estimated to be between 100 and 200.

31.2.5 Psychiatric Disorders

Psychiatric disorders, including schizophrenia, bipolar disorder, major depressive disorder, anxiety disorder, and panic disorders, are mostly multifactorial or polygenic. Genetic research of these diseases is especially difficult, since there are no quantifiable biological markers to classify or categorize the respective disorders. Twin studies point to a considerable genetic component in the etiology of certain psychiatric disorders (□ Table 31.3). Familial causes of psychiatric disease frequently manifest incomplete penetrance and variable expressivity even within a family. The same genetic defect may cause anxiety disorder in one family member and schizophrenia in another, illustrating the complex interplay of genetic predisposition, genetic modifier effects, and environmental influences.

Schizophrenia

With a lifetime risk of 1%, schizophrenic psychoses are frequent in the general population. Men and women are equally affected. Numerous twin and family studies have consistently shown that familial (i.e., genetic) factors are the strongest predisposing factors for schizophrenia. Current meta-analyses estimate the genetic contribution of schizophrenia at 80% to 85%. The concordance rate for monozygotic twins is three times higher than that for dizygotic twins. However, even in monozygotic twins, concordance is only 50%, illustrating the importance of environmental modification.

In the past, the accepted premise was that the vast majority of cases of schizophrenia were of **complex genetic inheritance**. Linkage analyses and genome-wide association studies have identified numerous chromosomal susceptibility regions and gene candidates for the development of schizophrenic psychoses. More recently, the use of DNA array analyses has identified microdeletions of 1q21, 15q13, or 3q29 in patients with schizophrenia. Interestingly, deletions of these regions are also found in children and adults with mild to moderate ID and/or autism.

■■■ **22q11 and Schizophrenia**

Region **22q11** is an example of a susceptibility region for schizophrenia. Not only is this region the area of a frequent microdeletion (Section 21.1), but it also contains the gene for catechol-*O*-methyltransferase (*COMT*), which has an important function in the catabolism of dopamine. In patients with microdeletion 22q11, the incidence of psychiatric disorders (e.g., schizophrenia, bipolar disorder, and anxiety disorder) is clearly elevated. Whether schizophrenia is associated with the loss of a *COMT* copy remains unknown. Another gene in the same region is *PRODH*, which codes for proline dehydrogenase. This enzyme is responsible for providing glutamate in the presynaptic neuron and therefore for the synthesis of the ligands of *N*-methyl-D-aspartate (NMDA) receptors.

□ **Table 31.3.** Estimated Genetic Component in the Etiology of Psychiatric Disorders

Disorder	Genetics (+)/Environment (−)	Genetic Component
Schizophrenic psychoses	+++++++++++++++++++−−−	82%–84%
Bipolar affective psychoses	++++++++++++++++++−−−−	80%
Endogenous depression	+++++++++−−−−−−−−−−−−	60%
Panic disorders	++++++++−−−−−−−−−−−−	40%
Phobic disorders	+++++++−−−−−−−−−−−−	35%
Generalized anxiety disorders	++++++−−−−−−−−−−−−	30%

Modified after Schumacher et al. (2002).

The lifetime risk for schizophrenic psychoses is 6% if one parent is affected, 9% if a sibling is affected, and 13% if a child is affected. If several family members are affected, the risk increases accordingly.

Bipolar Disorder

The lifetime risk for bipolar disorder in the general population is 0.5% to 1.5%. First-degree relatives of affected individuals, however, have a risk of 5% to 10%. If a monozygotic twin has bipolar disorder, the lifetime risk for the other twin is 40% to 70%. The genetic component of bipolar disorder is considered stronger than that of unipolar disorders (e.g., major depressive disorder or mania). Several chromosomal susceptibility loci for bipolar affective psychoses have been identified; the responsible genes, however, have not yet been identified.

31.3   Disorders of the Peripheral Nervous System

Depending on the damaged nerve fibers, peripheral neuropathies can be classified as motor, sensory, or autonomic. Heritable neuropathies are the most frequent cause of slowly progressing weakness in the distal extremities.

31.3.1   Hereditary Motor and Sensory Neuropathies

Also known as **Charcot-Marie-Tooth neuropathies**, these hereditary motor and sensory neuropathies (HMSNs) are the most frequent heritable disorders of the peripheral nervous system. They constitute a genetically heterogeneous group with an estimated total prevalence of 1 in 2,500. At least seven different types are clinically differentiated; each type is caused by mutations in several different genes and accordingly classified into a larger number of subgroups (labeled by different letters).

Hereditary Motor and Sensory Neuropathy Type I

This classic autosomal dominant disorder is the most frequent heritable neuropathy. It is characterized by progressive neural muscular atrophy.

Clinical Symptoms. In most cases, the clinical onset is between the ages of 5 and 20 years. It manifests itself as a slowly **progressing weakness of the feet, ankles, and calves,** as well as fatigue and **muscular pain** after physical exertion. Upon physical examination, there are depressed or absent deep tendon reflexes in the lower extremities and weakness upon dorsiflexion of the feet. Pareses of the peroneal muscles make it difficult to lift the feet when walking and require an unusual lifting of the knees. This is called *steppage gait*. Muscular atrophies result in foot deformities (**pes cavus** with hammer toes; ▢ Fig. 31.10). In adult patients, there is symmetric atrophy of the muscles below the knees (stork leg appearance) and atrophy of the intrinsic hand muscles. The sensory symptoms of HMSN type I are typically limited to a stockinglike

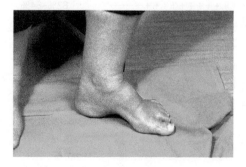

▢ **Figure 31.10. Hereditary Motor and Sensory Neuropathies Type I.** Pes cavus.

or glovelike distribution, and **sensations of vibration and position** in the respective areas are most severely affected. Physical examination reveals characteristic thickening of peripheral nerves, sometimes palpable subcutaneously (e.g., the ulnar nerve palpable at the olecranon groove and the greater auricular nerve running along the lateral aspect of the neck).

Diagnosis. Motor and sensory **nerve conduction velocity** in HMSN type I is typically markedly reduced, mostly to values below 20 m/s. Neuropathologically, the enlarged nerves show hypertrophy and **onion bulb formation**, which is thought to result from repeated demyelination and remyelination of Schwann cells wrapping around the individual axons.

Genetics. HMSN type I is genetically heterogeneous. In 70% to 80% of patients, there are heterozygous **duplications** of the *PMP22* gene on chromosome 17p12. This is called HMSN type Ia. One-third of these are de novo mutations.

∎∎∎ *PMP22* Mutations

PMP22 codes for peripheral myelin protein 22, a central component of the myelin sheath of peripheral nerves. Defects of peripheral myelination can be caused by changes in gene dosage as well as by point mutations in this gene. Sequence homologies in the environment of the gene on chromosome 17p12 often result in an unequal crossing over during meiosis. The resulting **duplication** causes a 1.5-fold overexpression of the protein, which causes demyelination and secondary loss of axons. It is by far the most frequent cause of HMSN type I. A **homozygous duplication** or some specific heterozygous **point mutations** in the gene result in a disease type that is clearly faster progressing and more severe, HMSN type III. A **deletion** of the gene, on the other hand, reduces gene expression by 50%, resulting in a completely different disease picture of **hereditary neuropathy with liability to pressure palsies** in which mechanical stress can trigger reversible palsies and paresthesias. Therefore, the pathogenesis of HMSN type Ia, and related disorders due to *PMP22* mutations, resembles the pathogenesis of Pelizaeus-Merzbacher disease and related disorders caused by *PLP1* mutations. An essential difference, however, is that HMSN affects the myelin sheaths of peripheral nerves, whereas Pelizaeus-Merzbacher disease affects the myelin sheaths of the white matter of the brain.

31.4 Hereditary Muscular Disorders

Muscular dystrophies are genetic disorders that primarily, but not exclusively, affect the skeletal muscles. They are characterized by progressive muscle weakness caused by muscle cell breakdown and fibrosis. More than 20 different types of muscular dystrophy are known, among them autosomal dominant, autosomal recessive, and X-linked disorders.

Duchenne and Becker Muscular Dystrophies

Duchenne muscular dystrophy (DMD) is the most frequent muscular dystrophy. It was first described by Duchenne in 1868 and by Gowers in 1879. Almost 100 years later (1955), Becker and Kiener described a milder type that (as we know today) is caused by allelic mutations in the same gene on the X chromosome. This milder type was named Becker muscular dystrophy (BMD).

Case History

Elias was found to have a muscular weakness around the age of 2 years, when in nursery school he had difficulty climbing stairs and a tendency to fall. Evaluation with his pediatrician revealed a highly elevated creatine kinase. The suspected diagnosis of Duchenne muscular dystrophy was confirmed by molecular genetic testing through identification of a deletion of exons 46 to 48 in the dystrophin gene. Currently, at age 3 years, Elias walks without support and can get up from a squat without having to support his legs. For mild speech delay, he was enrolled in speech therapy. His mother is heterozygous for the deletion that was detected in Elias; she was counseled that all future sons of hers have a 50% chance of being affected with DMD. Except for Elias, there is no family history of muscular weakness. Molecular genetic testing of at-risk individuals was recommended.

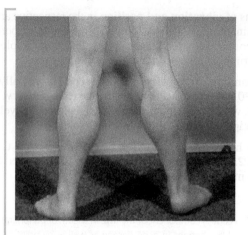

Figure 31.11. Pseudohypertrophy of the Calves in Duchenne Muscular Dystrophy. "Pseudo" implies there is no actual increase in muscle tissue. The striated muscle has been replaced by connective tissue and fat.

Epidemiology

Incidence of DMD is about 1 in 3,500 male newborns. BMD in male newborns is much rarer, with an incidence of 1 in 18,000.

Clinical Symptoms of Duchenne Muscular Dystrophy

Boys with DMD usually present with muscular weakness in early childhood, causing delayed motor milestones, and typically walk independently after the age of 18 months. Their gait remains unstable, yet clinical symptoms are so discreet that parents (and the pediatrician) frequently do not notice the motor weakness until age 3 or 4 years. The mean age of diagnosis is 4 years 10 months. Proximal weakness causes a waddling gait and difficulty climbing. The calves manifest a characteristic pseudohypertrophy and appear firm to palpation (Fig. 31.11).

A classic sign of Duchenne muscular dystrophy (and other muscular dystrophies) is the **Gower maneuver** (Fig. 31.12). When rising from the floor or from a squat, patients need to support themselves with their hands on knees and thighs, "climbing up on their own bodies." When walking, patients manifest the **Trendelenburg sign**: the pelvis drops on the side opposite to the weakness when the hip and knee of the normal side are flexed; this is clinically noted as "waddling gait." The cause for it is a muscular weakness of the gluteus medius muscle.

With increasing age, the motor handicap becomes more prominent. Due to shortened Achilles tendons, the boys increasingly walk on their toes. They develop significant lumbar hyperlordosis. Climbing stairs is only possible when they pull themselves up on the railing. Walking becomes increasingly difficult; as a rule, all patients with DMD are **wheelchair dependent** by the time they turn **13 years**. Cardiac symptoms occur (e.g., arrhythmias and cardiomyopathy) mostly between the ages of 14 and 18 years.

The most critical problem of progressive DMD is respiratory weakness. Chronic hypoxia, caused, for instance, by nocturnal hypoventilation, can cause secondary symptoms such as increasing tiredness, anxiety, depression, loss of appetite, dizziness, drowsiness, or lack of concentration.

Patients with DMD frequently have a mild, nonprogressive cognitive impairment. The average IQ is about 15 points lower than that of unaffected family members. The specific cognitive profile demonstrates deficits in working memory and executive function.

Clinical Symptoms of Becker Muscular Dystrophy

Becker muscular dystrophy is much rarer than DMD, and while the clinical signs and symptoms are similar to DMD, BMD manifests a milder phenotype with regard to age of onset and progression. **Loss of walking** occurs **after age 16 years** (walking loss between the ages of 13 and 16 years occurs for intermediate types). Intrafamilial variability is much larger in BMD than in DMD.

Figure 31.12. Gower maneuver in a female patient with limb girdle muscular dystrophy.

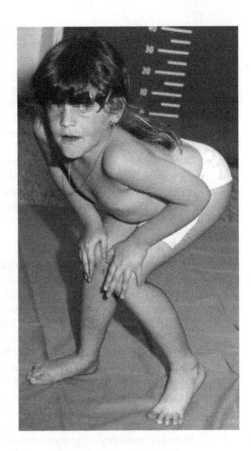

■■■ Females with Muscular Dystrophy

Heterozygous female carriers for DMD do not present with muscular dystrophy yet are at risk for cardiomyopathy and may have mild to moderate muscle weakness in adulthood. On muscle biopsy (not a recommended test), the muscle fibers display a mosaic pattern of dystrophin staining, and the creatine kinase level in the plasma may be elevated. Females who have symptoms that more closely resemble those of males with DMD require investigation for Turner syndrome (45,X) or X-autosomal translocation, or they may have skewed X inactivation.

Genetics and Etiology

DMD and BMD are allelic and are caused by mutations in the *DMD* gene on chromosome Xp21.2, which encodes for the protein **dystrophin**. This gene consists of 79 coding exons that cover more than 2,400 kb of genomic DNA. Seven different promoters are responsible for the transcription of the gene. Currently, it is the largest known human gene.

In **60%** of patients with DMD and BMD, a **deletion** of one or more exons can be detected, and in 5% to 10% of cases there are duplications. The remaining 30% of cases are mostly caused by point mutations or splice site mutations. Mutations that result in a complete loss of function of the protein always cause the severe phenotype (DMD). These are mostly deletions or duplications with shifts of the reading frame. Mutations that allow synthesis of some dystrophin result in the milder phenotype, BMD. This typically involves deletions that do not shift the reading frame.

Dystrophin is part of a protein complex that links the cytoskeleton with membrane proteins that, in turn, bind with proteins in the extracellular matrix, thereby stabilizing muscular sarcolemmas. In dystrophinopathies, this stability is disrupted. This results in focal tears of the plasma membrane and uncontrolled potassium influx into the muscle cell. In turn, endogenous proteases are activated, leading to premature apoptosis of the cell.

Diagnosis

The easiest and most sensitive screening test is **determination of creatine kinase** (CK) in plasma. In affected boys, it is almost always elevated to levels greater than 1,000 U/L. Female carriers usually (but not necessarily) have elevated CK levels greater than 100 U/L. The actual diagnosis of DMD/BMD is made by molecular genetic testing, which combines deletion/duplication testing and gene sequencing methods. Electromyography (EMG) is not necessary in the evaluation of DMD or BMD. Muscle biopsy with immunohistology is only advisable in cases where DNA analysis does not detect a mutation.

■■■ Histopathology of Muscular Dystrophies

In addition to endomysial fibrosis, foci of necrosis, and regeneration, muscular dystrophies distinguish themselves histopathologically through significant variation in fiber size. Centrally located muscle cell nuclei are visible. This allows an accurate differentiation from neurogenic muscular atrophies that reveal group atrophy of type I and type II fibers, as opposed to the normal checkerboard pattern.

Therapy

There is no definitive cure for dystrophinopathies, but physical therapy and medications can slow down the disease and help reduce complications. Over the past few years, it has been shown that early and consistent administration of **prednisone** can help treat the disease. It is thought that this is due to a membrane-stabilizing effect and perhaps an anti-inflammatory effect.

All patients with DMD/BMD, and all carriers of the disease, should be referred to cardiology. As ventricular remodeling occurs in males with DMD and BMD, early treatment with **angiotensin-converting enzyme (ACE) inhibitors** and/or beta-blockers is recommended. If overt heart failure develops, additional medications may be added.

Physical therapy is recommended for all individuals with DMD/BMD. Breathing exercises should also begin early. Active and passive physical therapy becomes increasingly important as the disease progresses. Intensifying training in active breathing techniques and regular drainages through body positioning are necessary in order to avoid complications of chronic hypoxia; possibly (nightly) mechanically assisted breathing devices may be considered for at-home treatment. Infections of the respiratory tract should be treated early with antibiotics. Pneumococcal and influenza vaccine are administered annually. Bone mineral density should be monitored, especially when the individual is nonambulatory, and treatment with calcium and vitamin D should be considered.

■■■ Experimental Therapy with Aminoglycosides

Approximately 15% of cases of DMD are caused by premature stop codons in the *DMD* gene. It has been shown, in cell culture and then mouse models of the disorder, that antibiotics of the aminoglycoside group allow **"read-through"** of premature stops. The treatment creates misreading of RNA and thereby allows alternative amino acids to be inserted at the site of the mutated stop codon. In the mouse model, treatment with gentamicin resulted in dystrophin expression at 10% to 20% of that detected in normal muscle.

Prognosis

Through optimal treatment, life expectancy for DMD can be extended from 18 to 25 years into the fifth decade of life. The main cause of death is respiratory insufficiency, frequently aggravated by recurrent pneumonias. The second most common cause of death is heart failure and cardiac arrhythmias. Average life expectancy for BMD patients had been 45 years but can now be significantly improved through optimal treatment.

Myotonic Dystrophy

Myotonic dystrophy is an autosomal dominant heritable multisystem disorder with muscular dystrophy and myotonia that results from a trinucleotide expansion in the 3′ untranslated region of the *DMPK* gene. See Section 3.6 for a detailed discussion of the disorder and the underlying molecular pathomechanism.

32 Neoplastic Diseases

LEARNING GOALS AND OBJECTIVES

1 Explain the concepts of the "two-hit hypothesis" and "loss of heterozygosity," using retinoblastoma as a clinical example. Explain general differences in the clinical presentation of sporadic versus hereditary cancers.

2 Discuss indications for molecular testing of *BRCA1* and *BRCA2* and management of an individual who harbors a mutation in one of these genes.

3 Contrast the clinical presentations of familial adenomatous polyposis (FAP) versus hereditary nonpolyposis colon cancer (HNPCC).

4 List the diagnostic criteria for neurofibromatosis type 1.

5 Describe three mechanisms of DNA repair.

32.1 Leukemias and Lymphomas

Scientific discoveries define typical chromosome abnormalities in the tumor cells of numerous leukemias and lymphomas. Moreover, specific cytogenetic abnormalities have been associated with morphologically and clinically distinct subsets of leukemias and lymphomas and often correlate with morphological, immunophenotypical, and clinical parameters.

Chronic Myeloid Leukemia

Chronic myeloid leukemia (CML) was the first malignant disease in humans for which a specific chromosomal abnormality was identified. This defect, called the **Philadelphia chromosome**, results from the reciprocal exchange between the long arm of chromosome 22 and the long arm of chromosome 9 (Sections 3.4 and 7.2; ◘ Fig. 3.2).

This **translocation**, designated **t(9;22)(q34.1;q11.2)**, leads at the molecular level to fusion of the initial part of the BCR gene on chromosome 22q11 with most of the ABL protooncogene (starting at exon 2) on chromosome 9q34. The resulting **BCR-ABL fusion gene** on the Philadelphia chromosome codes for a BCR-ABL fusion protein with tyrosine kinase activity that promotes cellular proliferation. In contrast, the reciprocal ABL-BCR translocation on chromosome 9q+ has no known functional significance.

A Philadelphia translocation is found in more than 90% of all patients with CML ("classic CML"). Atypical CML without t(9;22) is far less common. Many CML patients who are cytogenetically negative for the Philadelphia chromosome have a BCR-ABL recombination on molecular genetic testing. Individuals with CML without a BCR-ABL recombination tend to have a poorer prognosis.

Pathogenesis. CML develops in several stages, with translocation to the Philadelphia chromosome representing the initial step in most cases. The BCR-ABL fusion protein causes hematopoietic stem cells to acquire a growth advantage over other stem cells. The uncontrolled growth of the cell clone gives rise to additional chromosomal changes and an increasing dissociation between proliferation and differentiation. The clinical manifestation of maximal proliferation and minimal differentiation is the blast crisis that occurs in the advanced stage of CML.

> **Important**
>
> Tumor-specific balanced chromosome translocations may have considerable prognostic importance. They are found only in tumor cells and thus represent somatic mutations. A cytogenetic analysis of the abnormal cell line should be included in the standard workup of most leukemias and lymphomas and may supply information on treatment strategies.

Treatment. The clinical symptoms and the leukocytosis that occur during the chronic phase of CML can be treated with busulfan and hydroxyurea. Treatment with α-**interferon** induces a "hematological remission" in more than 50% of cases, marked by a normalization of the peripheral blood count and an improvement in clinical symptoms. However, a complete "cytogenetic remission" with the disappearance of a Philadelphia-positive cell clone is rarely achieved (less than 10% of cases). Better results have been obtained with **tyrosine kinase inhibitors (TKIs)** that selectively inhibit the aberrant BCR-ABL tyrosine kinase. Several of these have been developed (most notably imatinib, dasatinib, and nilotinib) and have been shown to produce up to 95% hematological remissions and 80% cytogenetic remissions during the chronic phase of CML. They have become the initial treatment of choice for most patients with CML. There are still only two curative treatment options for CML, however: **allogeneic bone marrow transplantation** and peripheral stem cell transplantation.

Acute Lymphoblastic Leukemia

Acute lymphoblastic leukemia (ALL) is not only the most common form of leukemia in children but also the most common malignant disease of childhood. It accounts for approximately 30% of all childhood malignancies. Approximately 2,500 to 3,500 new cases of ALL are diagnosed in children in the United States each year. The most common cytogenetic change in pediatric ALL is a t(12;21)(p13;q22) translocation, which generates a TEL-AML1 fusion gene (30% of cases).

The BCR-ABL fusion gene is also seen in ALL. The presence of this abnormality correlates with the age at diagnosis such that it is present in 5% of children, 35% of adults, and more than 50% of individuals over 60 years of age with ALL. The detection of a BCR-ABL translocation in ALL indicates a particularly malignant form of the disease. BCR-ABL translocation–positive patients have a median survival time of less than 9 months when treated with conventional ALL regimens because of a high early relapse rate.

The molecular detection of small numbers of residual leukemia cells (**minimal residual disease**) has prognostic implications in patients who are in remission from ALL. Patients with less than 1 tumor cell per 10,000 lymphocytes have a favorable prognosis, while patients with 1 or more tumor cells per 1,000 lymphocytes have an unfavorable prognosis.

32.2   Solid Malignant Tumors in Children

Solid tumors account for approximately 30% of all childhood cancers. Most of these manifest before the age of 5 years and a maximum incidence of embryonal tumors is found in this age group. The most common types of solid tumors in children include brain tumors, neuroblastoma, retinoblastoma, Wilms tumor, and lymphomas.

Retinoblastoma

Retinoblastomas are malignant eye tumors of infancy and childhood. Sixty percent occur sporadically, in which case they are generally unilateral and unifocal. Approximately 40% of retinoblastomas have a hereditary etiology. These tumors usually have an earlier onset and are frequently bilateral and/or multifocal.

Important
— **Sporadic retinoblastomas** are most commonly unifocal and unilateral. The average age at diagnosis is 24 months. — **Hereditary retinoblastomas** are more often multifocal and bilateral. The average age at diagnosis is 15 months.

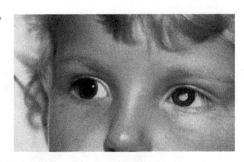

Figure 32.1. Leukocoria in Retinoblastoma. (Courtesy of Hj Müller, Department of Medical Genetics, University Children's Hospital Basel, Switzerland.)

Clinical Manifestations. Retinoblastoma usually presents initially as an abnormal white reflection in the iris of the affected eye (**leukocoria**; Fig. 32.1). The second most common presenting sign is strabismus, which may accompany or antedate the leukocoria. Visual deterioration is usually not noticed in small children. Less common clinical symptoms of retinoblastoma are uveitis, glaucoma, hyphema (blood in the anterior chamber of the eye), proptosis, and pain.

Genetics. The *RB1* **gene** on chromosome 13q14.1-q14.2 is crucial in the pathogenesis of retinoblastoma. It is considered the classic tumor suppressor gene. Based on a statistical analysis of retinoblastoma patients, Alfred Knudson formulated the **two-hit hypothesis** for tumorigenesis in 1971, stating that the inactivation of **both** *RB1* alleles in a retinoblast cell is necessary in order for a tumor to develop. In the case of hereditary retinoblastoma, one *RB1* germline mutation is already present in all cells of the body. A retinoblastoma develops when a "second hit" inactivates the second *RB1* allele in a retinoblast cell (**loss of heterozygosity**). This contrasts with the sporadic form of retinoblastoma, in which two independent somatic events must occur in the same cell (or successively in the same cell line) in order for a tumor to form.

Only 10% of children with retinoblastoma have a positive family history. Other cases of hereditary retinoblastoma are based on *de novo* mutations in the parental (usually paternal) germ line.

Patients with a hereditary *RB1* mutation have a greater than 95% chance of developing retinoblastoma, despite the fact that they inherit only one mutated allele of the tumor suppressor gene, which is recessive at the cellular level. This explains the **autosomal dominant** mode of inheritance of hereditary retinoblastomas.

More than 400 different mutations of the *RB1* gene have been described in retinoblastoma patients. The great majority of cases (85% to 90%) involve mutations that lead to a premature stop codon (nonsense, frameshift, or splice mutations).

Therapy and Management. Unilateral retinoblastomas are generally treated by enucleation of the affected eye, supplemented if necessary by adjuvant radiotherapy. Tumors of moderate size can be treated by radioactive plaque therapy (I-125 brachytherapy, which involves suturing of a radioactive plaque to the eye wall at the apex of the tumor). Only very small tumors are treatable by laser ablation or cryotherapy. In patients with bilateral retinoblastomas, the more severely affected eye is enucleated and the contralateral eye is treated with radiation. A permanent cure can be achieved in at least 80% of all children with retinoblastoma. Follow-up examinations should be continued for a number of years, given the increased risk of other primary ocular tumors and the potential for contralateral disease.

Complications. Patients with the hereditary form of retinoblastoma are at increased risk for developing other malignant tumors including osteosarcomas, soft tissue sarcomas, melanomas, and pinealomas.

Neuroblastoma

Neuroblastomas are embryonic tumors of the sympathetic nervous system (adrenal medulla, sympathetic trunk, sympathetic ganglia). They are among the most common solid tumors in children (Fig. 32.2). They are classified into four stages (I through IV), with stage IV having the worst prognosis.

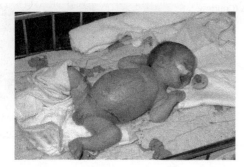

Figure 32.2. Massive Abdominal Swelling in a Newborn with Neuroblastoma. (Courtesy of University of Heidelberg Children's Hospital.)

Genetics. Overexpression of a specific gene of the *MYC* oncogene family is found in approximately 30% of all neuroblastomas. Designated *MYCN* because of its expression in neuroectodermal tissue, the gene maps to chromosome 2p24.1. Unlike the overexpression of the *MYC* gene in Burkitt lymphoma, which is caused by enhancer sequences of the immunoglobulin loci after translocation, overexpression of the *MYCN* gene in neuroblastoma is caused by the **amplification of *MYCN***. One tumor cell may contain up to 700 copies of the gene, some appearing as homogeneously staining chromosomal regions, others as small chromosome fragments separate from the other chromosomes ("double minutes"). *MYCN* amplifications are an important prognostic factor in neuroblastoma. While amplification of *MYCN* is very rarely found in stage I cases, it is detectable in 40% of patients with advanced stage III or IV disease. It is noteworthy that the amplification of *MYCN* is a prognostic parameter that is **independent of tumor stage**. For example, while stage II tumors have an inherently favorable prognosis, they are often refractory to treatment and have a poor prognosis in cases where *MYCN* amplifications are present.

Inherited forms of neuroblastoma are very rare.

Wilms Tumor (Nephroblastoma)

Wilms tumors are highly malignant embryonic tumors of the kidney. The incidence of Wilms tumor is 1 in 8,000 children. The average age at diagnosis is 3 years. Boys and girls are affected with equal frequency.

Etiology. A significant predisposing factor for the development of Wilms tumor is the persistence of renal blastema (primitive mesenchymal tissue), and the great majority of Wilms tumor predisposition syndromes are associated with **nephroblastomatosis**. The precise molecular mechanisms of tumorigenesis are understood in only a fraction of cases. Moreover, the exact function of the single known Wilms tumor gene, *WT1* (Wilms tumor 1), is not yet fully understood. The gene product plays an important role as a transcription factor in the differentiation of renal tissue at the junction of mesenchymal and epithelial tissue (glomerulus/nephron and the urinary tract).

Clinical Manifestations. Most Wilms tumors do not cause clinical symptoms. In 50% of cases, abdominal distention is noticed while the child is being dressed or bathed. In addition, nephroblastomas are often detected incidentally during routine examinations. Only 25% to 30% of children present with signs or symptoms such as abdominal pain, hematuria, or constipation. Approximately 5% to 10% of children with nephroblastoma have bilateral or multicentric tumors.

Genetics. Inactivating somatic mutations in the *WT1* gene are found in approximately 10% of Wilms tumors. The gene also has an important role in various syndromes:

— **WAGR syndrome** is characterized by a combination of **W**ilms tumor, **a**niridia, **g**enital anomalies, and mental **r**etardation. It is caused by a microdeletion of chromosome 11p13 with involvement of the *WT1* gene and *PAX6* gene.
— Patients with **Denys-Drash syndrome** have a 46,XY karyotype with female or ambiguous external genitalia, diffuse mesangial sclerosis, and Wilms tumors. The syndrome is caused by missense mutations (mainly exon 8 or 9) in the *WT1* gene.

— Point mutations at the donor splice site for intron 9 in the *WT1* gene lead to **Frasier syndrome**, in which a 46,XY karyotype is associated with ambiguous genitalia, focal segmental glomerulosclerosis, and gonadoblastomas.

An increased incidence of Wilms tumors (and other embryonal tumors) is found in genetic overgrowth syndromes. For example, it is not uncommon for patients with **Beckwith-Wiedemann syndrome** (Section 35.2) to have perilobar rests of renal blastema in their kidneys, and 5% of patients develop a Wilms tumor. Simpson-Golabi-Behmel syndrome (7.5%), Perlman syndrome (30%), and Sotos syndrome (less than 5%) are also associated with an increased risk of Wilms tumors.

Treatment. Surgical resection may be done primarily or may be preceded by neoadjuvant chemotherapy (e.g., with vincristine and actinomycin D), depending on tumor stage. Treatment almost always includes the complete removal of the tumor-bearing kidney (tumor nephrectomy). If complete resection cannot be achieved, surgery should be followed by radiotherapy. Wilms tumors are radiosensitive. The overall prognosis is good, and a permanent cure is achieved in more than 85% of children with Wilms tumors.

32.3   Breast and Ovarian Cancer

Breast cancer is the most common female cancer and the second most common cause of cancer death in women. The lifetime risk of developing breast cancer is up to one in six overall (and one in eight for invasive disease).

Large studies have shown that the risk of developing breast cancer is doubled in first-degree relatives of women with breast cancer. The observation that relatives of women with ovarian cancer also have a 30% to 60% greater risk of developing breast cancer suggests that some genetic risk factors predispose to both tumor entities. Approximately 5% to 10% of breast cancers occur in a person with an inherited predisposition to the disease. Two of these predisposition genes were discovered in 1990 and 1994 and have been designated ***BRCA1* and *BRCA2*** (breast cancer genes 1 and 2).

■■■ **Risk Factors for Breast Cancer**

While there are heritable disorders that predispose to breast cancer, the vast majority of cases have a multifactorial etiology. Risk factors for breast cancer include:

— Menarche before 12 years of age
— Menopause after 55 years of age
— Having a first child after 30 years of age
— Nulliparity
— Postmenopausal obesity
— Alcohol abuse
— Hormone replacement therapy
— Radiation exposure

Hereditary Breast and Ovarian Cancer

Case Study

Mrs. Dittner presents for genetic counseling because of a family history of breast cancer. Her mother was first diagnosed with breast cancer at age 45, and cancer was found in the contralateral breast at age 46. She died from the disease at 48 years of age. Mrs. Dittner's maternal aunt was diagnosed with breast cancer at age 58 and is currently 67 years old. Another maternal aunt and uncle are healthy at 73 and 78 years old, respectively. The maternal grandmother was diagnosed with ovarian cancer at age 71, and she died from the disease at age 72. Molecular testing is recommended and is performed in the aunt with breast cancer. Complete sequence analysis and deletion/duplication analysis of the *BRCA1* and *BRCA2* genes do not reveal a pathogenic mutation. Based on this result, Mrs. Dittner is not a candidate for predictive testing and is placed in an intensive screening program for high-risk patients pending further findings.

III

Genetics and Etiology

Only about 5% to 10% of all breast cancers are based on a genetic predisposition. A familial form should be suspected in cases of multiple breast cancers in the same family or the development of breast cancer at an early age. The prevalence of clinically relevant *BRCA1* mutations in the normal population is between 1 in 500 and 1 in 1,000. Reliable data are not yet available for *BRCA2*, but estimates are in the range of 1 to 2 persons per 1,000.

BRCA1 is located on chromosome 17q21 and *BRCA2* on chromosome 13q21. Both genes are tumor suppressor genes that code for proteins involved in **DNA damage repair** and are involved in cell cycle control and regulation of other proteins of DNA damage response. Familial breast cancer caused by mutations in *BRCA1* and *BRCA2* is transmitted in an **autosomal dominant** manner. Carcinogenesis is based on the "two-hit hypothesis," which requires inactivation of the second, normal allele by mutation or large deletion. Molecular genetic testing of the tumor tissue may demonstrate a loss of heterozygosity (LOH) in the corresponding chromosomal region.

Over 1,000 different mutations and variants in the *BRCA1* and *BRCA2* genes have been reported. Nonsense and frameshift mutations are clearly associated with disease, yet the pathological impact of many missense mutations is uncertain. These are **unclassified variants**, and thus cannot be used for susceptibility testing in other family members.

Clinical Features

Mutations in *BRCA1* and *BRCA2* lead to an increased risk of breast cancer as well as ovarian cancer (Table 32.1). An individual who harbors a *BRCA1* or *BRCA2* mutation has an increased susceptibility to disease; however, the penetrance is not complete. Some carriers develop multiple primary tumors before 50 years of age, whereas other people with the same mutation do not develop a single cancer past age 70. The lifetime risk for **breast cancer** in mutation carriers is 85%, and more than half of affected women will develop breast cancer before age 50. Carriers of *BRCA1* mutations have a significantly higher risk of developing **ovarian cancer** (44%) than carriers of *BRCA2* mutations (27%).

Men with mutations in *BRCA1* and *BRCA2* also have an increased cancer risk. *BRCA1* mutations are associated with an approximately threefold increase in the risk for **prostate cancer** but very rarely lead to male breast cancer. By contrast, a definite association exists between *BRCA2* mutations and **male breast cancer**, with carriers facing a cumulative risk of 7% by the age of 70 years. *BRCA2* mutations show less association with prostate cancer but have been linked (in both sexes) to tumors of the pancreas, larynx, esophagus, colon, stomach, and biliary tract, and to melanomas.

Diagnosis

The current recommendations (April 2009) of the American Congress of Obstetricians and Gynecologists (ACOG) state that further genetic risk assessment is recommended for women who have more than a 20% to 25% chance of having an inherited predisposition to breast or ovarian cancer. These women include:
— Women with a personal history of both breast cancer and ovarian cancer
— Women with ovarian cancer and a close relative—defined as mother, sister, daughter, grandmother, granddaughter, aunt—with ovarian cancer, premenopausal breast cancer, or both
— Women of Ashkenazi Jewish descent with breast cancer who were diagnosed at age 40 or younger or who have ovarian cancer

Table 32.1. Lifetime Disease Risk Associated with Pathogenic Mutations in *BRCA1* and *BRCA2*

	BRCA1	BRCA2
Female breast cancer	85%	84%
Ovarian cancer	44%	27%
Male breast cancer	Low	7%

— Women with breast cancer at age 50 or younger and who have a close relative with ovarian cancer or male breast cancer at any age
— Women with a close relative with a known BRCA mutation

Genetic risk assessment may also be appropriate for women with a 5% to 10% chance of having hereditary risk, including:
— Women with breast cancer by age 40
— Women with ovarian cancer, primary peritoneal cancer, or fallopian tube cancer or high-grade, serous histology at any age
— Women with cancer in both breasts (particularly if the first cancer was diagnosed by age 50)
— Women with breast cancer by age 50 and a close relative with breast cancer by age 50
— Women with breast cancer at any age and two or more close relatives with breast cancer at any age (particularly if at least one case of breast cancer was diagnosed by age 50)
— Unaffected women with a close relative that meets one of the previous criteria

Targeted mutation analysis may be offered to women of specific ethnic background, such as women of Ashkenazi Jewish heritage. It includes mutations known to be at greater frequencies because of founder effects. **Comprehensive analysis** includes full sequence analysis of *BRCA1* and *BRCA2* and testing for specific large genomic rearrangements of *BRCA1*.

Screening and Prevention

Women identified as belonging to a high-risk family should be offered a rigorous, close-interval screening program:
— **Breast:** Monthly breast self-examination starting in early adulthood, annual or semiannual clinical breast examination, and annual mammography starting at age 25 to 35 years or 5 years before the earliest age at diagnosis in the family. The National Comprehensive Cancer Network now recommends breast magnetic resonance imaging (MRI) as an adjunct to annual mammography and breast examination in *BRCA1/2* mutation carriers and their first-degree relatives who have not yet undergone testing (MRI is more sensitive but apparently less specific than mammography).
— **Ovary:** Annual or semiannual pelvic examination and transvaginal ultrasound with color Doppler and annual serum CA-125 concentration. All of these measures should start at the age of 25 to 35 years or 5 years before the earliest diagnosis in the family.

Every woman with a documented *BRCA1* or *BRCA2* mutation should be offered a **prophylactic mastectomy and oophorectomy** as a preventive measure. The decision to accept or decline surgery rests with the patient, but surgical prophylaxis is definitely associated with a better chance of survival. Two types of mastectomy are available:
— Subcutaneous mastectomy (approximately 5% residual tissue)
— Complete mastectomy (approximately 1% residual tissue)

A complete mastectomy reduces the risk for breast cancer by more than 90%. Oophorectomy should usually be considered in women older than 35 years of age or in cases where the patient does not desire future pregnancy. Both procedures are associated with a small (approximately 3%) residual risk of peritoneal cancer.

■■■ **Breast Cancer in Other Cancer Predisposition Syndromes**
During the clinical examination of patients with breast cancer, subtle external features may be noted that suggest the possible presence of a familial cancer predisposition syndrome:
— **Hyperkeratotic papillomas at the vermilion border of the lip** are found in **Cowden syndrome**, an autosomal dominant disorder characterized by the development of multiple hamartomas in various organs. Other features are disseminated intestinal polyposis and an increased risk of breast and thyroid cancer.
— **Mucocutaneous melanin pigmentation**, especially around the mouth, eyes, and nostrils; in the perianal area; and on the buccal mucosa, may be a sign of **Peutz-Jeghers syndrome**, another autosomal

dominant disorder associated with multiple hamartomas in the gastrointestinal tract. The polyps in this syndrome are potentially precancerous lesions with a 2% to 3% risk of malignant transformation. There is an increased likelihood for developing cancers of the breast, uterus, and pancreas.

Breast cancer may be a presenting tumor in Li-Fraumeni syndrome (see Section 32.8). Lobular breast cancer and diffuse gastric cancer are caused by mutations in the E-cadherin gene *CDH1*.

32.4 Colorectal Tumors

Colorectal cancers are the leading cause of cancer-related deaths in the nonsmoking population and thus pose one of the greatest challenges to our health care system. Several genes have been identified that predispose to colon cancer with moderate to high penetrance. The identification of individuals with predisposing gene mutations is one of the greatest and most economically important tasks in preventive medicine. Classic syndromes that predispose to colon cancer are familial adenomatous polyposis (FAP) and hereditary nonpolyposis colon cancer (HNPCC).

Familial Adenomatous Polyposis

Case Study

John Williams, age 19 years, presents at a genetics outpatient clinic with his parents and younger brother. He was diagnosed with anemia approximately 6 months earlier. This condition was investigated by gastroscopy, which revealed numerous polyps in the stomach. When the patient was reexamined 5 months later, the gastric polyps were essentially unchanged, but his hemoglobin level had fallen to 6.9 g/dL. Subsequent colonoscopy revealed several hundred polyps (histologically adenomas with no evidence of dysplasia) in the large bowel. Abdominal ultrasound showed no abnormalities except for a slightly enlarged spleen. John reports that he has noticed blood in his stool on several occasions. His parents recall that at 13 years of age, John was examined for bone changes ("osteomas" on the forehead and other sites) at a pediatric hospital, but that no diagnosis was made. They further state that several sebaceous skin tumors were removed. The family history is negative for polyposis. The father had already undergone a couple of gastroscopies and colonoscopies, which showed no abnormalities. The mother is scheduled for a colonoscopy. The mother's 55-year-old brother had several colon polyps removed and was advised to have yearly colonoscopies. There is no known family history of malignant bowel disease. Molecular genetic analysis of the *APC* gene in John shows heterozygosity for the c.4393_4394delAG mutation, a definite pathogenic deletion with a shift in the reading frame. This confirms the diagnosis of FAP. The mutation is not detectable in the parents, identifying it as a *de novo* mutation.

Epidemiology

FAP accounts for approximately 0.5% to 1% of all colorectal cancers in the population. The prevalence is approximately 3 in 100,000 individuals.

Clinical Features

The disease is defined by the presence of innumerable (at least 100, often more than 1,000) **colorectal adenomas**. They are always detectable at least by late puberty in affected individuals. These lesions follow the adenoma–carcinoma sequence, starting as benign epithelial tumors and developing over a period of years into epithelial dysplasia and finally to colorectal carcinoma (◘ Fig. 32.3). The average age of colon cancer diagnosis in untreated individuals with FAP is 39 years; 93% will develop colon cancer by the age of 50 years. FAP is therefore classified as an **obligate precancerous lesion**.

In addition to colon lesions, patients with FAP also have **extracolonic manifestations** (◘ Fig. 32.4), which include:
- **CHRPE** (85% of cases) = **c**ongenital **h**ypertrophy of the **r**etinal **p**igment **e**pithelium. This finding in the optic fundus, while harmless, is still a useful source of diagnostic information.
- **Duodenal adenomas** and gastric glandular cysts (80% of cases). The risk of developing duodenal cancer is approximately 10%.

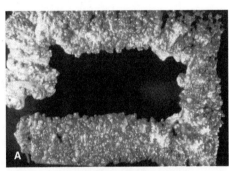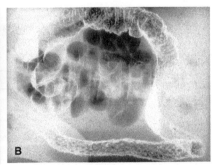

Figure 32.3. **Familial Adenomatous Polyposis. A.** Specimen. **B.** Radiographic appearance.

- Osteomas of the mandible and skull (more than 90% of cases, clinically irrelevant and benign)
- Epidermoid cysts (60%), which are mainly a cosmetic problem
- Semimalignant desmoid tumors (5% to 10%), which are the leading cause of death in FAP patients who undergo colectomy
- Increased risk for the following tumors: papillary thyroid cancer, medulloblastomas (the association of FAP and central nervous system [CNS] tumors is known as **Turcot syndrome**), sarcomas, and hepatoblastomas in children

---

Important

Attenuated FAP. This is a variant of FAP in which the number of polyps is far less than 100 (30 on average). It produces clinical manifestations much later than classic FAP, with colorectal cancer usually developing in the fifth decade. Attenuated FAP is still associated with a high cancer risk, however.

Genetics and Etiology

FAP and attenuated FAP are caused by heterozygous mutations in the **APC gene** (adenomatous polyposis coli) on chromosome 5q21-q22. Most confirmed mutations lead to a truncation of the gene product, either by point mutations or by deletion/insertion with a frame shift, resulting in

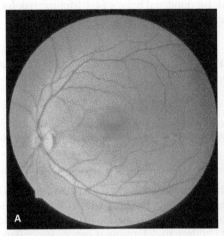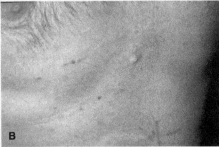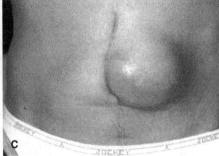

Figure 32.4. **Extracolonic Manifestations of Familial Adenomatous Polyposis (FAP).**
A. Congenital hypertrophy of the retinal pigment epithelium (CHRPE). **B.** Epidermoid cyst. **C.** Desmoid tumor of the abdominal wall. (Courtesy of M. Kadmon, University of Heidelberg, Department of Surgery.)

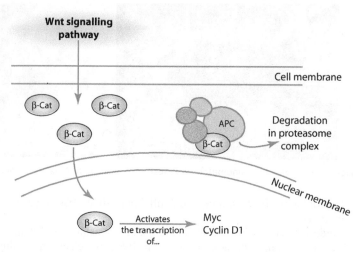

Wnt signalling
pathway

Cell membrane

β-Cat   β-Cat

β-Cat

APC

β-Cat

Degradation
in proteasome
complex

Nuclear membrane

β-Cat   Activates
the transcription
of...

Myc
Cyclin D1

Figure 32.5. APC and the β-Catenin Signal Pathway. (Modified from Farrington and Dunlop, 2004.)

a **premature stop codon** downstream from the mutation. There are also a substantial number of missense mutations, whose pathogenic relevance is unclear and which are described as unclassified variants. FAP has an **autosomal dominant** mode of inheritance, but approximately one-fourth of patients represent *de novo* cases.

Functionally competent APC protein binds to β-catenin and is part of a protein complex whose actions include the breakdown of β-catenin in the proteasome complex (Fig. 32.5). When APC is absent, β-catenin remains in the cytoplasm in an unbound state. It can easily enter the cell nucleus, where it activates the transcription of several oncogenes including MYC and cyclin D1. Owing to these pathophysiological relationships, *APC* is classified as a **tumor suppressor gene**.

An **autosomal recessive** form of attenuated polyposis may be caused by mutations in the *MUTYH* **gene** coding for a DNA glycosylase involved in oxidative DNA damage repair. Molecular testing for this condition, denoted **MAP** (MUTYH-associated polyposis), is indicated in all individuals with a high number of colonic polyps but no mutation in the *APC* gene. Affected persons also have an increased risk for duodenal polyps (4% lifetime risk for duodenal cancer) and some extraintestinal malignancies.

Diagnosis

Colonoscopy is the main tool for the diagnosis of colonic adenomas. Rectal adenomas can also be detected by endorectal ultrasound.

> **Important**
>
> Whenever a single colorectal adenoma is detected, the entire colon should be scrutinized for possible additional adenomas (complete colonoscopy) because at least one more adenoma is present in up to 30% of cases!

A detailed **family history** should be taken in all patients with colon cancer. A molecular genetic analysis of the *APC* gene can be performed in individuals with a clinical diagnosis of FAP and in at-risk family members. Because malignant transformation may occur in adolescents, molecular testing is recommended in at-risk children to determine if cancer surveillance is necessary.

Therapy and Management

Prophylactic proctocolectomy (sphincter-preserving ileoanal pouch surgery) is recommended for individuals with classic FAP once adenomas emerge. Colectomy may be delayed depending on the number and size of polyps. Colectomy is usually advised when more than 20 or 30 adenomas or multiple adenomas with advanced histology have developed. **After colectomy**, it is possible for new adenomas to form in the rectal stump. Studies indicate that long-term therapy with nonsteroidal anti-inflammatory drugs, especially sulindac, will reduce this risk.

Individuals with FAP must also undergo regular **screening examinations for extracolonic manifestations**. Gastroduodenoscopy with inspection of the papillae should begin at age 25 and should be repeated at least every 3 years.

Lynch Syndrome (Hereditary Nonpolyposis Colon Cancer)

Case Study

Mrs. Byers presents for genetic counseling. One year ago, at age 43, she was diagnosed with endometrial cancer. Because she had other family members with cancer, she wanted to learn about the cancer risk in her two children. The father of Mrs. Byers was diagnosed with transverse colon cancer at age 68 and died 1 year later. One of her father's brothers had ureteral cancer at age 53 and also developed bowel cancer at age 63. Two other of her father's siblings are healthy. Her paternal grandfather died during World War II, and her grandmother died from pneumonia while in her 80s. There is no known cancer history in Mrs. Byers' mother or her family. The patient's personal and family history meet the Amsterdam criteria, justifying a clinical diagnosis of Lynch syndrome. (Incidentally, Mrs. Byers herself and her uncle would also meet the Bethesda criteria even if there had been no cancer in other family members.) Analysis of tumor tissue from Mrs. Byers reveals microsatellite instability and the absence of MLH1 protein based on immunohistochemical testing. A subsequent analysis of genomic DNA reveals a pathogenic frameshift mutation in the *MLH1* gene. The same mutation is detected in a stored DNA sample from her father. In addition to lifelong follow-up examinations, Mrs. Byers should take part in an intensive cancer screening program for Lynch syndrome patients. Given the autosomal dominant nature of Lynch syndrome, each of her children is at 50% risk of inheriting the mutation in *MLH1*.

Epidemiology

With an incidence of 1 in 1,000, HNPCC accounts for approximately 5% of all colorectal cancers.

Clinical Features

The cardinal feature of Lynch syndrome, also known as hereditary nonpolyposis colon cancer, is the **familial occurrence of colon cancer** or certain other cancers at a relatively **young age**. The median age at onset of colorectal cancer in Lynch syndrome is 45 years. These cancers very rarely occur before age 25. Unlike sporadic cancers, Lynch syndrome–associated colon cancers are frequently (in more than 50% of cases) located in the right side of the colon, and so cancers at that location are always suspicious for HNPCC. The lifetime risk of developing colorectal cancer is as high as **80%** in male carriers of the HNPCC mutation. Female carriers have a 50% lifetime risk for colon cancer and a 60% risk of developing **endometrial cancer**. **Extracolonic neoplasms** that have been linked to Lynch syndrome include cancers of the stomach (10% to 20% lifetime risk), ovaries (12%), biliary tract (7%), small intestine (4%), urothelium, pancreas, and CNS. As with FAP, the combination of HNPCC with brain tumors is classified as **Turcot syndrome**. The combination with sebaceous gland tumors (which may undergo malignant transformation) is known as **Muir-Torre syndrome**.

Important

Features of Lynch syndrome–associated colorectal cancers compared with sporadic cancers:
- Earlier age at diagnosis (average 44 years)
- More frequent involvement of the proximal colon
- Increased likelihood of multiple colorectal cancers (synchronous or metachronous)
- Better prognosis for the individual tumor

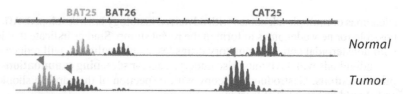

Figure 32.6. Microsatellite Instability in Lynch Syndrome. Microsatellites are common repetitive sequences of two to four nucleotides that may show different repeat counts on different alleles (Section 2.3). As a rule, the repeat count (or genotype) is the same in all cells from a given individual. But when the repair of base pair mismatches is defective (DNA mismatch repair defect), an instability develops in which the number of repeats of certain microsatellites may change with cell division. In the example shown here, different lengths (repeat counts) of the microsatellites BAT25, BAT26, and CAT26 were found in DNA samples from colon cancer cells compared to blood cells (leukocytes) taken from the same individual. Thus, the cancer cells display a clonal change consistent with a failure of the DNA mismatch repair system. This is considered strong evidence of Lynch syndrome. (Courtesy of M. Kloor, Department of Pathology, University of Heidelberg.)

Genetics and Etiology

Lynch syndrome is heterogenous and generally has an **autosomal dominant** mode of inheritance. It is caused by mutations in the genes of the **DNA mismatch repair system**. Usually these involve mutations in the *MLH1 or MSH2* genes, which together account for approximately 90% of cases with a detectable mutation. Other Lynch syndrome–associated genes are *MSH6*, *PMS1*, and *PMS2*. Like other DNA repair genes, these are tumor suppressor genes. Inherited heterozygous mutations are not sufficient by themselves to produce a clinical phenotype. A "second hit" on the healthy allele is necessary to cause a complete loss of functional protein, resulting in defective DNA mismatch repair. This triggers an avalanche of mutations in numerous genes including some that are important for normal cell function. This hypermutability of a cell clone may be recognized on the basis of **microsatellite instability** (MSI; Fig. 32.6).

Diagnosis

The diagnosis of Lynch syndrome is based on the **Amsterdam II clinical criteria** (1999). All of the following criteria must be met:
— At least three family members must be diagnosed with colon cancer or another Lynch syndrome–associated cancer.
— One of the three family members must be a first-degree relative of the other two.
— At least two successive generations must be affected.
— At least one of these relatives was diagnosed before age 50.
— FAP has been excluded.
— Cancers have been histopathologically confirmed.

The **molecular detection rate** is 50% to 70% in cases where the Amsterdam criteria are fulfilled.

The Amsterdam criteria are more specific than the **Bethesda criteria**, which allow a presumptive diagnosis to be made also in individuals or small families. According to these criteria, screening for MSI should be recommended in patients who are diagnosed with colorectal cancer or endometrial cancer before 50 years of age. This also applies to cases where two Lynch syndrome–associated cancers are found in the same individual (regardless of age), when there are two relatives with a Lynch syndrome–associated cancer, or when there is one relative with diagnosis before 50 years of age.

Microsatellite instability in tumor material is an important diagnostic criterion (Fig. 32.6). It should be noted, however, that approximately 10% to 15% of sporadic colorectal cancers are MSI positive, while only 10% of Lynch syndrome–associated colorectal cancers are MSI negative. **Immunohistochemical** testing can be done to determine which protein of the DNA mismatch repair system (e.g., MLH1 or MSH2) is absent in the tumor tissue (Fig. 32.7). This allows for targeted sequencing of the presumably affected gene.

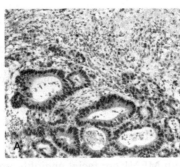
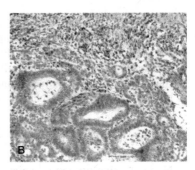

MLH1 MSH2

Figure 32.7. Immunohistochemistry of Lynch Syndrome. MLH1 protein is clearly detectable histochemically in the tumor cells (reddish brown stain in **A**), while MSH2 protein is absent (light blue stain in **B**). A mutation in the *MSH2* gene was detectable by molecular genetic analysis. (Courtesy of M. Kloor, Department of Pathology, University of Heidelberg.)

Treatment

Once a diagnosis of Lynch syndrome has been made, two main treatment options are available.

— **Screening examinations** once a year starting at age 20 to 25. Each examination should include **colonoscopy**, abdominal ultrasound, physical examination, and transvaginal ultrasound in women. The standard follow-up protocol for sporadic tumors, consisting of colonoscopy every 3 to 5 years, is inadequate for patients with Lynch syndrome due to the typically rapid progression from adenoma to carcinoma in this subgroup. Yearly esophago-gastroduodenoscopy may also be recommended, especially in patients who have multiple family members with stomach cancer. Annual urinary cytology was formerly recommended but has poor sensitivity.

— Some patients opt for a **prophylactic subtotal colectomy**. Because the distal colon is rarely affected by Lynch syndrome, proctectomy with ileostomy is generally not indicated because the remaining colonic segment can be adequately monitored by flexible sigmoidoscopy every 1 to 2 years. The screening program for other organ manifestations should be conducted without change.

32.5 Multiple Endocrine Neoplasia

Multiple endocrine neoplasia (MEN) encompasses two tumor predisposition syndromes with an autosomal dominant inheritance, each characterized by variable combinations of primary endocrine tumors. They are caused by mutations in two different genes.

Important
Typical features of multiple endocrine neoplasias:
— MEN1: hyperparathyroidism, endocrine pancreatic tumors, prolactinoma
— MEN2: medullary thyroid cancer, pheochromocytoma, hyperparathyroidism

Multiple Endocrine Neoplasia Type 1

Multiple endocrine neoplasia type 1 (MEN1), also called Wermer syndrome, is caused by mutations of the MEN1 gene on chromosome 11q13 and is transmitted in an **autosomal dominant** manner. The tumors that occur in MEN1 (except for gastrinomas) do not metastasize.

— **Primary hyperparathyroidism** is present in 90% of patients with MEN1 by 20 to 25 years of age. The resulting hypercalcemia leads to the clinical manifestations of lethargy, depression, anorexia, constipation, nausea and vomiting, hypertension, prolonged

QT interval, diuresis with dehydration, and calciuria with urolithiasis. Increased osteoclast activity increases the risk of fractures in affected patients.

— **Pancreatic tumors**, most notably gastrinomas and insulinomas, are found in 50% of MEN1 patients. Gastrinomas present clinically as Zollinger-Ellison syndrome (symptoms: diarrhea, peptic ulcers), while insulinomas present as hypoglycemia. Less common pancreatic tumors in MEN1 are glucagonomas and VIPomas.

— Approximately 30% of patients with MEN1 develop **pituitary tumors**, usually prolactinomas. Prolactinomas in women lead to oligomenorrhea or amenorrhea, possibly accompanied by galactorrhea. In males, sexual dysfunction is usually the only clinical manifestation of a prolactinoma.

— Nonendocrine tumors associated with MEN1 are facial angiofibromas, collagenomas, lipomas, meningiomas, ependymomas, and leiomyomas.

Genetics. *MEN1* is a tumor suppressor gene. The MEN1 gene product **menin** controls the transcription of various genes and has important functions in regulating cell proliferation, apoptosis, and genome stability. The precise molecular mechanisms are still poorly understood, however. Ten percent of patients with MEN1 have a negative family history, but even in these cases it is common to detect germline mutations in *MEN1*.

Multiple Endocrine Neoplasia Type 2

Multiple endocrine neoplasia type 2 (MEN2) is one of the few familial disorders caused by dominant mutations in a **protooncogene**. These are "gain-of-function" mutations in the *RET* gene, which codes for the RET receptor tyrosine kinase. The principal tumor is **medullary thyroid cancer** (C-cell carcinoma), which accounts for 10% to 25% of all thyroid cancers. One-fourth of medullary thyroid cancers occur in a setting of hereditary MEN2. The subtypes of MEN2 and their manifestations are reviewed in ◘ Table 32.2.

Multiple Endocrine Neoplasia Type 2A. Index patients within a family usually present at 15 to 20 years of age with a palpable thyroid nodule. By this time most patients already have bilateral or multifocal medullary thyroid cancer, which has metastasized to cervical lymph nodes in 50% of cases. Fifty percent of patients develop **pheochromocytomas**, which are bilateral in a significant number of cases. While these tumors rarely metastasize, they often cause hypertension that is difficult to control with medications. Approximately 15% to 30% of patients have **primary hyperparathyroidism**. Most patients have mutations in one of six cysteine codons in the extracellular domain of the RET protein, which lead to dimerization and constitutive activation.

Multiple Endocrine Neoplasia Type 2B. In addition to medullary thyroid cancer, this subtype features characteristic mucosal neuromas involving the lips and tongue, ganglioneuromas of the gastrointestinal tract, and a marfanoid habitus. Forty percent to 60% of patients develop pheochromocytomas; hyperparathyroidism is rare. Multiple endocrine neoplasia type 2B (MEN2B) has a poorer prognosis due to its earlier manifestations and the metastasis of thyroid cancer. Ninety-five percent of patients with MEN2B are found to have point mutations in the intracellular tyrosine kinase domain in exon 16 of the RET protooncogene.

◘ **Table 32.2.** Subtypes of Multiple Endocrine Neoplasia Type 2: Relative Frequency and Tumor Types

	MEN2A	MEN2B	FMTC
Relative frequency of MEN2	80%	5%–6%	15%
Medullary thyroid cancer (histologic)	95%	100%	100%
Primary hyperparathyroidism	20%–30%	Rare	0%
Pheochromocytoma	50%	50%	0%
Mucosal neuromas and ganglioneuromatosis	0%	>98%	0%

Familial Medullary Thyroid Cancer. Familial medullary thyroid cancer (FMTC) is diagnosed clinically when four or more cases of medullary thyroid cancer are present within one family and are not associated with pheochromocytoma or primary hyperparathyroidism. Ninety percent of these cases have detectable mutations in the *RET* gene, which have less activating effects than the mutations found in multiple endocrine neoplasia type 2A (MEN2A).

■■■ Hirschsprung Disease and Papillary Thyroid Cancer

Other diseases associated with mutations in the *RET* protooncogene are Hirschsprung disease and papillary thyroid cancer. The pathogenic mechanisms are different for those two disorders:

— **Hirschsprung disease** is caused in 20% to 40% of all cases by inherited (and possibly familial) germline mutations with inactivation of the RET gene.

— Forty percent of all patients with **papillary thyroid cancer** are found to have clonal somatic rearrangements in which fusion of the tyrosine kinase domain of *RET* with the 5′ region of a different gene leads to RET activation.

Management of Multiple Endocrine Neoplasia Type 2. Given the prophylactic and therapeutic implications of familial medullary thyroid cancer, predictive molecular genetic testing should be scheduled at an early age, preferably before 6 years. Molecular genetic testing in MEN2B should be done at the earliest possible age. Prophylactic thyroidectomy is recommended to mutation-positive individuals, and should be performed before the child enters school, even during the first year of life in the case of MEN2B. Follow-up tests include annual urinary catecholamine assays (in MEN2A and MEN2B) and annual serum assays of calcium and parathormone (in MEN2A).

Genetics. RET is a receptor tyrosine kinase, which conveys signals important for cell growth and differentiation from the cell membrane to intracellular signal cascades. An important effector in this process is the G-protein RAS. RAS activates the RAF-MEK-ERK cascade, which has been a subject of intense investigation. Abnormal RAS activation is also found in many other genetic diseases such as neurofibromatosis type 1 (Section 32.6).

■■■ Protein Kinases

It is estimated that 1.7% of all human genes code for protein kinases, which are key components of signal transduction pathways in man. Twenty percent of these proteins are tyrosine kinases, which are located within the cytoplasm or on the cell membrane. The activation of protein kinases is an important mechanism of carcinogenesis. For example, activation of the cytosolic tyrosine kinase ABL in the Philadelphia chromosome is a key factor in the pathogenesis of chronic myeloid leukemia (Section 32.1). **Receptor tyrosine kinases** are an important group of transmembrane proteins in which the binding of specific extracellular ligands leads to the activation of a catalytic domain and to the subsequent autophosphorylation of tyrosine residues. The resulting phosphotyrosines serve as docking sites for other proteins, which act through various mechanisms to trigger an intracellular signal cascade. The end result of this process is a modification in the expression of specific genes. Receptor tyrosine kinases thus have an important role in conveying signals from the cell membrane to the nucleus. The activity of receptor tyrosine kinases is strictly regulated under normal circumstances. Not infrequently, their genes are protooncogenes, which contribute to tumor formation when activating mutations are present.

32.6 The Hamartoses

Hamartomas are focal tumors composed of mature local cells that grow concurrently with the parent organ but lack the normal structural organization of the organ tissue. They are not neoplasms in the true sense because they do not have a potential for excessive growth. Hamartomas occur in a great variety of tissues, are generally benign (malignant transformation results in hamartoblastomas), and are usually occult unless visible externally. Hamartomas may cause clinical problems when located at certain sites. This may occur with large intracranial tumors or tumors that impinge on surrounding structures. When visible externally, hamartomas may be cosmetically objectionable to the patient and may cause significant emotional distress.

Hamartoses are a group of **autosomal dominant** diseases characterized by the presence of multiple hamartomas in various organs. Their common pathogenic mechanism is based on the inactivation of tumor suppressor genes. Another expression is **phakomatoses**, a collective term for **neurocutaneous syndromes** coined by the Dutch ophthalmologist van der Hoeve in the 1920s. This class of disorders includes neurofibromatosis type 1 and tuberous sclerosis, which are characterized by similar spots or lens-shaped patches visible on the optic fundus.

Multiple hamartomas are also found in **Cowden syndrome** and **Peutz-Jeghers syndrome**, which are associated with an increased risk of breast cancer (Section 32.3).

Neurofibromatosis Type 1 (von Recklinghausen Disease)

Case Study

Mrs. White presents with her two children aged 17 and 19 years for genetic evaluation and consultation. She has a more than 30-year history of neurofibromatosis type 1 (NF1), and her children would like to learn about their personal risk of having the disease and transmitting it to their offspring. Mrs. White was diagnosed at age 12 based on the presence of numerous café-au-lait spots, freckles, and cutaneous neurofibromas. Since then she has noticed a gradual increase in her neurofibromas, several of which have been surgically removed and histologically examined. On current physical examination of Mrs. White, axillary freckling and Lisch nodules of the irises are noted. Mild scoliosis is present. Physical examination (including an ophthalmic examination) of the children shows no abnormalities. These findings exclude NF1 in the children, and their offspring will not be at increased risk for the disease. Molecular analysis is not necessary as the diagnosis of NF1 can be made by clinical criteria.

Epidemiology

NF1 is one of the most common monogenic diseases known, with an incidence of 1 in 3,000 newborns. Males and females are affected equally.

Clinical Features

The typical clinical manifestations of NF1 develop with age and often a definitive diagnosis cannot be made in early childhood. The condition is diagnosed based on the presence of two or more well-defined **major criteria** (hereafter shown in boldface).

The hallmark of NF1 is the presence of **at least six café-au-lait spots** (▢ Fig. 32.8). These circumscribed, light brown hyperpigmented macules on the skin must measure at least 0.5 cm

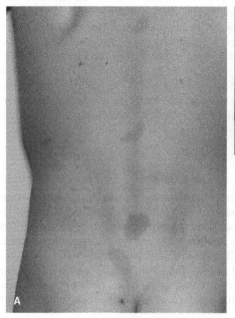
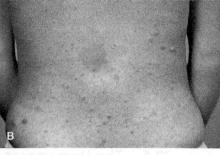

▢ Figure 32.8. Neurofibromatosis Type 1.
A. Café-au-lait spots in a 6-year-old child. **B.** Multiple hyperpigmented macules and neurofibromas in an adult woman.

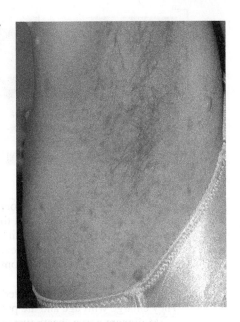

Figure 32.9. Neurofibromatosis Type 1. Axillary freckling in a 41-year-old woman.

in diameter before puberty or 1.5 cm after puberty to meet the major criterion for NF1. More than 99% of children with NF1 have numerous café-au-lait spots by their second birthday, and often this will prompt their initial referral to a geneticist. The macules become larger and more numerous as the patient nears puberty.

Another common pigmented skin lesion (present in 40% of patients) is **axillary or inguinal freckling** (Fig. 32.9).

Neurofibromas, from which the disease derives its name, are benign tumors of the peripheral nervous sheath. Often they do not develop until after puberty but are present in more than 99% of adults with NF1 (Fig. 32.10). **Plexiform neurofibromas** arise from large visceral

Figure 32.10. Cutaneous Neurofibromas in Neurofibromatosis 1. Neurofibromas may not be present at the time of diagnosis, especially in a child, but increase in size and number with age. (Photo courtesy of Rick Guidotti, www.positiveexposure.org.)

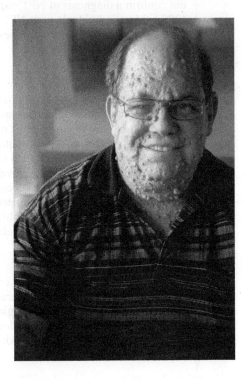

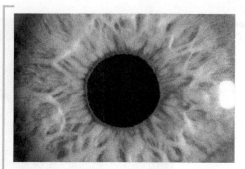

Figure 32.11. Neurofibromatosis Type 1 (NF1). Lisch nodules are benign, dome-shaped, avascular melanocytic hamartomas located on the surface of the iris stroma. Often tan, they may vary in color from glassy-translucent to dark brown. Among all persons with NF1 from birth to age 5 years, about 35% will have Lisch nodules, increasing in probability and number with age. By midteens, about 98% of persons with NF1 will manifest Lisch nodules. (Courtesy of R. Lewis, Baylor College of Medicine, Houston, Texas.)

nerve trunks and are usually congenital. Massive enlargement of these tumors often causes severe cosmetic problems, and they can impinge on or displace adjacent organs. Plexiform neurofibromas have an approximately 5% risk of undergoing malignant transformation (to malignant peripheral nerve sheath tumors). Nonplexiform neurofibromas do not have this tendency. Plexiform neurofibromas are found in 30% of patients with NF1 and are highly specific for this disease.

Hamartomas of the iris, called **Lisch nodules**, are pathognomonic for NF1 (◻ Fig. 32.11). They enlarge with age and are present in nearly all adult patients with NF1.

Malignant nerve sheath tumors are the most frequent malignant neoplasia associated with NF1, occuring in approximately 10% of affected individuals. Other malignancies include juvenile myeloid leukemia, rhabdomyosarcoma, and pheochromocytoma. The most common intracerebral tumors in NF1 are **optic gliomas**, which are found in up to 15% of all NF1 patients. Most are asymptomatic and detected incidentally. Approximately 70% of all optic gliomas are attributable to NF1. When they are bilateral, it is virtually certain that the patient has the disease.

The major criteria for NF1 also include typical skeletal deformities (thoracic deformities, kyphoscoliosis, curvature of the long bones in early childhood, **sphenoid dysplasia**, or **tibial pseudarthrosis**). Additionally, there are other symptoms and findings that support but do not confirm a diagnosis of NF1, especially macrocephaly (45%) combined with short stature (30%). Most individuals with NF1 have normal intelligence, but 20% of children with NF1 have significant learning disabilities and up to 80% have variable cognitive deficits. Epilepsy may also be attributable to NF1.

Genetics and Etiology

NF1 is an **autosomal dominant** disorder with variable expression but complete penetrance after childhood. It is caused by mutations in the *NF1* gene on chromosome 17q. *De novo* mutations are present in 50% of cases. Most of the mutations in *NF1* are point mutations, but deletions, duplications, insertions, splice mutations, and others have also been described.

NF1 codes for a protein called neurofibromin, which is an intracellular signaling molecule of the RasGAP (Ras GTPase activating protein) signal cascade. When a congenital mutation of *NF1* exists, only half of the necessary protein is present within the cell. Like other dominant neoplasias, however, NF1-associated tumors are caused by a "second-hit" loss of the normal allele. ◻ Figure 32.12 shows simplified diagrams illustrating the physiology and pathophysiology of neurofibromin within the cell.

Diagnosis

NF1 is a **clinical** diagnosis based on the 1997 revision of the diagnostic criteria. Sequencing of the neurofibromin gene is generally not indicated. However, there is at least one important differential diagnosis of NF1: **Legius syndrome**, caused by mutations in the *SPRED1* gene. Its phenotype includes a high incidence of café-au-lait macules and axillary/inguinal freckling, but no neurofibromas or Lisch nodules. This condition seems to be much rarer than NF1 but

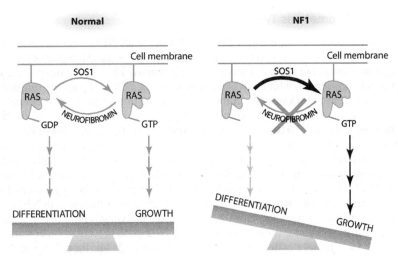

Figure 32.12. Physiology and Pathophysiology of Neurofibromin in the Cell. (Modified from Viskochil 2005.)

should always be considered, specifically in adults who have no features of NF1 other than café-au-lait macules and freckling.

Important

According to National Institutes of Health (NIH) diagnostic criteria, a patient has NF1 when two or more of the following features are present:

- Six or more café-au-lait spots greater than 5 mm in diameter, or greater than 15 mm after puberty
- Two or more neurofibromas or at least one plexiform neurofibroma
- Axillary or inguinal freckling
- Optic glioma
- Lisch nodules
- Sphenoid dysplasia
- NF1 diagnosed in a first-degree relative

Treatment

Causal therapy is not available. Treatment is symptomatic and is best accomplished by a multidisciplinary team of physicians including an ophthalmologist, a geneticist, and a neurosurgeon. Many findings and symptoms do not require treatment (including most optic gliomas). Large or cosmetically objectionable neurofibromas can be surgically removed but will often recur. The excision of large plexiform neurofibromas is technically difficult because they are often fused to other organs and cannot be completely removed.

Neurofibromas are associated with extensive mast cell proliferation and often cause severe itching, which can be relieved by treatment with mast cell stabilizers (e.g., ketotifen).

■■■ Novel Therapeutic Approaches to Neurofibromatosis Type 1

Figure 32.11 depicts neurofibromin's involvement in the RAS signaling cascade. Several experimental therapeutic approaches to NF1 target this specific molecular function of the neurofibromin protein.

- To be active, Ras must be anchored in the cellular membrane by addition of a farnesyl group. Small molecule inhibitors of farnesylation were designed to inactivate Ras even in cells deficient of neurofibromin protein.
- Statins (HMG-CoA reductase inhibitors) disrupt cholesterol synthesis needed for farnesylation of Ras. Treatment with lovastatin was able to reverse learning deficits in a mouse model of NF1.

Plexiform neurofibromas frequently demonstrate extensive mast cell invasion, which is mediated by c-kit signaling. Treatment with imatinib (Gleevec), an inhibitor of c-kit, has been shown to decrease the size of plexiform neurofibromas in a mouse model of NF1. Clinical trials in children with plexiform neurofibromas are now under way.

Neurofibromatosis Type 2

Neurofibromatosis type 2 (NF2) is much rarer than NF1, with an incidence of 1 in 25,000. The term *neurofibromatosis* is actually misleading, because the primary tumors in NF2 are not neurofibromas but schwannomas or meningiomas. The classic tumors are **bilateral vestibular schwannomas**, which are present in more than 80% of patients (unilateral in 6%) and are derived from Schwann cells in the vestibular portion of the eighth cranial nerve (hence they are not acoustic neuromas). Clinical symptoms include **tinnitus and dizziness**, **progressive hearing loss**, and **vertigo**. On average, clinical manifestations appear between 18 and 24 years of age. In addition to vestibular schwannomas, many NF2 patients also have involvement of other cranial nerves and peripheral nerves. When subcutaneous peripheral nerves are involved, the schwannomas may present clinically (not histologically) in a similar manner as peripheral neurofibromas in NF1, but this is the only real clinical similarity between NF1 and NF2. Subcapsular posterior **cataracts** are a common finding in **children** with NF2 and may suggest the correct diagnosis. Approximately half of affected individuals have one to three café-au-lait spots; it is rare to encounter more than three. The *NF2* gene is located on chromosome 22q12.2 and codes for a protein called **merlin** or neurofibromin 2. Merlin belongs to a family of proteins that connect the actin cytoskeleton to the cell membrane and it seems to regulate growth-factor signal transduction and cellular adhesion. NF2 is inherited in an **autosomal dominant** fashion, with 50% of cases classified as *de novo* mutations.

Tuberous Sclerosis (Bourneville-Pringle Disease)

Tuberous sclerosis is an autosomal dominant disorder of the skin, brain, kidneys, and heart. It is among the most common neurocutaneous syndromes, with an incidence of 1 in 20,000.

Clinical Manifestations. The disorder often presents in early childhood with refractory epilepsy and psychomotor retardation. A diagnosis of tuberous sclerosis is suggested by typical skin changes:

— **Ash-leaf spots** are small, usually elliptical hypopigmented areas on the skin that are clearly visible under Wood light (ultraviolet [UV] light with a wavelength of 360 nm). They are often detectable at birth (■ Fig. 32.13A).

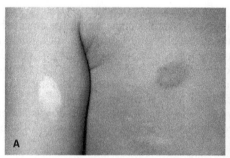

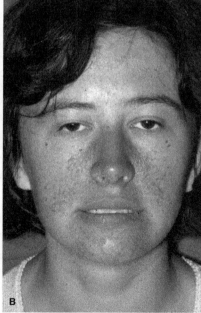

■ **Figure 32.13. Tuberous Sclerosis.**
A. Hypopigmented macules of the skin.
B. Sebaceous adenoma in an adult woman.
(Courtesy of V. Voigtländer, Ludwigshafen Hospital.)

- **Facial angiofibromas** (yellowish red papules arranged in a butterfly pattern on the cheeks, also called adenoma sebaceum; Fig. 32.13B) usually develop during childhood or adolescence. Unlike acne, they persist at the same site and do not involve sebaceous glands.
- **Subungual or periungual fibromas** (also known as Koenen tumors) are present in most adult patients. Some lesions may cause painful tearing of the nail.

Other cutaneous manifestations are fibrous, leathery plaques occurring in the lumbar region (Shagreen patches) or on the forehead. Funduscopic examination reveals characteristic retinal hamartomas in 50% of patients. Typical CNS lesions are subependymal glial nodules and cortical **tubers** (focal lesions typically located at the gray/white matter junction). Other common organ manifestations are **rhabdomyomas of the heart**, which are generally detectable at birth and later regress, as well as **angiomyolipomas of the kidneys**.

Approximately 60% to 80% of affected children have **epilepsy**, which is sometimes refractory to treatment, and only 50% have normal intelligence (including most patients without seizures). Mental retardation is sometimes present and may be so severe that active speech is not attained. Many affected children manifest autistic or disruptive behavior and sleep disorders.

Genetics. Mutations in two different genes, *TSC1* and *TSC2*, may lead to tuberous sclerosis. *TSC1* is located on chromosome 9q and codes for the protein hamartin. *TSC2* is located on 16p and codes for tuberin. Within the cell, hamartin and tuberin form heterodimers and are prime regulators of the AKT signaling pathway. The known disease-associated mutations of *TSC1* and *TSC2* have a penetrance of 100% with highly variable expressivity. Some patients are found to have a contiguous gene syndrome based on a large deletion of *TSC2* and the adjacent *ADPKD1* gene for autosomal dominant polycystic kidney disease.

32.7 Disorders of DNA Repair

Eukaryotic cells have a sophisticated system for monitoring the integrity of the genome and repairing damaged DNA. Tumor suppressor genes that participate in DNA repair are called **caretaker genes**. Loss-of-function mutations in both copies of caretaker genes compromise the ability of the cell to repair damaged DNA. This can lead to the activation of protooncogenes and/or the inactivation of other tumor suppressor genes. Hereditary syndromes based on congenital defects of DNA repair are consequently associated with a markedly increased risk of developing cancer (cancer predisposition syndromes).

■■■ **Types of DNA Repair in Eukaryotic Cells**

- **Mismatch repair systems** are active in the identification and repair of base pair mismatches. One of the most common mutations in humans is the GC→AT transversion, which may develop in various ways. For example, methylated cytosine (e.g., in CpG dinucleotides) may undergo hydrolytic deamination to uracil, which pairs with adenine. If the single base mismatch is not promptly recognized, the result is a C→T mutation or a G→A mutation on the complementary strand. DNA mismatches in humans are usually detected by the proteins MSH2 to MSH6 as well as MLH1 and PMS2. Germline mutations in the corresponding genes cause Lynch syndrome (Section 32.4). Once a base pair mismatch has been recognized, the free deoxyribose is excised by endonuclease; the correct sequence is restored by a DNA polymerase and returned to the double strand by a DNA ligase.
- **Base excision repair** is an important mechanism for the removal of DNA bases that have been altered by oxidation or alkylation. For example, reactive oxygen species lead to the oxidative modification of guanine to 8-oxoguanine, which pairs with adenine instead of cytosine. If this was not repaired, a GC pair would be replaced by an AT pair in both daughter strands. The enzyme glycosylase (deficient in MUTYH-associated polyposis; Section 32.4) can recognize the altered base and remove it while preserving the ribose-phosphate backbone of the DNA. Exonucleases, polymerases, and ligases are then responsible for excising the defect and resynthesizing and ligating the DNA strand.
- In **nucleotide excision repair**, special helicases and endonucleases excise an approximately 26- to 28-bp-long segment from a single strand that contains damaged DNA. The resulting gap is closed again

by polymerases and ligases. This method is particularly effective for the repair of relatively complex damage (e.g., crosslinks) in a single strand like that caused by UV radiation exposure or certain chemical carcinogens. Examples of diseases resulting from defective nucleotide excision repair are xeroderma pigmentosum (Section 20.1) and Cockayne syndrome (see below).

— **Recombination repair** is a process for repairing DNA double-strand breaks and crosslinks (covalent crosslinks in the double strand), which are typically caused by ionizing radiation or the action of chemotherapeutic agents such as cisplatin or mitomycin C. Various mechanisms of recombination repair are known, including **homologous recombination** (the intact homologous chromosome or sister chromatid serves as a template for repairing the defective DNA strand), **nonhomologous end joining** (fragments are prepared by exonuclease activity and then covalently joined by ligase), and **single-strand annealing** (homologous sequences of double-strand breaks with sticky ends are recognized and correctly assembled). Diseases that result from recombination repair defects are Fanconi anemia, Bloom syndrome, and Nijmegen breakage syndrome.

Cockayne Syndrome

Cockayne syndrome is caused by mutations in the genes involved in nucleotide excision repair: *ERCC8* (Cockayne syndrome A, 25%) or *ERCC6* (Cockayne syndrome B, 75%). Cockayne syndrome is an autosomal recessive, progressive neurodegenerative disorder of early childhood marked by postnatal growth failure and abnormal photosensitivity of the skin. Light-exposed skin areas develop erythematous and verrucous eruptions that usually heal to leave hyperpigmented patches. Premature hair loss (alopecia) and deep-set eyes due to subcutaneous fat loss give the patient an aged appearance. Cataracts, optic atrophy, and retinitis pigmentosa are typical ophthalmological manifestations.

Fanconi Anemia (Fanconi Pancytopenia Syndrome)

Fanconi anemia is characterized by malformations, short stature, bone marrow failure, and an increased susceptibility to cancer. The incidence is approximately 1 in 100,000. The carrier frequency in the Ashkenazi Jewish population is approximately 1 in 90.

Clinical Manifestations. Most patients with Fanconi anemia present at birth with congenital malformations, specifically radial ray anomalies and/or other skeletal malformations (Fig. 32.14), and malformations of internal organs (kidney, heart). Other clinical hallmarks are prenatal and postnatal growth deficiency and microcephaly. Only few children show mental retardation, but minor cognitive deficiencies are common. Typical hematological features (aplastic anemia, leukocytopenia, and thrombocytopenia) typically manifest after 3 years of age and before age 12. The median age at diagnosis is 8 years. Twenty five percent to 40% of patients with Fanconi anemia have no morphological abnormalities, and the disease should be included in the differential diagnosis of childhood pancytopenia even in the absence of dysmorphic changes. The predisposition to cancer includes a particularly high risk of myeloid leukemias (in 9% of all patients, usually AML), myelodysplastic syndrome (7%), and squamous cell carcinomas (skin, gastrointestinal tract). The average life expectancy is 20 to 30 years. **Heterozygous carriers** have a slightly increased risk of malignancy.

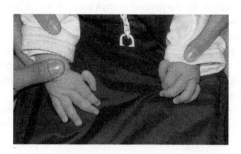

 Figure 32.14. Fanconi Anemia. Bilateral malformations of the thumbs.

Diagnosis. The diagnosis of Fanconi anemia is based primarily on the cytogenetic detection of **increased chromosome fragility** in cultured leukocytes or fibroblasts following the application of alkylating agents (cross-linkers such as diepoxybutane). Molecular genetic testing is complicated by the marked heterogeneity of the disease.

Genetics. Fanconi anemia can be caused by mutations in **15 currently known genes**, which are designated *FANCA, FANCB, FANCC*, etc. At least some of the gene products form a common nuclear protein complex that is involved in the repair of DNA crosslinks and double-strand breaks. All forms of Fanconi anemia have an **autosomal recessive** inheritance except FANCB, which is located on the X chromosome and results in an X-linked mode of inheritance. FANCD1 is the tumor suppressor gene BRCA2, whose mutations predispose to hereditary breast and ovarian cancer in heterozygous cases (Section 32.3) and cause Fanconi anemia in homozygous (or compound heterozygous) cases.

Ataxia Telangiectasia

Cerebellar ataxia, oculocutaneous **telangiectasia**, and **immune deficiency** make up the clinical triad of this autosomal recessive disease, which is described more comprehensively in Section 31.1.2.

Bloom Syndrome

This syndrome usually presents in childhood with prenatal and postnatal **growth retardation**, a sun-sensitive **erythematous skin lesion** in "butterfly distribution" on the face, and increased **susceptibility to bacterial infections** (immunodeficiency). The cancer risk is markedly increased and shows no predilection for particular tumors. Bloom syndrome has an **autosomal recessive** inheritance and is caused by mutations in the *BLM* gene on chromosome 15. Cytogenetic tests show an increased frequency of chromosome breaks and chromosomal rearrangements. It is particularly common to find an increased rate of sister chromatid exchanges and reunion figures between homologous chromosomes.

Nijmegen Breakage Syndrome

The clinical hallmarks of this syndrome are **growth retardation**, progressive **microcephaly**, characteristic facial features, and recurrent sinopulmonary **infections**. Most patients have learning disability or psychomotor retardation. The increased cancer risk relates mainly to leukemias and lymphomas (lifetime risk approximately 35%). The disease has an **autosomal recessive** inheritance and is caused by mutations in the *NBS1* gene. The deletion of five base pairs in exon 6 of the gene is the most common mutation identified in individuals with Nijmegen breakage syndrome. The gene product **nibrin** is involved in the repair of DNA double-strand breaks, particularly those following exposure to ionizing radiation.

32.8   Other Familial Cancer Predisposition Syndromes

Li-Fraumeni Syndrome

This rare cancer predisposition syndrome has an **autosomal dominant** inheritance and is characterized by an increased risk of developing many types of cancer: soft tissue sarcomas, breast cancer, leukemias, osteosarcomas, melanomas, and tumors of the colon, pancreas, adrenal cortex, and brain. One-half of affected individuals have a tumor by 30 years of age, and this increases to 90% by age 65. Patients are at high risk for developing multiple primary tumors.

The classic **diagnostic criteria** described by Li and Fraumeni in 1969 are as follows:
- A bone or soft tissue sarcoma occurring before age 45 **and**
- a first-degree relative with any cancer before age 45 **and**
- a first- or second-degree relative with cancer before age 45 or a sarcoma at any age

Less stringent diagnostic algorithms define "Li-Fraumeni-like syndrome." The **Manchester criteria** are among the most commonly used:

— Cancer occurring in childhood, or a sarcoma, brain tumor, or adrenocortical cancer occurring before age 45 **and**
— a first- or second-degree relative with a typical Li-Fraumeni tumor before age 60

More than 50% of patients with a clinical diagnosis of Li-Fraumeni syndrome are found to have germline mutations of the tumor suppressor gene *TP53* on chromosome 17p13.1. The **tumor suppressor p53** serves a key function as gatekeeper of the genome. If DNA damage is recognized at the G_1/S checkpoint of the cell cycle (i.e., before DNA replication), p53 induces cell death by activating the transcription of apoptosis-related genes. A small percentage of cases of Li-Fraumeni syndrome result from germline mutations in the *CHEK2* gene on chromosome 22q. *CHECK2* codes for a serine/threonine kinase that is part of the p53 signaling cascade.

Predictive testing for Li-Fraumeni syndrome is problematic since strategies for prevention or early detection of tumors are limited and of unproven value.

> **Important**
>
> **Somatic** mutations of the *TP53* tumor suppressor gene are found in at least half of all malignant tumors. Thus, *TP53* is the most commonly mutated gene in human malignancies.

Gorlin Syndrome (Nevoid Basal Cell Carcinoma Syndrome)

Mutations in *PTCH* (protein patched homolog 1) on chromosome 9q cause this **autosomal dominant** condition, which is characterized by multiple basal cell carcinomas occurring predominantly in the face and also on the trunk and limbs (◻ Fig. 32.15). The first basal cell carcinomas usually appear at about 20 years of age. Some 70% to 80% of patients with Gorlin syndrome have a positive family history, while 20% to 30% of cases probably represent de novo mutations.

Von Hippel-Lindau Syndrome

Von Hippel-Lindau syndrome (VHL) is characterized by a predisposition to numerous, otherwise rare tumors. It is caused by mutations in the *VHL* tumor suppressor gene on chromosome 3p25 and has an **autosomal dominant** mode of inheritance. Twenty percent of cases are *de novo* mutations. Most patients become symptomatic during the second decade of life, typically presenting with vision problems or cerebellar symptoms. Characteristic tumors, which develop in 70% to 90% of patients by age 60, are as follows:

— **Retinal angiomas**, which should be treated promptly (e.g., by laser ablation) to avoid blindness

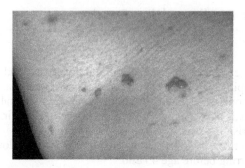

◻ **Figure 32.15. Nevoid Basal Cell Carcinoma in Gorlin Syndrome.** (Courtesy of V. Voigtländer, Ludwigshafen Hospital.)

- **Hemangioblastomas of the CNS (especially the cerebellum)** or spinal cord, which are often multiple or recurrent and, while primarily benign, are still a potential cause of mortality because of their location
- **Renal cell carcinomas**, which are frequently associated with renal cysts, are often multifocal or bilateral, and are the leading cause of mortality (average age at diagnosis 44 years)

Approximately 20% of patients develop a **pheochromocytoma** (VHL type II). The risk of developing this tumor depends partly on the underlying mutation.

Approaches to Clinical Problems

33 Infertility and Sterility

LEARNING OBJECTIVES

1 Discuss the importance of a pedigree analysis in the assessment of a couple with infertility.

2 Give examples of male-specific and female-specific causes of sterility or infertility as well as causes that can be identified in males or females.

3 Describe the clinical features of Klinefelter syndrome, and explain the rationale for obtaining a chromosomal analysis for a male with infertility.

4 Identify at least three monogenic disorders that may present with infertility, and explain the pathogenesis of each.

Sterility is defined as the inability of a couple to reproduce within a period of 1 year despite having frequent, unprotected intercourse. After successful conception, **infertility** is defined as the inability of a **woman** to carry a pregnancy to term and to give birth. In standard medical usage, however, the terms are frequently used synonymously.

Worldwide, one in seven couples remains unintentionally childless. The causes can be either sterility or infertility and can be caused by "female factors," "male factors," or a combination thereof (□ Fig. 33.1).

Investigating sterility or infertility involves the evaluation of both partners. It begins with a consultation concerning the detailed medical histories. Besides the general medical histories, this consultation should cover the woman's gynecological history as well as a history of her menstrual cycles. Both partners should be assessed for sexually transmitted diseases, many of which are associated with infertility. The evaluation should also address possible problems during intercourse, including those of an emotional nature. Also, it is important to obtain a detailed medication history, since some medications can result in sterility (often reversible) or erectile dysfunction (e.g., dopamine antagonists). The pedigree analysis should pay special attention to couples who have no children (which can be due to infertility or choice), miscarriages, early childhood or infant deaths, and congenital anomalies among relatives, since these may indicate a chromosomal abnormality (translocation) in the family.

33.1 Male Infertility

Male infertility can have numerous causes. For an overview, see □ Figure 33.2.

General Physical Examination. There are several relevant clinical features in a male that may indicate an underlying basis for infertility/sterility. Abnormal fat distribution and/or an abnormal body hair pattern with or without gynecomastia may indicate a relative hyperestrogenemia caused by severe damage of liver cells or hypergonadotropic hypogonadism (e.g., Klinefelter syndrome; 47,XXY).

Examination of the Genitalia. Genitourinary abnormalities, such as micropenis, hypospadias, cryptorchidism, or small testes (measured by comparing palpation with a Prader orchidometer), may indicate hypovirilization. Inflammation of the glans penis (balanitis) can indicate infection, trauma, or environmental irritation. Abnormal consistency or mass of the testes may indicate the presence of a neoplasm. Ultrasonography is performed to evaluate for an asymptomatic varicocele.

Semen Analysis. This is the most important diagnostic tool for determining male infertility, as it detects abnormalities of sperm density, movement, and morphology (oligoasthenoteratospermia [OAT]), as well as the amount and pH of the ejaculate. After 2 to 3 days of ejaculation abstinence, fresh sperm obtained by masturbation is examined under the microscope for quantity, density, and motility of the spermatozoa. □ Table 33.1 lists normal spermiogram

Table 33.1. Normal Semen Analysis Values (According to World Health Organization Guidelines)	
Criterion	Normal Value
Quantity of the ejaculate	2–6 mL
pH value	7.2–7.8
Spermatozoal density	$>15 \times 10^6$/ml
Motility	>50% spermatozoa with normal motility
Morphology	<20% malformed spermatozoa

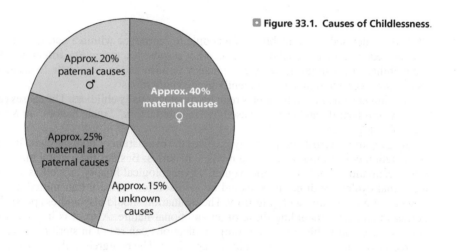

Figure 33.1. Causes of Childlessness.

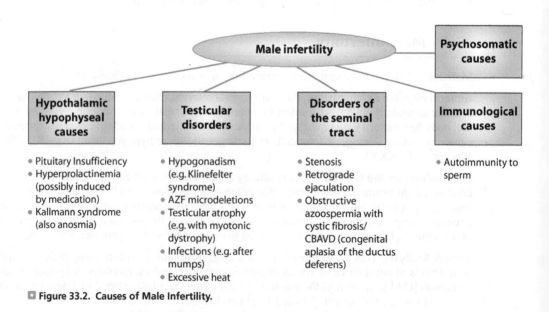

Figure 33.2. Causes of Male Infertility.

◻ Table 33.2. Semen Analysis Pathology

Name	Finding
Aspermia	No sperm
Azoospermia	No spermatozoa in the ejaculate
Oligospermia	$<15 \times 10^6$/ml
Asthenospermia	<50% spermatozoa with normal motility
Teratospermia	>50% malformed spermatozoa

values according to World Health Organization (WHO) guidelines. ◻ Table 33.2 lists possible pathological findings.

Hormone Analyses. Determining the plasma values of follicle-stimulating hormone (FSH) and testosterone permits the differentiation between hypergonadotropic hypogonadism (FSH ↑, testosterone ↓) and hypogonadotropic hypogonadism (FSH ↓, testosterone ↓).

Male Infertility in Human Genetics

Chromosome Abnormalities. A chromosome disorder should be suspected especially in patients with oligospermia. Studies have shown that 5% to 15% of all patients with oligospermia have an abnormal chromosome complement. Generally, **the lower the number of spermatozoa in the ejaculate, the higher the probability of a chromosome disorder**. Patients with oligospermia typically have structural abnormalities (especially robertsonian translocations). Patients with nonobstructive azoospermia are more likely to have abnormalities in their sex chromosomes.

Men with sex chromosome disorders typically have small, firm testes and hypergonadotropic hypogonadism; they frequently have gynecomastia and, in most cases, azoospermia or severe oligospermia. By far, the most frequent disorder is **Klinefelter syndrome**, with the chromosome complement 47,XXY or a mosaic of 46,XY/47,XXY.

Klinefelter Syndrome

Case History

Mr. Goode is 19 years old; recently he changed his primary care provider (PCP), who noted unusually small testicles on physical examination. The PCP referred him to the genetics clinic with a suspicion of Klinefelter syndrome. Mr. Goode is of tall stature and has excessive fat in the abdominal and hip areas. He reports that he entered puberty relatively late and that he only needs to shave once a week. He has a high school degree but states that he struggled during senior years and required tutoring. The physical examination reveals mild gynecomastia, sparse body and facial hair, and small testes. Chromosome analysis revealed a 47,XXY complement, which confirms the diagnosis of Klinefelter syndrome. Mr. Goode is referred to an endocrinologist for initiation of testosterone treatment.

Epidemiology

Klinefelter syndrome is the most frequent aneuploidy of the sex chromosomes. The incidence is estimated to be between **1 in 500** and **1 in 1,000** male neonates. It is the most frequent cause of male hypogonadism and is a common cause of male infertility. It is found in 10% to 15% of men with azoospermia and in 5% of men with oligospermia.

Clinical Features

Before puberty, boys with 47,XXY have no physical abnormalities. The diagnosis is usually made after the age of 12 years, except for those cases that are diagnosed prenatally (e.g., following an amniocentesis in the setting of advanced maternal age). Many patients are seen in the clinic for delayed puberty and gynecomastia, or the diagnosis isn't made until adulthood during an evaluation of infertility.

Men with Klinefelter syndrome tend to be tall. They have reduced facial and body hair, and usually only shave once or twice a week. **Hypergonadotropic hypogonadism** manifests itself by breast enlargement, a female pattern of hair growth, small testes, and a relatively small penis. Without treatment, men with Klinefelter syndrome are at increased risk for osteoporosis.

Klinefelter syndrome does **not cause intellectual disability**; however, the IQ of affected men is roughly 10% to 15% below the familial average. Verbal IQ, on average, is lower than functional IQ. Not infrequently, there is mild dyslexia. Psychosocially, men with Klinefelter syndrome sometimes appear insecure, shy, and immature. This can result in difficulties being accepted and can lead to social isolation.

Diagnosis

The suspected clinical diagnosis is confirmed by chromosome analysis. This should be followed up with endocrinological assays, which will reveal hypergonadotropic hypogonadism: the average testosterone values are half of normal, while FSH and luteinizing hormone (LH) levels are elevated. The semen specimen reveals azoospermia.

Cytogenetics

Approximately 75% of men with Klinefelter syndrome have the karyotype **47,XXY**. Other anomalies, such as 48,XXXY, 48,XXYY, or 49,XXXXY, are much more rare. One in five men with Klinefelter syndrome has a mosaic chromosomal complement, which can result from several possibilities: 47,XXY/46,XY, 47,XXY/46,XX, 47,XXY/46,XY/46,XX, or 47,XXY/46,XY/45,X. In 51% of cases, the additional chromosome is of maternal origin; the remaining 49% of cases are of paternal origin.

Therapy and Management

An early diagnosis (i.e., before the onset of puberty) is beneficial for the outcome of hormone therapy. In such cases, **testosterone replacement** is started between ages 11 and 12 years. Treatment results in a more masculine body habitus, more facial and pubic hair, more self-confidence, less fatigue and increased libido, more muscle strength, and better bone density. Even if testosterone therapy is not started until the ages of 20 to 30 years, it still proves clinically beneficial. Gynecomastia is seen in 30% of all men with karyotype 47,XXY. It has been noted that these men have an increased risk of developing breast cancer. While it is true that, compared with 46,XY men, the risk of cancer development increases 20-fold, its incidence is only 1 in 5,000. Therefore, routine screening mammography is not recommended.

Other Chromosomal Abnormalities

Males with a **46,XX** chromosomal complement should undergo fluorescence in situ hybridization (FISH) analysis for the *SRY* gene, which, in a 46,XX male, will be translocated to the X chromosome. Assisted reproductive techniques, such as intracytoplasmic sperm injection (**ICSI**), in which seminal or testicular spermatozoa are used for in vitro fertilization of the oocyte, have enabled men with oligospermia and/or immotile sperm to father children.

Hypogonadotropic Hypogonadism. Patients with idiopathic hypogonadotropic hypogonadism (IHH) have defective secretion of gonadotropin-releasing hormone (GnRH). IHH in combination with anosmia (i.e., loss of smell) is known as **Kallmann syndrome**; with an incidence of 1 in 10,000 individuals, it is one of the more frequent monogenic disorders in men. There are autosomal recessive, autosomal dominant, and X-chromosomal types of Kallmann syndrome. The *KAL1* gene is located in the pseudoautosomal region of the X chromosome; it is responsible for the majority of cases. In addition to considering Kallmann syndrome, one should also consider **Prader-Willi syndrome** (incidence 1 in 10,000), especially if hypogonadotropic hypogonadism occurs together with obesity and intellectual disability (ID).

Azoospermia. The most frequent causes for azoospermia or severe oligospermia with a normal chromosome analysis are **microdeletions of the AZF region** on the long arm of the Y chromosome (Yq). There are more than two dozen *AZF* genes, and deletions can be confirmed with array

DNA analysis or other methods. Another cause for the absence of sperm in the spermiogram is an obstruction of the seminal pathways (**obstructive azoospermia**). **Congenital bilateral aplasia of the vasa deferentia (CBAVD)** is characterized, as the name indicates, by a bilateral absence of the spermatic ducts, which results in a blockade of transport of spermatozoa from the epididymis to the distal genital tract. This type of obstructive azoospermia is observed in most males with cystic fibrosis, but rarely is the only clinical feature in a male with compound heterozygous or homozygous *CFTR* mutations (Section 22.1). CBAVD is responsible for 1% to 2% of all cases of male infertility. A low seminal pH value (less than 7.2) is also seen in CBAVD and is a clue to the diagnosis and should prompt mutation analysis of the *CFTR* gene (being sure to note the indication of "infertility" or "suspected CBAVD" on the laboratory requisition).

An overview of genetic causes of male infertility is found in ◻ Table 33.3.

◻ **Table 33.3.** Male Infertility: Important Genetic Causes

Name	Frequency	Clinical Features	Hormones	Semen Analysis	Karyotype	Causes of Infertility
Klinefelter syndrome	1:1,000 in males	Male phenotype, hypogonadism	↑ FSH, LH ↓ T, ↑ estrogen	Azoospermia, OAT	47,XXY mosaics	Disruption of spermiogenesis
XX sex reversal	1:20,000	Male genitalia to intersex; hypogonadism, gonadal dysgenesis	↑ FSH, LH ↓ T, ↑ estrogen	Azoospermia	46,XX	80% SRY translocation onto the X chromosome
Chromosome translocations	1:1,000 in males	Male phenotype	—	OAT or NS		Disruption of spermiogenesis
Kallmann syndrome	1:10,000	Delayed puberty, anosmia	↑ FSH, LH ↓ T GnRH test inconclusive	Azoospermia	46,XY	For example, *KAL1* gene defect leading to abnormal neuronal migration
Prader-Willi syndrome	1:10,000	Male phenotype, ID, obesity, hypogonadism	↓ FSH, LH ↓ T	Not reported	46,XY	Unknown
CBAVD/cystic fibrosis	1:2,500	Male phenotype	Normal	Obstructive azoospermia; low pH	46,XY	Bilateral aplasia of the vasa deferentia through *CFTR* mutations
Mild androgen insensitivity syndrome (MAIS)	Not determined	Male phenotype, undervirilization, gynecomastia,	Normal or ↑ T Normal or ↑ LH	Oligospermia/ azoospermia	46,XY	Defective androgen binding in target tissues due to mutations in androgen receptor gene
Yq microdeletions	? 1:400 in males	Male phenotype	Normal	Azoospermia, OAT	46,XY	Missing spermatogenesis through AZF microdeletions

T, testosterone; NS, normospermia; AZF, azoospermia factor.
After Lissens et al. (2002).

33.2 Female Sterility/Infertility

While men's fertility remains relatively stable from puberty through age 60 years, women are most fertile between ages 20 and 24 years, have a slow decline in fertility to age 34 years, and have a rapid decline in fertility after age 40 years. Causes for female sterility are classified into the following groups (◻ Fig. 33.3):

- Hypothalamic pituitary (approximately 30%)
- Ovarian (approximately 30%)
- Tubal (approximately 15%)
- Uterine (uncommon)
- Cervical/vaginal (undetermined)
- Psychiatric/psychosocial
- Extragenital endocrine

Genetic causes of female infertility are mostly associated with anovulatory cycles or amenorrhea. More than 50% of cases of infertility in women who experience delayed puberty and primary amenorrhea are caused by **chromosomal abnormalities**, the most frequent being 45,X, or Turner syndrome. The likelihood of a chromosomal abnormality is substantially less in cases of secondary amenorrhea; however, a chromosome analysis is still indicated.

Diagnostic Measures for Female Sterility. Similar to the evaluation of the male partner, medical history, physical examination, and diagnostic studies are essential in the process of determining the etiology for female sterility or infertility. Detailed documentation of the woman's menstrual cycle is necessary and often paired with hormonal assays such as thyroid function studies, androgens (testosterone and dehydroepiandrosterone [DHEA] in serum), and prolactin. The anatomy is further assessed with vaginal ultrasound, which is of special importance for determining the condition of the endometrium (which, before ovulation, should be 8 to 10 mm in thickness), and pelvic ultrasound to visualize the ovaries (which are abnormal in gonadal dysgenesis and polycystic ovary disease). Additional imaging techniques (e.g., hysterosalpingography) and

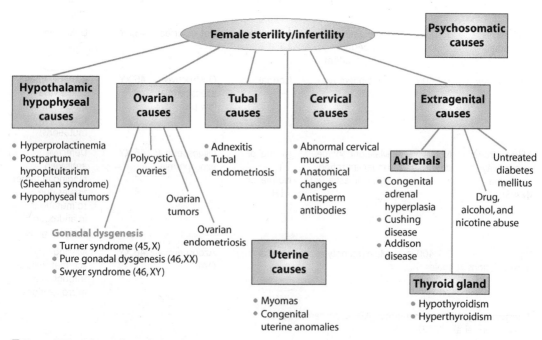

◻ Figure 33.3. Causes of Female Sterility.

possible invasive measures (e.g., endometrial biopsy, hysteroscopy, and diagnostic laparoscopy) are sometimes necessary.

Female Gonadal Dysgenesis. Gonadal dysgenesis in the female is characterized by markedly reduced or absent follicle content and an increase in fibrous tissue and ovarian stroma (manifest as "streak gonads"). The müllerian structures (e.g., uterus, fallopian tubes, and upper vagina) and external genitalia are structurally normal but may be hypoplastic due to hypogonadism (hypergonadotropic type).

There are **three major causes** for female gonadal dysgenesis:

— **Turner syndrome:** 45,X or another similar chromosomal disorders (Section 19.1)
— **Pure gonadal dysgenesis:** 46,XX, but with a mutation in the FSH receptor gene
— **Swyer syndrome:** 46,XY disorder of sex development (DSD; Chapter 28), which results from one of several mechanisms including (a) *SRY* mutations (Y chromosome), (b) *DSS* (dosage-sensitive sex reversal gene, X chromosome) duplication, and (c) mutations or rearrangements in other X-linked or autosomal loci. Because of the risk of gonadoblastoma, resection of the gonads is indicated.

Hypothalamic Causes of Female Sterility. As with males, mutations of the *KAL1* gene can lead to an X-chromosomal form of hypogonadotropic hypogonadism with accompanying anosmia (**Kallmann syndrome**). The KAL1 protein participates in the neuronal migration of the GnRH neurons and olfactory neurons. Hypogonadotropic hypogonadism with resulting female sterility can also be caused by gene mutations in *AHC* (adrenal hypoplasia congenita), the leptin gene, and the leptin receptor gene.

Congenital adrenal hyperplasia (CAH), caused by deficiency of the enzyme 21-hydroxylase, is an autosomal recessive condition caused by mutations in the *CYP21A2* gene (Section 25.2). The mild end of the spectrum (also referred to as nonclassic CAH) may present as primary or secondary amenorrhea and elevated testosterone in a woman with hirsutism. Approximately 60% of adult women with nonclassic CAH have only hirsutism; however, many will develop polycystic ovaries.

34   Miscarriage and Fetal Demise

LEARNING OBJECTIVES

1 Differentiate between a spontaneous miscarriage and stillbirth in terms of gestational age and common etiologies.

2 Identify three major causes of embryonic or fetal demise, and give at least two examples of each.

3 Explain the rationale for obtaining parental chromosome analysis in recurrent pregnancy loss (RPL).

The loss of an embryo, the demise of a fetus, or the occurrence of a stillbirth carries a diagnostic burden to the obstetrician, pathologist, and geneticist. Even greater is the burden to the parents, who mourn the death of their child, whether born or unborn.

A **miscarriage** or **spontaneous abortion** is the unintended loss of a pregnancy up to 20 weeks' gestation. Approximately 15% of all clinically recognized pregnancies end in miscarriage; however, total reproductive loss from conception is actually closer to 50% to 60%. Miscarriage is the most common complication of pregnancy, yet most couples experience only a sporadic loss. **Recurrent pregnancy loss** (RPL) is defined as three or more consecutive pregnancy losses before 20 weeks' gestation; this affects nearly 1% of couples. **Stillbirth** is defined as the death of a fetus after 20 weeks' gestation. Over time, the envelope of viability is being pushed to lower gestational ages, yet presently, viability is generally agreed to be 24 weeks after conception or 500 grams.

> *"It seems evident that most of 'humanity' dies before, not after birth and that perhaps only one-third survive from earliest beginnings until birth or the end of the first year of life."*—John M. Opitz

Clinical symptoms of miscarriage include bleeding, cramping, and abdominal pain, followed by the expulsion of tissue and amniotic fluid (later gestations). Later in gestation, the cessation of fetal movement would call attention to the possibility of fetal demise. Occasionally, the demise is not recognized by the mother but rather is diagnosed by fetal ultrasound. The etiology of spontaneous abortion and fetal demise is diverse and includes genetic disorders of the fetus, maternal anatomical abnormalities, and systemic maternal disease (◘ Fig. 34.1). Genetic disorders of the fetus (e.g., chromosomal imbalance) are more commonly identified in early gestations, whereas maternal illness, anatomical abnormalities, or infection is more likely to be the cause of a late fetal demise or stillbirth. Pathological examination of the embryo or of the fetus and placenta is an essential component in ascribing an etiological diagnosis of any pregnancy loss.

Chromosome Disorders. Fetal aneuploidy is the most frequent cause of early (less than 10 weeks) spontaneous abortion and is found in approximately 60% of all abortions. With an incidence of more than 50%, **autosomal trisomies** are the most frequent cause of spontaneous abortions caused by chromosome disorders (◘ Fig. 34.2). Advanced maternal age is the most important risk factor owing to meiotic *nondisjunction* in oogenesis. **Trisomy 16** is the most frequent autosomal trisomy of all abortuses (up to 30%); however, these conceptuses never survive to term and typically are miscarried by the 12th week of pregnancy. Interestingly, **autosomal monosomies**, which are also associated with advanced maternal age, are only rarely found in abortuses because these are miscarried early—even prior to implantation—and never recognized as a pregnancy.

As opposed to autosomal monosomy, **X-chromosomal monosomy** is compatible with life (Turner syndrome). Yet, 99% of X-chromosomal monosomies result in miscarriage, accounting for nearly 20% of all miscarriages in the first trimester and making it the second most frequent

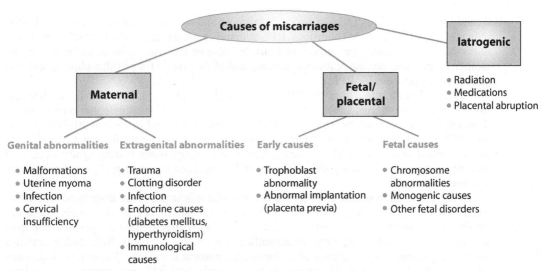

Figure 34.1. Causes of Spontaneous Abortions and Fetal Demise.

chromosome abnormality found in spontaneous abortions. Unlike the autosomal monosomies, 45,X is not associated with maternal age.

Triploidies constitute 15% of all cytogenetically abnormal abortions. The clinical findings depend on whether the additional chromosome complement comes from the mother (digynic triploidy) or the father (diandric triploidy, two-thirds of the cases) (Section 3.3). **Tetraploidies** are found in 5% of all miscarriages with chromosome aberrations, while 2% of the cases reveal unbalanced structural chromosome abnormalities.

Recurrent Pregnancy Loss

Whereas 25% to 50% of all women experience at least one miscarriage, only 1% of couples are affected by the loss of three or more consecutive pregnancies prior to 20 weeks' gestation. Following a miscarriage, the risk of spontaneous abortion for each subsequent pregnancy increases to 24%. After three miscarriages, the risk is 32%; after six miscarriages, it is 53%.

Figure 34.2. Frequency of Chromosome Abnormalities in Spontaneous Abortions.

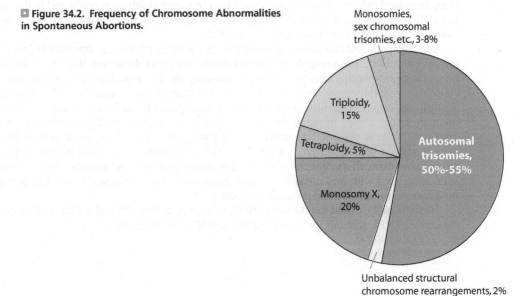

Examination of the fetus and placenta for chromosomal aberrations or other abnormalities is indicated for all spontaneous abortions. RPL demands not only an examination of the products of conception, including the embryo or fetus, but also an extensive clinical evaluation of the mother for possible uterine or medical disease and of the couple for possible chromosomal or genetic predisposition for RPL.

Maternal anatomical abnormalities may be congenital or acquired. **Uterine malformations** (e.g., septate uterus, subseptate uterus, arcuate uterus, and bicornate uterus) are among the most frequent causes for RPL. Such malformations are found in 15% to 30% of patients with RPL (compared to 0.5% to 2% in the general population). Surgical correction increases the likelihood of a successful pregnancy. **Cervical incompetence** is a recognized cause of recurrent pregnancy loss in the second trimester. Cervical cerclage may prolong the pregnancy in some cases.

In regards to **chromosomal aberrations**, sporadic miscarriages are associated with autosomal trisomy, triploidy, and monosomy X. However, in cases of RPL in which a chromosomal abnormality is present, it is more likely to be due to a **rearrangement** of the genome. A parent who has a balanced **chromosomal translocation** is at risk for infertility, RPL, and/or having a child with multiple congenital anomalies due to chromosome imbalance. The exact risk depends on the specific chromosomal abnormality. In 5% of couples with RPL, one partner proves to have a balanced chromosome aberration. These aberrations are typically reciprocal or robertsonian translocations that confer an increased risk of an unbalanced chromosomal complement in the embryo and, consequently, the risk of miscarriage. As the chromosomally unbalanced ovum is more likely to be fertilized than a chromosomally unbalanced sperm is to fertilize, it is observed that the mother is the translocation carrier in approximately two-thirds of the cases.

Numerous **monogenic disorders and malformation syndromes in the fetus** can also lead to spontaneous abortions. Again, examination of the fetus (ideally via a formal autopsy) is essential in determining a specific etiology, recommending diagnostic analyses (which can be used as a basis for prenatal diagnosis in subsequent pregnancies), and ascribing a recurrence risk. If recurring pregnancies manifest similar fetal anomalies and the parents are not affected, there is a strong likelihood of an autosomal recessive disorder with a recurrence risk of 25% for either a miscarriage or a liveborn child with similar anomalies.

All couples who experience RPL should be given a **genetic consultation (genetic counseling)**, which will include a detailed reproductive history of pregnancies with fetal pathological findings if possible, construction of a three- to four-generation pedigree, and a subsequent chromosome analysis of both parents. If the chromosomes of both parents are normal, there is **no** increased risk for chromosome aberrations in future children as compared to the general population; however, one must recognize that monogenic disorders will have normal chromosomes yet may pose a substantial recurrence risk.

While genetic and chromosomal disorders are the focus of this text, other etiologies of RPL are also prevalent. For example, **maternal immunological disorders** that cause the formation of antiphospholipid antibodies (lupus anticoagulants) or anticardiolipin antibodies can cause recurrent thromboses and infarctions of the placenta that eventually lead to miscarriage. **Antiphospholipid syndrome** involves arterial and venous thromboses; in addition, recurrent pregnancy loss and/or immune thrombocytopenia and antiphospholipid antibodies may be involved. To avoid placental thromboses during pregnancy, *low-dose* aspirin as well *low-dose* heparin should be administered. A similar pathomechanism is suspected in other nonimmunological **clotting disturbances** of the mother (procoagulatory and anticoagulatory) that have been associated with miscarriages. Among these are factor V diseases, factor XII deficiency, prothrombin mutations, and protein C defects.

Unfortunately, even after the couple undergoes a complete medical and genetic evaluation, the cause of RPL remains undetermined in over 50% of the cases.

35 Growth Disturbances

LEARNING OBJECTIVES

1 Differentiate between proportionate and disproportionate short stature and give at least one example of each.

2 List at least three conditions that are associated with tall stature and/or overgrowth.

3 Identify at least three features in the developmental history and/or physical examination that would be expected in an individual with (a) Prader-Willi syndrome and (b) Beckwith-Wiedemann syndrome.

In general, environmental and genetic factors influence linear and ponderal growth in a multifactorial manner, often making it difficult to separate one influence from another. However, there are many recognizable genetic disorders that affect these growth parameters. This chapter delineates the process of evaluating abnormal growth and focuses on selected mendelian and chromosomal disorders that affect growth.

The evaluation of an individual with a suspected growth disturbance requires documentation of height in first-degree relatives (parents and siblings) and other family members, if possible, to determine a familial basis for abnormal growth. The individual's weight and height (length for infants) should be plotted on standardized growth curves from birth to evaluation to distinguish between prenatal and postnatal growth disturbances and to determine if linear growth is maintained on a specific percentile or if there is substantial growth deceleration or acceleration. Physical examination of the patient with abnormal stature includes anthropomorphic measures of arm span, upper and lower body segments, hand and finger lengths, and head circumference. These measurements can help distinguish between proportionate growth abnormalities and localized growth abnormalities (e.g., **overgrowth**) that affect one-half of the body or a single limb. Diagnostic imaging, including bone age and skeletal survey, and laboratory analysis of specific growth factors may be needed to further define the patient's phenotype.

Chromosome analysis and molecular analysis of specific genes, when available, are employed to confirm a clinical diagnosis. More recently, various pathogenic genomic copy number variants (CNVs) have been identified in children with growth disturbances. These CNVs may also be associated with intellectual disability or other abnormalities in later childhood and adulthood. Thus, a DNA array analysis is indicated in the evaluation of all children with unexplained growth disturbance, in particular when associated with developmental delay or intellectual disability.

35.1 Short Stature

Short stature is defined as body height **below the third percentile for age and gender**. Important factors in the evaluation of an individual with short stature include family history, personal growth history, and body proportion. Diagnostic imaging and laboratory analyses help to delineate specific abnormalities and assist in determining an underlying cause.

Disproportionate Short Stature. Typically, disproportionate short stature results from an underlying skeletal dysplasia affecting growth and maturation of the limbs and/or vertebrae. Skeletal dysplasias are categorized by the location of growth disturbance. Rhizomelic, mesomelic, and acromelic describe linear growth deficiency of the proximal, middle, and distal extremities, respectively. The term "spondylo" is used when the spine is also involved (◻ Fig. 35.1).

A classic genetic condition characterized by disproportionate short stature is **achondroplasia** (Section 26.1.2), which is characterized by **rhizomelic** short stature, macrocephaly, and distinctive facial appearance. Nearly all individuals (99%) with achondroplasia harbor one of two point mutations in the *FGFR3* gene (fibroblast growth factor receptor 3). **Hypochondroplasia**

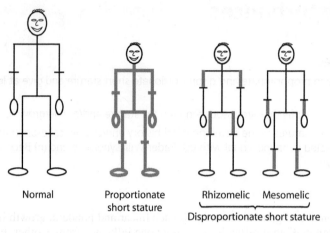

Figure 35.1. Different Forms of Short Stature. (Modified from Menger and Zabel 1998.)

Normal

Proportionate short stature

Rhizomelic   Mesomelic

Disproportionate short stature

and **thanatophoric dysplasia** are also caused by mutations in the *FGFR3* gene. Hypochondroplasia is clinically less severe than achondroplasia, whereas thanatophoric dysplasia is lethal because of severe impairment of thoracic growth. Skeletal dysplasias are described more fully in Section 26.2.

Proportionate Short Stature. In the investigation of proportionate short stature, it is important to distinguish between prenatal and postnatal growth restriction. Prenatal growth restriction may have exogenous causes, such as intrauterine infection, alcohol, and other teratogenic agents, or endogenous causes (genetic disorders). A syndromic etiology should be considered when short stature is accompanied by other anomalies (■ Table 35.1). For example, many **chromosomal**

■ Table 35.1. Syndromes Associated with Proportionate Short Stature

Syndrome	Prenatal or Postnatal	Clinical Features	Gene(s)	Mutation Type, Inheritance
Cornelia de Lange syndrome	Prenatal	Typical facies (synophrys [fused eyebrows]), micromelia, microcephaly, ID	NIPBL, SMC1A	Usually sporadic
Rubinstein-Taybi syndrome	Postnatal	Typical facies (beaked nose), broad thumbs and toes, microcephaly, ID	CREBBP, EP300	Usually sporadic
Russell-Silver syndrome	Prenatal	Small, triangular face with a normal-sized cranium; asymmetry of limbs; ID	H19; matUPD (7); (epi)genetic mutations of 11p15.5	Usually sporadic
Williams syndrome	Prenatal	Supravalvular aortic stenosis, typical facies ("elfin face"), mild microcephaly, ID, strong verbal and weak spatial skills	Microdeletion at 7q11.23; ELN, etc.	~95% de novo
Dubowitz syndrome	Prenatal	Microcephaly, ptosis, broad nose, pediatric eczema	Unknown	AR
Bloom syndrome	Prenatal	Telangiectatic butterfly erythema, hirsutism, microcephaly	BLM (RECQL3)	AR

ID, intellectual disability; matUPD (7), maternal uniparental disomy of chromosome 7; AR, autosomal recessive.

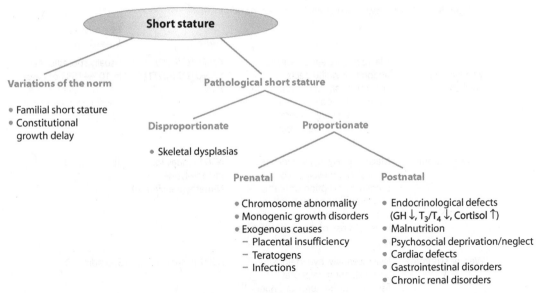

Figure 35.2. Algorithm for the Differential Diagnosis of Short Stature.

disorders are characterized by proportionate short stature. Although Turner syndrome (45,X; Chapter 19) often presents in the neonatal period due to cardiovascular anomalies, individuals with this condition may also present for evaluation of short stature later in childhood. Haploinsufficiency of the *SHOX* gene is implicated in the short stature of Turner syndrome, and treatment with growth hormone is effective in increasing final adult height in these patients.

Proportionate short stature that develops postnatally in the absence of other obvious abnormalities is likely to have an **endocrine** basis. For example, short stature may be the dominant feature of hypothyroidism, hypercortisolism, or growth hormone (GH) deficiency. Proportionate short stature may also be due to effects of malnutrition. Many of such children will show marked rebound growth with adequate caloric and nutritional supplementation. The **laboratory workup** of short stature should include hormone assays and a chromosome analysis and may include testing for mutations or deletions of the *SHOX* gene in cases in which a specific dysmorphic syndrome is not suspected.

The differential diagnosis of short stature is summarized in ◘ Figure 35.2.

> **Important**
>
> "Placental insufficiency" is often cited as an explanation for prenatal growth retardation. It should be noted that placental insufficiency does not exclude a genetic cause, and the insufficiency itself may have a genetic etiology. Newborns with growth retardation due to intrauterine malnutrition often exhibit rebound growth after birth.

35.2 Tall Stature

Tall stature is a term applied when body height is above the 97th percentile for age and gender. As with short stature, the evaluation of an individual with tall stature requires documentation to determine if the tall stature has a familial basis. In addition, the clinician should determine if the overgrowth is localized (e.g., affecting a single limb or side of the body) or general. Diagnostic imaging is usually limited to bone age for individuals with tall stature, but skeletal survey may be useful in some cases. Laboratory analysis of specific growth factors, chromosomal complement, and molecular analysis of specific genes, when available, are employed to confirm the clinical diagnosis.

IV

◘ Table 35.2. Overgrowth Syndromes with Prenatal Onset

Syndrome	Clinical Features	Gene(s)	Mutation Type, Inheritance
Beckwith-Wiedemann syndrome	Macroglossia, ear creases, abdominal wall defects, visceromegaly, hemihypertrophy, neonatal hypoglycemia, increased risk of malignant abdominal tumors, mental development often normal	*CDKN1C (KIP2)*, *KCNQ1OT1 (LIT1)*, *H19*	Usually sporadic; AD in 10%–15% of cases, usually with maternal transmission (imprinting of 11p15)
Sotos syndrome	Macrocephaly, hypertelorism, downslanting eyelid folds, premature eruption of teeth, accelerated bone maturation, large hands and feet, hypotonia, increased risk of malignant tumors, ID	*NSD1* (codes for histone-lysine N-methyltransferase)	Sporadic, AD
Weaver syndrome	Macrocephaly, hypertelorism, down-slanting palpebral fissures, contractures of fingers (camptodactyly), loose skin, ID.	*NSD1* in some cases	Sporadic, AD
Simpson-Golabi-Behmel syndrome	Macrocephaly, coarse facial features (broad short nose, macrostomia, macroglossia), postaxial polydactyly, syndactyly of second and third digits, cryptorchidism, polycystic kidneys, gastrointestinal anomalies, ID	*GPC3* (codes for glypican-3) and others	X linked (females with mild phenotype)
Proteus syndrome	Regional gigantism of hands and/or feet, asymmetry of limbs, hemangiomas, lipomas, lymphangiomas, etc; occasional ID	*PTEN* and others	Sporadic

AD, autosomal dominant; ID, intellectual disability.

A distinguishing feature of overgrowth syndromes is that some are associated with an **increased risk of neoplastic diseases** relating to an overexpression of growth factors or a deficiency of growth suppressors. The term *overgrowth syndromes* refers not only to tall stature but also to excessive growth in general, including localized areas of increased growth affecting one or more parts of the body.

As the etiologies often differ, it is important to distinguish between **primary and secondary overgrowth**. Primary forms are attributable to intrinsic, cellular hyperplasia whereas secondary forms have an endocrine/humoral cause (outside the skeletal system).

As with short stature syndromes, a distinction is made between **prenatal** and **postnatal** causes of tall stature. Most primary overgrowth syndromes such as Beckwith-Wiedemann syndrome and Sotos syndrome are apparent at birth (◘ Table 35.2). The most frequent cause of prenatal secondary overgrowth is maternal diabetes mellitus leading to diabetic macrosomia of the fetus (Fig. 13.9).

Postnatal overgrowth, unlike prenatal overgrowth, is much more likely to have a secondary cause such as precocious puberty (increased estrogens or androgens), acromegaly (increased GH), or hyperthyroidism (increased triiodothyronine [T_3]/thyroxine [T_4]). Some genetic diseases feature a predominantly postnatal, primary growth increase. These include conditions with additional sex chromosomes (XYY, poly-X females, Klinefelter syndrome) as well as Marfan syndrome and homocystinuria. Some children with fragile X syndrome exhibit a relatively tall stature. With syndromic tall stature, a marked difference is usually noted between the height of the child and his or her parents. At the same time, the growth rate is generally normal as it is in familial tall stature, with height gains paralleling the percentile lines on growth charts.

A few disorders are characterized by **regional overgrowth**. Examples are Klippel-Trenaunay-Weber syndrome, Maffucci syndrome, and Proteus syndrome. The pathogenic mechanism underlying these diseases is not fully understood. They are presumably based on somatic mutations of growth-promoting genes or somatic loss of a normal second allele in individuals with a heterozygous mutation in a growth control gene. Hence, they occur sporadically with rare familial cases and generally become symptomatic after birth.

> **Important**
>
> — Prenatal overgrowth: frequent primary cause (genetic)
> — Postnatal overgrowth: frequent secondary cause (endocrine)

35.3 Obesity

Obesity refers to an excessive accumulation of body fat. Because the actual measurement of body fat content is a technically complex process, the usual practice is to determine the body mass index (BMI) and define obesity as a **BMI above the 97th percentile**.

However, body fat content during childhood varies greatly with age. Body fat content rises steadily during the third trimester of pregnancy, peaks toward the end of the first year of life, declines for some years thereafter, and then rises again during adolescence and adulthood.

A basic distinction is drawn between primary and secondary obesity. **Secondary obesity** is present when the patient is found to have an underlying endocrine disorder or a causative central nervous system (CNS) lesion (usually involving the hypothalamus). Most patients have **primary obesity** with a multifactorial etiology. Adverse environmental factors (e.g., low socioeconomic status, fatty diet, lack of exercise) may lead to obesity in genetically disposed individuals. In addition, several rare, monogenic forms of early-onset obesity have been described in recent years, such as those relating to mutations in the **leptin gene**. A deficiency of leptin, secreted by adipocytes, leads to obesity, hyperphagia, infertility, and immune defects. The phenotype is completely reversible with the administration of leptin. Other examples of genes whose mutations can lead to early-onset obesity are the leptin receptor, proopiomelanocortin, and melanocortin-4 receptor genes. Proopiomelanocortin induces a feeling of satiety by binding to the melanocortin-4 receptor (◻ Fig. 35.3).

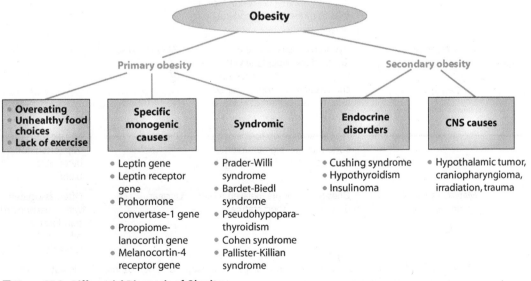

◻ **Figure 35.3. Differential Diagnosis of Obesity.**

In some cases, primary obesity is part of a genetic syndrome. A well-characterized example is **Prader-Willi syndrome (PWS) (Section 4.3)**. Individuals with PWS typically present with severe infantile hypotonia and feeding difficulties, prompting feeding tube placement in the neonatal period. Untreated, infants with PWS fall far below the normal growth curve and are diagnosed with failure to thrive. Interestingly, as the dysphagia resolves (usually just after 12 months), children with PWS become hyperphagic and are at risk for morbid obesity in early childhood. Although behavior contributes substantially to obesity in PWS, intrinsic factors such as short stature and low metabolic rate are also implicated. Behavioral and dietary therapy in conjunction with exercise and growth hormone therapy have proven successful in the amelioration of obesity in PWS. Other features of PWS and methods of diagnosis are detailed in Section 4.3.

Any individual with obesity and intellectual disability or behavioral abnormalities should undergo an evaluation to determine if an underlying syndromic diagnosis is present. Chromosomal microdeletion disorders such as Smith-Magenis syndrome (Section 19.2) are associated with obesity as are single-gene disorders such as Bardet-Biedl syndrome and Cohen syndrome (◘ Table 35.3).

◘ Table 35.3. Differential Diagnosis of Syndromic Obesity

Syndrome	Clinical Features	Gene(s)	Mutation Type, Inheritance
Prader-Willi syndrome	Marked hypotonia, small hands and feet, hypogonadism, hypopigmentation, mild to moderate ID, feeding difficulties in infancy, later hyperphagia and truncal obesity	Loss of the *HBII-85* snoRNA cluster in the *SNURF-SNRPN* transcript on the paternal allele	Loss of paternal 15q11-q13; 75% deletion, 20% matUPD (15), 5% imprinting defect
Bardet-Biedl syndrome	Ocular manifestations (myopia, nystagmus, retinal dystrophy), postaxial polydactyly, renal anomalies, hypogonadism, obesity by 2–3 years of age, reduced intelligence (especially verbal IQ)	*BBS1, BBS2, ARL6, BBS4, BBS5, MKKS, BBS7, TTC8, B1, BBS10, TRIM32, BBS12, MKS1, CEP290*	AR/triallelic; 14 different gene loci currently known
Pseudohypoparathyroidism Albright hereditary osteodystrophy	Short metacarpals and metatarsals (especially in fourth and fifth rays), with or without hypocalcemia and hyperphosphatemia, round face, mild to moderate ID, moderately severe obesity	*GNAS* (codes for α-subunit of G_s protein)	AD
Cohen syndrome	Hypotonia, usually severe ID, maxillary hypoplasia with very prominent incisor teeth, chorioretinal dystrophy, truncal obesity (usual onset at age 5–6 years)	*COH1* (*VPS13B*)	AR
Pallister-Killian syndrome	Typical facies (high forehead), abnormal skin pigmentation (mosaicism), possible obesity, ID	Unclear	Mosaic tetrasomy 12p (often not detectable in blood)
Maternal UPD-14 syndrome	Obesity, hypotonia, delayed motor development, short stature	Unclear	Often associated with robertsonian translocation, otherwise sporadic

ID, intellectual disability; matUPD (15), maternal uniparental disomy of chromosome 15; AR, autosomal recessive; AD, autosomal dominant.

35.4   Failure to Thrive

A prolonged deficiency of energy and/or protein intake, especially in children, leads to malnutrition, which when present over a prolonged period is associated with failure to thrive. With today's adequate food supply, severe malnutrition in developed countries is usually a **result of disease, neglect, or the imposition of an extreme diet**.

Three main groups of diseases can lead to malnutrition. One group consists of **maldigestion and malabsorption** syndromes, which are characterized by an inadequate uptake of ingested nutrients. Another group consists of various **chronic diseases**, in which nutrients are inadequately utilized by metabolic processes, or energy intake is outstripped by energy consumption (a good example is Huntington disease in adults). Finally, severe **hypotonia** with or without disorders of the swallowing process can lead to feeding difficulties and malnutrition in infants.

Clinical Manifestations

The earliest sign of malnutrition is a fall in the percentile curve for weight. The weight percentile in malnourished children often falls well below the percentile for body length. Severe malnutrition is also marked by stunted longitudinal growth accompanied by normal head circumference. Malnutrition presents clinically with loss of subcutaneous fat. Typical areas of involvement are the buttocks ("wrinkled buttocks"), inner thighs, and abdominal skin. Protein deficiency leads to edema and ascites due to reduced serum colloid osmotic pressure.

Malabsorption and maldigestion syndromes typically present with chronic diarrhea, bloating, and flatulence. The color and consistency of the stool vary with the underlying enzyme deficiency (e.g., fatty stools in cystic fibrosis). Malabsorption syndromes are usually associated with iron deficiency anemia, and a deficiency of fat-soluble vitamins is common in cystic fibrosis (e.g., coagulation problems due to a vitamin K deficiency). Not infrequently, malnutrition in children also leads to psychomotor retardation and delays in developmental milestones.

36 Abnormal Head Size

LEARNING OBJECTIVES

1. Distinguish between primary and secondary microcephaly.
2. Identify maternal, environmental, and intrinsic fetal etiologies for microcephaly.
3. List three disorders that are associated with macrocephaly.
4. Describe three features that would support a diagnosis of either familial microcephaly or familial macrocephaly.

36.1 Microcephaly

Microcephaly is defined as a head circumference (occipitofrontal circumference [OFC]) less than two standard deviations below the mean for gender and age; it is found in 2.5% of the population. As there is a close link between **brain and cranial growth**, microcephaly may be a sign of abnormal brain development. **Primary microcephaly** reflects poor cranial growth in utero. Additional studies may be indicated when microcephaly is observed in a newborn, although familial microcephaly should also be considered. Insufficient head growth that occurs over time is termed **secondary microcephaly** (also referred to as **acquired microcephaly**) and should prompt additional diagnostic studies, as it often reflects an underlying central nervous system disorder. Observing the head circumference during the first several months of life also assists in determining prognosis; slow or no growth typically indicates a poorer prognosis.

Microcephaly may occur as an isolated finding (except for variable intellectual disability) or with additional features in the context of a genetic syndrome. Many chromosomal anomalies and monogenic syndromes are associated with microcephaly. ◻ Table 36.1 lists selected disorders that are important for a differential diagnosis. Classic chromosome disturbances associated with microcephaly, such as trisomy 13 and 18, are not listed. In addition to primary genetic disorders, the differential diagnosis of microcephaly includes maternal metabolic diseases (e.g., phenylketonuria [PKU]), poorly managed diabetes mellitus, congenital infections (e.g., rubella, cytomegalovirus, and herpes), and teratogenic effects of alcohol consumption, medications (e.g., phenytoin and aminopterin), or illicit substance use.

Important	

Diagnoses that need to be considered in cases of microcephaly:
- Maternal metabolic disease (e.g., maternal PKU)
- Teratogenic effects of infection, medication, alcohol, and drugs
- Chromosomal abnormality
- Craniosynostosis

Important tests:
- Maternal blood phenylalanine content
- TORCH (**t**oxoplasmosis, **r**ubella, **c**ytomegalovirus, and **h**erpes) analysis for congenital infection (performed at birth)
- DNA array analysis
- Cranial computed tomography (CT) with three-dimensional reconstruction
- Brain magnetic resonance imaging (MRI)
- Ophthalmological evaluation

Diagnostic Evaluation. The evaluation of a patient with microcephaly requires a complete obstetrical and birth history, family history, and physical examination. The head circumference of both parents should be recorded. The underlying diagnosis is further refined through

◻ Table 36.1. Syndromes with Microcephaly

Syndrome	Clinical Symptoms	Gene(s)	Inheritance
Angelman syndrome	Absent speech development, ataxia, seizures, typical facies, macrostomia, moderate to severe ID	*UBE3A*	Imprinting defect
Cornelia-de-Lange syndrome	Synophrys (fusion of the eyebrows), thin upper lip, micromelia, microcephaly, ID	*NIPBL* (*nipped-B–like*), *SMC1A*	AD, mostly sporadic
Deletion 4p (Wolf-Hirschhorn syndrome)	Hypertelorism, growth retardation, broad beaked nose, cranial asymmetry, low-set ears, preauricular tag or pit, severe ID, seizures	Unknown	Mostly sporadic
Dubowitz syndrome	Short stature, ptosis, broad nasal tip, infantile eczema, mild ID	Unknown	AR
Fetal alcohol syndrome	Pre- and postnatal growth retardation, cardiac defects, smooth philtrum, thin upper lip, ID	Unknown	—
Meckel-Gruber syndrome	Prenatal growth deficiency, cerebral and cerebellar hypoplasia, encephalomeningocele, microphthalmia, polydactyly, renal anomalies, ID	*MKS1*, *TMEM216* (*MKS2*), *TMEM67* (*MKS3*), and others	AR
Miller-Dieker syndrome	Severe ID, seizures, bitemporal cranial narrowing, high forehead, small nose, late eruption of primary teeth, short stature; lissencephaly on MRI	*LIS1*, etc.	Microdeletion 17p13.3, mostly sporadic
Rubinstein-Taybi syndrome	Typical facies (beaked nose), broad thumbs and toes, short stature, ID	*CREBBP* (coding for the CREB-binding protein), *EP300*	AD, mostly sporadic
Smith-Lemli-Opitz syndrome	Dysmorphic facial features, growth retardation, hypotonia, syndactyly of second and third toes, cataract, brain malformations, ID	*DHCR7* (coding for 7-dehydrocholesterol reductase)	AR
Williams syndrome	Supravalvular aortic stenosis, peripheral pulmonary stenosis, typical facies (full cheeks), ID, specific cognitive profile	*ELN* (coding for elastin), etc.	Microdeletion 7q11.2, mostly sporadic

ID, intellectual disability; AD, autosomal dominant; AR, autosomal recessive.

diagnostic imaging (usually an MRI), which may reveal additional anomalies of the central nervous system (CNS; e.g., holoprosencephaly [Section 31.2.1], defective development of cortical gyri/lissencephaly, myelination disturbances, and many others). Intracranial calcifications may indicate intrauterine exposure to an infectious agent; however, the calcifications can also be caused by genetic diseases (e.g., pseudo-TORCH syndrome) or perinatal asphyxia. In order to confirm a suspicion of an infectious etiology for microcephaly, serological and/or microbiological tests should be done as early as possible. Microcephaly also indicates an **ophthalmological examination**, as the presence of coloboma, cataract, chorioretinopathy, or megalocornea (among other abnormalities) may help to establish an underlying diagnosis.

Autosomal Recessive Primary Microcephaly. Primary, severe microcephaly without other malformations (previously also referred to as "true microcephaly" or "microcephaly vera") may be caused by mutations in a number of genes and is inherited as an autosomal recessive trait. Incidence is generally low, but may reach 1 in 10,000 in some consanguineous communities. The diagnosis may be made if there is (a) congenital microcephaly with a head circumference at least two standard deviations (SD) below age and gender means at birth and at least three SD below the mean after age 6 months; (b) intellectual disability but no other neurological findings such as spasticity or progressive cognitive decline (epileptic seizures are unusual, but do not exclude the diagnosis); and (c) normal height or mildly short stature and appearance (apart from severe microcephaly), as well as normal brain scans (apart from reduced brain size). Based on the function of the causative genes identified to date, autosomal recessive primary microcephaly (MCPH) appears to be a primary disorder of cell division (mitosis) in neural precursors and not one of neural migration, neural apoptosis, or neural function.

The genetic basis of autosomal dominant or "familial" isolated microcephaly is poorly defined; it may be associated with variable intellectual deficiencies and may be a multifactorial trait similar to body size (◘ Fig. 36.1).

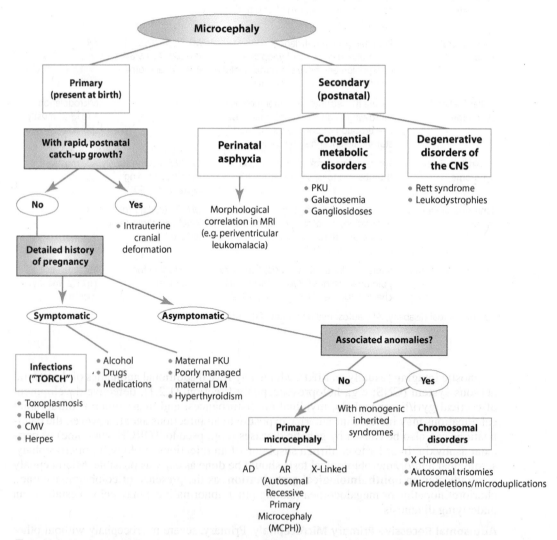

◘ **Figure 36.1. Causes of Microcephaly.** *A diagnosis of perinatal asphyxia needs to be substantiated by medical documentation and confirmed by MRI (hypoxic ischemic encephalopathy with periventricular leukomalacia). PKU, phenylketonuria; AD, autosomal dominant; AR, autosomal recessive.

36.2 Macrocephaly

Macrocephaly is defined as an OFC greater than two standard deviations above the mean for gender and age and, by this definition, is found in 2.5% of the population. As for microcephaly, one distinguishes between a condition present at birth or acquired over time and places particular importance on the rate of growth over several weeks to months. Macrocephaly may be inherited as an autosomal dominant trait without functional significance (**benign macrocephaly**); thus, family history and parental OFC measurements are essential as part of the initial evaluation.

The majority of cases of macrocephaly are caused by expansive processes in the cranial cavity. In infants, the most frequent cause of macrocephaly (prenatal or postnatal onset) is **hydrocephalus** with dilation of the ventricular system. Other expansive processes that can result in abnormal cranial growth include arachnoid cysts, brain tumors, subdural bleeding, and abscesses. Urgent cerebral imaging is imperative for differential diagnostic clarification. If the anterior fontanel is open, a head ultrasound can be performed relatively quickly. Additional imaging may be necessary to further define an underlying abnormality. In true **megacephaly**, however, the ventricular system is not enlarged, and there are no intracranial tumors or other expansive structures. Cranial MRI should be performed in all children in whom a primary neurogenetic disorder is suspected.

In children with **skeletal dysplasia** such as achondroplasia, macrocephaly can be primary or may be a secondary phenomenon due to hydrocephalus. Even without hydrocephalus, the cranial circumference in children with achondroplasia is typically more than two standard deviations above the average at birth; it continues to increase during the first year. The posterior cranial fossa is flat with hypoplastic foramina. Small jugular foramina restrict venous drainage, and a hypoplastic foramen magnum inhibits the flow of cerebrospinal fluid, resulting in increased intracranial pressure, enlarged ventricles, and open fontanels.

Several **metabolic disorders** are associated with an increased head circumference. **Glutaric aciduria type 1** should be considered in all infants with progressive macrocephaly and possibly minor neurological abnormalities such as hypotonia. Early diagnosis by acylcarnitine analysis (increasingly part of neonatal screening) or urinary organic acid analysis allows for adequate treatment; this may prevent the devastating metabolic crisis with destruction of the basal ganglia, which is otherwise typical for this condition. Urine organic acid analysis should also detect **Canavan disease**, one of the leukodystrophies associated with macrocephaly. Lysosomal storage disorders, such as **mucopolysaccharidoses**, may also have macrocephaly as a physical finding, in addition to an enlargement of other organs (e.g., liver and spleen) and a coarse facial appearance.

As can be expected, some **overgrowth syndromes** are associated with prenatal macrocephaly. A classic example is macrocephaly in **Sotos syndrome**, also called *cerebral gigantism syndrome*. Approximately 50% of the children manifest a macrocephaly at birth; at the age of 1 year, this is increased to 100%. In these cases, the ventricles are only slightly dilated. In the other "classic" overgrowth syndrome, Beckwith-Wiedemann syndrome, macrocephaly occurs only in some of the patients.

A relatively large cranial circumference also occurs in fragile X syndrome and in neurofibromatosis type 1. In both cases, however, the values usually remain within the age-specific norm, whereas individuals with mutations in the *PTEN* gene may have OFCs three to five standard deviations above the mean.

| Important | |

The following tests should be considered for children with intellectual disability and macrocephaly:
- Urinary organic acid analysis
- Urinary mucopolysaccharides and oligosaccharides
- Skeletal survey
- Brain MRI
- Molecular studies for fragile X syndrome
- DNA array analysis

37 Immunodeficiency Syndromes

LEARNING OBJECTIVES

1. List three features that would prompt an investigation for an immunodeficiency syndrome.
2. Compare and contrast X-linked and autosomal recessive combined immunodeficiency.
3. Explain the benefits and limitations of bone marrow transplantation in ataxia telangiectasia.

During the first year of life, the human immune system undergoes major maturational changes. While infants and toddlers are susceptible to **physiological immune deficiencies** due to the partial immaturity of their immune systems, this susceptibility decreases significantly by the time a child enters kindergarten. Pathological immune deficiency should be suspected if any of the following are present:

- Infections occur **more than eight** times per year.
- Infections occur as distinctly **polytopic** (e.g., skin, respiratory tract, intestinal tract, urinary tract, or central nervous system [CNS]).
- Infections tend to become **chronic** despite adequate treatment.
- Infections are caused by **opportunistic pathogenic agents**.
- Infections progress **atypically** (e.g., if severe abscesses occur without elevated systemic temperature).

Primary immunodeficiencies are congenital and usually have a genetic basis. Various components of the immune system can be affected, including the T and B lymphocytes, monocytes, granulocytes, and/or the complement system. **Secondary immunodeficiencies** are acquired as sequelae of other diseases or conditions (e.g., leukemias, HIV infections, malnutrition, severe liver damage, or as the result of immunosuppressive medication). Information on the most important genetic immunodeficiencies follows.

Severe Combined Immunodeficiency

Severe combined immunodeficiency (SCID) is the most severe and most rapidly progressive primary immunodeficiency syndrome; it is characterized by serious defects of the **cellular** and **humoral immune systems**. In the first few months of life, affected individuals present with severe bacterial, viral, and/or fungal infections. Typically, there is a generalized candidiasis, and frequently, there are chronic pneumonias because of infection with *Pneumocystis jiroveci* (previously *Pneumocystis carinii*). Patients can have chronic and severe diarrhea triggered by a wide variety of pathogens. Immunization with a live vaccine can be fatal. The clinical evaluation of SCID patients reveals severe hypoplasia of lymphatic tissues such as the thymus, lymph nodes, and tonsils, as well as leukopenia and hypogammaglobulinemia. The majority of cases of SCID are **X linked** and **B-cell positive**—the T lymphocytes are absent and the B lymphocytes are deficient. **Adenosine deaminase deficiency** is an autosomal recessive form of combined immunodeficiency (CID) and was the first disorder to be treated successfully in humans with gene therapy. Generally, treatment of SCID/CID is only possible through bone marrow transplant. Other therapies are either experimental (gene therapy) or symptomatic/prophylactic (e.g., antibiotic prophylaxis, immunoglobulin [Ig] administration, and isolation). Without treatment, SCID results in death within the first 2 years of life.

Agammaglobulinemia

X-linked (**Bruton**) agammaglobulinemia is the classic example of an isolated B-cell defect. It is caused by mutations in the *BTK* gene, which codes for a tyrosine kinase required for B-cell maturation. During the first months of life, affected individuals are usually healthy because of protection through placental IgG. Beginning between the ages of 6 months and 1 year, frequent pyogenous bacterial infections, involving the respiratory tract and skin, occur and are often complicated by meningitis and septicemia. Viral or gram-negative infections are rare. Diagnosis is supported by finding a severe deficiency or lack of IgG, IgM, and IgA using immunoglobulin titers and confirmed by immunoelectrophoresis. The therapy of choice is lifelong administration of intravenous immunoglobulin and antibiotic therapy, as needed, for bacterial infections. Heterozygous females are usually asymptomatic but can be identified through skewed X inactivation limited to B cells.

Selective Immunoglobulin A Deficiency

Selective immunoglobulin A deficiency is the most frequent immunodeficiency. Studies in healthy blood donors showed a prevalence of 0.1% to 0.2%, indicating that this deficiency is subclinical in most "affected" individuals. The mode of inheritance has not been determined; however, among first-degree relatives, the incidence of IgA deficiency increases 14-fold.

Microdeletion 22q11 (Thymic Hypoplasia)

In 1965, Angelo DiGeorge described a patient with **hypoparathyroidism** and cellular immuno-deficiency as a result of **thymic hypoplasia**. Within a short time, a large number of additional patients with similar symptoms were reported. It turned out that the complete clinical picture included additional defects, which embryologically can be attributed to the **third and fourth branchial arches**; the defects include cardiovascular malformations involving the arterial system (e.g., truncus arteriosus and interrupted aortic arch), hypocalcemia due to absence of the parathyroid glands, and craniofacial abnormalities. **DiGeorge syndrome** is the eponym that applies to the most severe end of the clinical spectrum of a **microdeletion of chromosome 22q11.2** (Section 21.1). Another manifestation of the same genetic defect is velocardiofacial syndrome, or Shprintzen syndrome, with typical craniofacial malformations (e.g., cleft palate or a prominent nose with hypoplastic nares). Neonates with classic DiGeorge syndrome can manifest with seizures or tetanic spasms that result from hypocalcemia. After the neonatal period, life-threatening infections affect the prognosis; typical are fungal infections of the gastrointestinal tract, *P. jiroveci* pneumonias, and therapy-resistant diarrhea. The peripheral blood contains a lower than normal number of T lymphocytes; often, immature T-precursor cells are present. Immediate therapy involves the surgical correction of life-threatening cardiac defects, correction of the immunodeficiency with fetal thymic or bone marrow (more reliable) transplant, and administration of calcium. Without therapy for the immunodeficiency, the life expectancy of children with complete DiGeorge syndrome is markedly decreased, with a mortality rate of 80% within the first year.

Wiskott-Aldrich Syndrome

This X-linked disorder is characterized by the triad of **thrombocytopenia, chronic eczema**, and **recurring opportunistic infections**. It is caused by mutations in the *WAS* gene, whose product belongs to a family of proteins involved in signal transduction from the cell surface to the actin cytoskeleton. At birth, the children have petechial hemorrhages. Additional infections aggravate the thrombocytopenia, with gastrointestinal and intracranial hemorrhages. The infections are mostly caused by pyogenic pathogens with polysaccharide capsules; typical are pneumococcal, meningococcal, *Haemophilus*, and *P. jiroveci* infections. The number of B lymphocytes is normal; IgA and IgE are often elevated, while IgM is lower than normal. The isoagglutinin titer (anti-A and anti-B) is low or absent. Therapy is symptomatic (e.g., antibiotics and platelet concentrates) or causal (bone marrow transplant). Human leukocyte antigen (HLA)-identical transplants have a success rate of over 90%. Untreated patients typically die from serious infections (60%), although less frequently death results from hemorrhages (30%) or lymphoreticular malignancies (5%). Heterozygous females are usually asymptomatic but can be identified through skewed X inactivation limited to peripheral blood T cells, granulocytes,

□ Table 37.1. Immunodeficiency Syndromes

Category	Syndrome	Inheritance	Number of T Cells	Number of B Cells	Ig Level
Combined T- and B-cell immunodeficiency	SCID (severe combined immunodeficiency)	X	↓	Normal or ↑	All ↓
	Adenosine-deaminase deficiency	AR	Progressive ↓	Progressive ↓	All ↓
	Hyper-IgM syndrome	X	Normal	Normal	IgM normal to ↑, IgA ↓, IgG ↓
	DiGeorge syndrome	AD	Normal to ↓	Normal	Normal to ↓
Antibody deficiency	X-linked (Bruton) agammaglobulinemia	X	Normal	↓↓ or –	↓↓ or –
Phagocyte defects	Chronic granulomatous disease	AR, X	Normal	Normal	Normal
	Leukocyte adhesion defect	AR	Normal	Normal	Normal
Other syndromes with immunodeficiencies	Wiskott-Aldrich syndrome	XR	Normal to ↓	Normal	Normal, sometimes IgM ↓
	Louis-Bar syndrome	AR	Normal	Normal	Normal
	Bloom syndrome	AR	Normal	Normal	Normal

X, X chromosomal; AR, autosomal recessive; ↓, low; ↑, elevated; ↓↓, very low; –, undetectable.

and B cells. Mutations in the *WAS* gene may also cause isolated X-linked **thrombocytopenia** or **neutropenia**.

Ataxia Telangiectasia (Louis-Bar Syndrome)

This autosomal recessive syndrome (Section 31.1.2) also has a classic triad of symptoms: **cerebellar ataxia**, **oculocutaneous telangiectasia**, and **recurring bronchopulmonary infections**. The repeated bronchopulmonary infections lead to bronchiectatic changes in the lungs. The condition is caused by mutations in the *ATM* gene, which is involved in DNA repair. The ATM protein senses double-stranded DNA breaks, coordinates cell cycle checkpoints prior to repair, attaches near damage sites, and recruits other repair proteins to damaged sites. Ataxia telangiectasia is one of the chromosome instability syndromes. Presently, no curative therapy is available; a bone marrow transplant only corrects the immunodeficiency.

Additional chromosome instability syndromes with immunodeficiency are **Nijmegen breakage syndrome** and **Bloom syndrome** (□ Table 37.1; Chapter 32).

Living with Genetic Disorders: Patient Reports

38   Reports of Patients and Their Families

LEARNING OBJECTIVES

1 Try to perceive the uncertainty of having a child with intellectual disability and not knowing the cause. Discuss the positive and negative effects for the family that can be associated with establishing a diagnosis.

2 Empathize with an adult individual who was recently diagnosed with a hereditary disorder. Describe how this may affect self-esteem, self-perception, social interactions, and future planning.

38.1   Felix

Late in my pregnancy with Felix, a routine ultrasound showed that he had a rare but serious heart defect. The news was upsetting, but we learned that the defect (truncus arteriosus) could be repaired with surgery. Felix was born on August 13, 1998, after a complicated vaginal delivery. He was taken from us immediately, sent to intensive care, and placed in an incubator, and had heart surgery 4 weeks later. By then he had lost more than a pound, and even after surgery he needed to be fed through a tube because he couldn't suck well from the bottle. When he was 8 weeks old we were finally allowed to take him home, and for the first time, our older daughter Sophie was able to hold him in her arms.

Felix's doctors told us that because of the heart defect and surgery he would take extra time to catch up with other babies his age, so we weren't worried when he didn't react to noises like Sophie had or that he seemed to turn his head in an awkward way. We were happy that he was finally gaining weight without a tube! Shortly before Christmas during a well-child visit, his doctor noticed that Felix's muscle tone was low and that he wasn't hearing or seeing well. The doctor ordered a magnetic resonance image (MRI), which showed that Felix had a small cerebellum. Although my husband and I were devastated by this news, the pediatrician told us not to panic. He recommended an eye examination and scheduled a return visit to see him in 8 weeks. We left his office dumbfounded.

The next day my husband and I took Felix to an emergency room at a children's hospital. We wanted to know right then and there what was wrong. At the same time, however, we were hoping that nothing was wrong with our baby boy. Between December 1998 and March 1999, Felix was hospitalized several times, confirming all of the things his first doctor noticed yet not pinpointing a cause. The doctors and nurses recommended therapies for Felix to help him reach his developmental milestones, and we enrolled him in a special program; however, we still wanted to know more. We wanted to know why Felix was having problems. I worried that I had done something wrong during my pregnancy with Felix or that somehow I had caused him not to develop properly.

My husband and I took Felix to see a pediatric neurologist. They suspected that Felix had a condition known as "a congenital disorder of glycosylation" or CDG. After some testing, this diagnosis was confirmed. We were shattered when we received the information booklet from the family network for children with CDG. Not one doctor, nurse, or therapist had warned us that the prognosis for Felix was so terrible. At the time we were sorry that we had agreed to the heart surgery that kept Felix alive. We had huge problems in trying to cope and felt totally isolated. It would have been really important for our family to have psychological counseling at the time, but none of the doctors showed any concern for us.

We were extremely depressed, and it took months until we realized that we had to accept Felix the way he was, that we could not change him. There was nothing we could do, and comparing him to other children was totally useless. On the contrary: it was unfair to Felix, and it only made us more angry and unhappy. That is the most important thing we have learned over the last 2 years.

Felix is now 3 years old and for a while has been attending a school for children with special needs. Fortunately, many of the frequent symptoms described in the brochure by the family network did not materialize. So far he has had no seizures or palsies. The orthopedic doctor has not detected any contractures. His hearing and vision have luckily improved quite a bit; he needs no glasses, and we could also discontinue the hearing aids. Whether Felix will ever walk, we don't know. Yet, the most important thing for us is that we have a happy and curious child who is very much loved by everyone in our family. No one can laugh as spontaneously and heartily as Felix. It has been a rough road up to this point and will be rough in the future. However, we have learned a lot, and we no longer pay so much attention to the "norms" that our society imposes on us. We look to the future with courage and hope, for we know that Felix is happy with us, no matter what the future may bring.

38.2   On the 50th Birthday of a Woman with Triple X Syndrome

I was born in Germany in 1955, when people were still trying to cope with the events of the postwar period. My parents were struggling to make ends meet, and although I didn't walk until I was 3 years old, most everyone thought that was due to malnutrition. No one even considered another explanation. In fact, my parents thought the milk and butter that they eventually were able to feed me helped strengthen my muscles so I could stand on my own!

I remember quite well the first day of school. I looked no different from other children, but I remember that I did not feel comfortable with them. I still don't know why. First grade was hell for me. Learning was hard, because I felt so different and insecure at school. I had no problem with what we were studying and was a good student. It is hard to describe how I felt then; a child of 6 to 10 years is never too sure what is going on and cannot always find the words to describe her thoughts or feelings. All I remember is, "I just felt somehow different." Even my mother used to say, "Why can't you be like other children?" Both of my parents expected me to be like "other children." Whatever they meant by that, I didn't know. In school, I was very good in German, and I also was good at languages. Math was more of a problem, even though I later passed my accounting exams with honors.

After I finished school, I completed an apprenticeship as a legal assistant. Even then I felt that somehow I did not fit into the circle of young people. At the age of 16 years, I took a course in ballroom dancing. I liked moving with the music. To this day, I like to dance whenever I have a chance. Still, being around young men made me feel uneasy—I felt awkward. As a young girl, I was socially awkward, and being with people my age was difficult. Looking at old photographs, I would say that I was pretty. Outwardly, nothing made me different from other women.

I married in 1978. In May of 1982, my handicapped daughter was born—she was born with hydrocephalus. In December of 1982, I separated from my husband; we were later divorced. Problems with her shunt were and are a source of great worry to us. In addition, there were numerous other problems that seemed to have nothing to do with hydrocephalus. In July 1999, she underwent a genetic test. She was diagnosed with a genetic defect 46,XX, del 21q. At that time I wanted to find out if I had the same genetic defect and if I had transmitted it to my daughter. So I was tested as well.

It turned out that I have triple X syndrome. The doctor who informed me of the findings over the telephone added, "But don't tell anyone about this genetic defect." Of course she meant well, because in the literature some of these women are also somewhat mentally handicapped.

For the last 5 years I have had problems with my menstrual cycle. It is said that women with this syndrome could possibly have an early menopause. Could this be the case with me? I don't know. Other women tell me they have similar problems. Since I have seen quite a few doctors in the last few years, I did tell them about my triple X syndrome, against the advice of the doctor who had informed me of it years ago. Some doctors did not react. Others showed a sudden interest in how my sex life would be affected.

I am now looking back on 50 years. Until 1999, I felt totally unburdened. Knowing that I have an extra X chromosome did make me feel insecure. I read up on the medical descriptions of people with triple X syndrome. Some do apply to me. Muscular development can be late. Social behavior and perception is not totally normal. Fine motor skills have never been my forte. My IQ was tested because of a request for a school change. The results proved that I did not have any learning disability. At the time, I took the test to start training as a nurse. Looking back, I would say that it was good for me that, until 1999, I knew nothing about my genetic defect. Had I known, I would have probably, with the help of some medical dictionary, tried to see whether I was conforming to the norm. Early support, as it exists now, was not available in the fifties. Would physical therapy have helped my muscular development? It is also possible that people would have expected me to be mentally handicapped. Would they have given me the chance to make it in a regular school environment? My life probably would have been much different.

Regarding the genetic defect of my daughter, this has nothing to do with me. As far as I am concerned, I see myself as a woman who is different in many respects. I feel that the people who wrote the medical dictionary forgot to mention possible talents and positive attributes, of which I do have some. "To have a defect does not mean that one is defective." This is how I look at it. For I do not feel defective. I am a special person!

38.3 Simon

Simon was born on October 29, 1998. He weighed 7 lbs. 13 oz. and was 20 inches long. Everything seemed normal. Yet, the midwife became suspicious because no matter how hard she tried, she could not get Simon to cry. I put him to my breast, but he appeared too tired to drink. The physician who examined him a second time suggested that Simon probably did not feel like crying, that everything was OK. He did start to cry several hours later, but very faintly. From the first moment, I felt that Simon had not quite arrived in the world. I also realized very rapidly that he was very different from his sister. The pediatrician kept saying that he needed more time than others, that I should be patient. At 3 months, he could still not hold up his head that I considered very large and heavy. My sister-in-law (who has three almost-grown children and works with people with disabilities) suspected early on that something was wrong and told me that she worried it could be something "serious." I preferred to listen to the pediatrician that everything would be all right. When Simon was 6 months old, we started with physical therapy since his muscles were very weak. At 10 months, he was enrolled in an early childhood intervention program, and from then on he had occupational therapy as well. When Simon was barely 1 year old, a developmental delay was obvious. He was unable to sit and very weak. The pediatrician finally suggested that we go to see specialists to have his condition clarified. Simon had a normal-sized head but his body did not fit. It was much too small and weak. I nursed Simon until he was 1 year and also began adding solids. It worked, yet he ate only small amounts. When we got to the clinic, several tests were performed on Simon. The doctors suspected that something was wrong with his head. This suspicion, however, was not confirmed, for nothing remarkable was found.

The last thing they did was to take a blood sample for a chromosome analysis. The result showed a partial trisomy of chromosome 5 with deletion on chromosome 18. We had no idea what that meant. The doctor said she could not say much about it either, for they had never had a case like this. Simon would learn everything a bit later than other children. While I thought that would not be such a big deal, I could not get rid of the feeling that this wasn't all there was to it. We went to see another doctor who consulted with us for a very long time. He also could not tell us how Simon would develop, but he was certain that Simon would, at some time, learn to walk. Yet he told us explicitly that, while Simon could receive support and learn lots of things, we should realize that he would always be disabled. It was not nice to hear the word *disabled*, but I was relieved to finally know what was wrong, although in the beginning I was having a lot of self-doubts. I had no experience with handicapped persons and felt totally insecure. How does one deal with such people? A friend told me, "Every soul chooses its parents, and Simon has known why he chose you." Somehow I found this comforting, and I thought that if Simon thinks I can handle this, I can give it a try. My husband considered Simon his beloved son from

V

day one, no matter whether he was healthy, sick, strong, weak, or handicapped. He loved him, and I sensed that Simon, too, had a very strong affection for his Dad.

Now Simon is 6 years old. He walked on his own at age 2½. Feeding him was, at times, very difficult, since he ate very little. I remember days when I fed him nothing but noodle soup. Fortunately, this has significantly improved. He eats with us at the table. His large and fine motor skills are not very well developed; therefore, he is often quite clumsy. Unfortunately, he also continues to fall. Since September 2002, he has been going to the local school. He was integrated into the school and gets special support, and he is obviously happy there. Since Simon is quite fearful, he always used to be afraid of other children. However, this fear is gone now. When Simon learned to walk, we stopped physical therapy. Soon after, we began with speech therapy. Now he can speak a few words, though not quite clearly. Still, persons who know him can understand him quite well. He learned most words and syllables during the last few months, which may have to do with the fact that his little brother was learning to speak, and suddenly Simon too began to utter sounds.

Simon has no feeling for time. He never is in a hurry. He lives so totally in the here and now that I sometimes envy him for that. We often have appointments, and we should be on time. If I begin to hurry, Simon often does not know what this is all about; he will look where the bird was flying or at a car driving by, and then he forgets everything around him. Although Simon can see, hear, smell, and feel just as we can, I am certain that he lives in a world that is totally different from our world of "normal" persons. He probably processes his perceptions in a totally different way. For him the world is interesting, mysterious, and unpredictable.

Simon is disabled, yet I believe that he is a special gift. He is healthy, and he never had to have surgery. Occasionally, he has had diarrhea, and we had to go to the hospital for that. Also, he is more prone to infections than my other two children. However, everything is manageable. Simon is unique, but I believe that every child and every human being is unique and should be considered as such. While Simon's being "different" is sometimes difficult for us, and his lack of understanding and his fears of many everyday situations sometimes tax my patience, we all love him very much and would not want to miss him!

Glossary

Acrocentric chromosomes: The centromere is positioned at the end of the chromosome, separating a normal long arm from a short arm that contains only multiple (many hundred) copies of ribosomal RNA (rRNA) genes (chromosomal satellites).

Allele: One of two or more variants of a gene; the term may be used in connection with various denominators such as a particular DNA sequence (e.g., polymorphism), a combination of genetic markers (haplotype), functional characteristics (wild type vs. disease causing), or parental origin (maternal or paternal).

Allelic heterogeneity: The phenomenon that different mutations in the same gene (allelic mutations) may cause the same disorder.

Amelia: Absence of a limb.

Aneuploidy: The number of chromosomes varies from that of a normal diploid chromosome sequence (e.g., 47,XY,+21).

Anticipation: The phenomenon that the symptoms become more severe or start at an earlier age as a disease is passed on to the next generation.

Capping: The attachment of 7-methylguanosine to the 5' start of mRNA.

Centromere: The element of a chromosome that serves as anchor point for the spindle apparatus during cell division; it contains repetitive α-satellite DNA sequences and divides the chromosomes into a short arm **p** (for "petite") and a long arm **q** (the letter that follows p in the alphabet).

Chromatid: One of the two identical copies of DNA, attached at the centromeres, making up a duplicated chromosome during mitosis.

Chromatin: The combination of DNA and (histone and nonhistone) proteins that makes up a chromosome.

Coding region: The part of the gene that is translated into protein.

Codominance: The phenomenon that two distinct phenotypes associated with two different genetic variants are both found in a compound heterozygous individual.

Conditional probability: The chance of something occurring, assuming that each event is true (e.g., the chance of a mother having four unaffected sons, assuming that she is a carrier for X-linked hemophilia A, is equal to $1/2 \times 1/2 \times 1/2 \times 1/2 = 1/16$).

Contiguous gene syndrome: The presence of several distinct (dominant inherited) monogenic disorders, caused by a deletion affecting several neighboring genes, can occur in the same patient.

Digenic: A disease that is caused by the combined effect of mutations in two different genes.

Dizygotic twins (DTs): Twins that result from simultaneous yet independent maturation, ovulation, and fertilization of two ova.

Dominant: A genetic variant that causes a recognizable phenotype in the heterozygous state, or the phenotype caused by this type of variant.

Epigenetic factors: Hereditary factors that are independent of the actual DNA sequence.

Epistasis: The phenomenon in which the effects of one gene are modified by one or several other genes.

Euchromatin: Relatively loosely packed chromatin that represents transcriptionally active DNA or may be recognized as light bands during chromosome analysis (G-banding).

Euploidy: A normal diploid chromosome complement (2n) of 46 chromosomes (46,XX or 46,XY).

Exons: Coding sequences in the pre–messenger RNA (pre-mRNA) that are separated by noncoding introns.

Expressivity: The variable phenotypic manifestation caused by a genetic variant.

Frameshift mutation: The deletion or insertion of coding nucleotides in a number not divisible by three, which destroys the reading frame beyond the mutation and leads to a completely wrong protein.

Gain-of-function mutation: A mutation that causes increased or novel function of the gene.

Gene: A functional unit in the genome that contains the genetic information for one or more gene products.

Genetic heterogeneity: The same disorder can be triggered by mutations in different genes. For example, Lynch syndrome can result from mutations in *MLH1, MSH2, PMS1, PMS2,* or *MSH6.*

Genotype: The total genetic information available to an organism or a cell, either as a whole or with regard to a specific function.

Helicases: Enzymes that start replication by unwinding the DNA bidirectionally, leading to the separation of the hydrogen bonds and, in effect, the two chains. This results in the creation of two so-called replication forks.

Hemizygous: A genetic variant on a gene of which there is only a single copy.

Heterochromatin: Highly condensed chromatin that represents transcriptionally inactive (often repetitive) DNA or may be recognized as dark bands during chromosome analysis (G-banding).

Heteroplasmy: A mitochondrial DNA (mtDNA) variant is found only in a portion of the cell's mitochondria.

Heterozygous: A genetic variant/sequence on only one of the two copies of a gene.

Histones: Specific evolutionarily conserved proteins that are used to package the DNA strand in a chromosome.

Homoplasmy: All mtDNA copies have the same sequence (e.g., all mtDNA copies contain a particular mutation).

Homozygous: A genetic variant/sequence on both copies of a gene.

Hypomorphic mutation: A mutation that causes only partial loss of function of the gene.

Imprinting: Expression of a gene is inhibited by epigenetic factors. An imprinted gene is not expressed and thus is inactive.

In cis: Two different variants of a gene that occur beside each other on the same chromosomal strand and not on the homologous chromosomal strand.

In trans: Two different genetic variants of a gene that occur on the two homologous chromosomal strands.

In-frame mutation: The deletion or insertion of coding nucleotides in a number divisible by three, which leaves the reading frame intact.

Interspersed repeats: Identical elements linked to mobile genetic elements that are scattered throughout the genome.

— **Copy number variants (CNVs):** Chromosomal regions with a size ranging from 1 kb to many Mb that occur in variable copy number in the general population.

— **DNA-Transposons:** Mobile DNA fragments with a length of approximately 1.2 to 3 kb that encode for a transposase, which cuts out a transposon and inserts it elsewhere.

— **Low copy repeats (LCRs):** Duplicated or multiplicated chromosomal regions of 1 to 400 kb; they facilitate the generation of chromosomal rearrangements through nonhomologous pairing and recombination during meiosis.

— **Retrotransposons:** DNA sequence elements multiplied through reverse transcription of mRNA into complementary DNA (cDNA).

Introns: Noncoding sequences in a gene that are positioned between coding sequences (exons) and are removed by splicing from the pre-mRNA transcript.

Joint probability: The prior probability multiplied by the conditional probability.

Ligases: Enzymes that splice cut DNA pieces (e.g., during replication).

Locus heterogeneity: The phenomenon that some clinically defined disorders may be caused by a deficiency of different genes (loci), meaning the absence of different proteins causes the same phenotype.

Lyon hypothesis: In somatic cells of female mammals, only one X chromosome is transcriptionally active. Additional X chromosomes are randomly inactivated during early embryogenesis; once established, the X-inactivation pattern will be passed on to daughter cells during mitosis.

Malignant transformation: The change from controlled to uncontrolled growth of a cell that is caused by mutations in oncogenes or tumor suppressor genes.

Metacentric chromosomes: The centromere is positioned in the middle of the chromosome.

Missense mutation: A point mutation that causes the substitution of an amino acid with a different amino acid in the protein.

Monogenic: A disease that is caused by mutations in a single gene.

Monosomy: One copy of a chromosome.

Monozygotic twins (MTs): Twins that result from the fertilization of one ovum by one sperm and the subsequent division into two zygotes.

Mosaic: The occurrence of two or more genetically different cell lines within a tissue or within an organism.

Multifactorial: A disease that is caused by the combined effect of multiple genetic and non-genetic factors.

Mutation: The occurrence of a change in the genomic sequence, or the resultant change itself. The term is generally used for disease-causing genetic variants.

Noncoding RNA: Various types of RNA molecules that do not carry sequence information for protein synthesis.

Nonsense mutation: A point mutation that leads to a stop codon.

Nonsense-mediated decay: A quality-control mechanism that selectively degrades mRNAs that contain premature stop (nonsense) codons.

Nucleosome: The basic packaging unit in a chromosome that consists of 8 core histones and 146 base pairs of DNA.

Null mutation: Any type of mutation that causes complete loss of function of the gene.

Penetrance: The likelihood with which a genetic variant causes any kind of phenotypic manifestation.

Peromelia: Congenital malformation of a limb (general term).

Pharmacodynamics: The effects the drug has on the body, or more exactly, the target tissue.

Pharmacogenetics: The study of the impact of single genetic variants on drug metabolism.

Pharmacogenomics: The study of drug metabolism in relation to the whole genome or the individual's overall genetic constitution.

Pharmacokinetics: The representation of the body's action on the drug.

Phase I reactions: Modification of a chemical, usually rendering it (more) polar.

Phase II reactions: The attachment of a polar, ionizable group to the respective molecule.

Phenocopy: A particular phenotype that is caused by exogenous factors (such as teratogens) and resembles the phenotype caused by genetic factors (such as a monogenic disorder).

Phenotype: The physical manifestation of the genetic information.

Phocomelia: Extreme shortening of the long bones of a limb, with a hand or foot close to the shoulder or hip.

Pleiotropy: Different mutations in the same gene can be responsible for the development of different disorders. For example, mutations in the lamin A/C gene can result in several different disorders, including mandibuloacral dysostosis, Charcot-Marie-Tooth disease, familial lipodystrophy, and progeria.

Point mutation: A mutation that affects one single base pair; most frequently refers to a single nucleotide substitution, but the term also describes single nucleotide insertions or deletions.

Polyadenylation: The attachment of multiple adenylate residues to the $3'$ end of mRNA.

Polygenic: A disease that is caused by the combined effect of mutations in multiple genes.

Polymerases: Enzymes that synthesize DNA or RNA strands.

Polymorphism: A genetic variant where the rarer allele in a population occurs with a frequency of at least 1%, independent of the functional or pathogenetic relevance of this alteration.

Polyphenism: The phenomenon in which the effects of one gene are modified by external factors.

Polyploidy: Multiples of the haploid chromosome complement of greater than 2n.

Posterior probability: The probability of the event after taking into account additional information. It is calculated as the quotient of the joint probability divided by the sum of all of the joint probabilities.

Prior probability: The probability of an event **before** taking additional information into account.

Progeria syndromes: Syndromes that recapitulate the phenotype of the aging person in an accelerated manner.

Protooncogenes: Genes that, through (dominant) activating mutations, can be turned into oncogenes. Oncogenes facilitate malignant transformation by synthesis of structurally altered or defective proteins.

Pseudoautosomal regions: The distal ends of the X and Y chromosomes that contain homologous gene sequences, pair in meiosis, and experience obligatory crossing over.

Pseudogenes: DNA sequences that have all the characteristics of a potential encoding transcription unit but which encode for no functional product.

RNA interference (RNAi): A natural mechanism of eukaryotic cells by which short RNA fragments, denoted small interfering RNA (siRNA), identify and cleave mRNAs if the respective sequence is perfectly complementary.

Recessive: A genetic variant that causes a recognizable phenotype only in the homozygous state, or the phenotype caused by this type of variant.

Riboproteins: Complexes of proteins and RNA molecules that carry out various functions in the cell.

Ribozymes: RNA molecules that catalyze enzymatic reactions in cellular metabolism.

Semidominance (incomplete dominance): The phenomenon that a genetic variant causes a recognizable phenotype in the heterozygous state and another (usually more severe) phenotype in the homozygous state.

Silent mutation: A mutation that has no functional effects.

Single nucleotide polymorphism (SNP): A polymorphism where the alleles vary within one single nucleotide base.

Sirenomelia: The fusion of the legs, creating the appearance of a mermaid's tail.

Sister chromosomes: During mitosis the two identical DNA copies after their separation at the centromeres.

Splice mutation: A mutation that alters the sequence of an intron–exon transition or another relevant sequence in a way that prohibits or impairs correct splicing.

Splicing: Removal of noncoding introns positioned between coding exons in the pre-mRNA transcript.

Submetacentric chromosomes: The centromere is positioned between the middle and the end of the chromosome.

Tandem repeats: The presence of a number of identical elements in a row.

— **Minisatellites (variable number tandem repeats, or VNTRs):** Tandem repeats with a unit size of 10 to 60 nt.

— **Satellite DNA:** Repetitive units of 60 to 200 nt that constitute important chromosomal structures, such as the centromeres.

— **Short tandem repeats (STRs):** Tandem repeats with a unit size of 2 to 6 nt.

Telomere: The ends of the chromosomes that consist of numerous tandem repeats of 5′-TTAG-GG-3′ sequences.

Tetraploidy: A quadruple chromosome complement.

Topoisomerases: Enzymes that prevent a supercoiling of the DNA helix during unwinding and separation because they are capable of cutting individual strands, permitting them to unwind.

Transition: The substitution of a purine (A, G) for a purine, or of a pyrimidine (C, T) for a pyrimidine.

Translation: The mechanism of protein synthesis in the ribosomes that translates the language of nucleic acids into the language of polypeptides.

Transversion: The substitution of a purine for a pyrimidine or vice versa.

Triploidy: Triple chromosome complement (3n) (e.g., 69,XXX).

— **Diandric triploidy:** The origin of the additional set of chromosomes is paternal.

— **Digynic triploidy:** The origin of the additional set of chromosomes is maternal. This results in partial mole.

Trisomy: Three copies of a chromosome.

Tumor suppressor genes: Genes that are relevant for the regulation of growth, repair, and cell survival, with malignant transformation supported through (recessive) loss-of-function mutations on both copies of the gene. They typically include DNA repair genes that are responsible for detecting and repairing genetic damage within a cell.

Untranslated region (UTR): The part of the gene that is transcribed and included in the mature mRNA but is not translated into protein. The 5′ UTR denotes the translated sequences prior to the start codon, while the 3′ UTR denotes the translated sequences after the stop codon.

Variable expressivity: The same mutation can result in variable clinical phenotypes.

Index

Note: Page locators followed by f and t indicate figure and table, respectively.

N